ADVANCE PRAISE
THE HPV VACCINE ON TRIAL

"The reader will see the truth: the side effects are underreported by medical personnel, while there are a growing number of parents suing manufacturers and governments for inducing lifelong handicaps, even death, of their loved ones. In fact, this is the tragic example of various segments of our society, worldwide, placing economic interests before the health and protection of our younger generation. I congratulate the authors of this book, who are showing the world this scandal." —Luc Montagnier, MD, Nobel Prize winner for discovery of the HIV virus

"I have voiced concerns about this vaccine from the time it first got fast tracked through the system and even spoke out about it on an *Oprah* appearance years ago. Finally the whole story is revealed in this book. It is high time." —Christiane Northrup, MD, Author of *Women's Bodies, Women's Wisdom*

"This book is the most informative source you will find on the sordid machinations that went into convincing the public that Human Papillomavirus (HPV) vaccination is a wise health choice. The clinical trials never showed that it protects from cervical cancer. There is overwhelming evidence that the vaccine causes harm, both in terms of autoimmune disease and infertility or even death in rare cases. Please read this gripping book before deciding whether to allow your son or daughter to receive the HPV vaccine." —Stephanie Seneff, PhD, Senior Research Scientist, MIT

"Having worked with HPV-vaccination studies in Denmark and subsequently with severely disabled patients attributing their disorder to possible side effects of vaccination, it is both fascinating and scary to read such a thorough unraveling of the faulty processes and the hidden facts behind the development and marketing of the vaccine. A real page-turner that anyone ought to read before considering vaccination." –Jesper Mehlsen, MD, Senior Medical Consultant, Denmark

"Vaccines are one of the most important revolutions in medicine, leading to reduced morbidity and mortality, as well as the eradication of some deleterious viral and bacterial-associated diseases. Yet to expect that injecting foreign substances, especially immersed in adjuvants, will not cause any side effects in some genetically prone individuals is a historical mistake. This book, written in clear language, explains how the US government has given vaccine manufacturers almost blanket liability protection, leading to unreasonably risky vaccines, including HPV vaccines. This book should lead regulatory institutions and medical journals to recognize vaccine adverse effects more completely." –Professor Yehuda Shoenfeld, MD, Sheba Medical Center, Tel Aviv University

"For most people, quarantine conjures up a set of procedures put in place to avoid people with the Plague or Ebola infecting the rest of us. In extreme cases, anyone escaping from the Hot Zone might be killed. It has a new meaning. Quarantine now means what Government and Business put in place to contain anyone who has been injured by a vaccine or a drug from infecting the rest of us, in extreme cases . . . Read this measured but compelling book from inside the Hot Zone and find out." –David Healy MD, author of *Pharmageddon* and *Let Them Eat Prozac*

"Living in the 'Aluminum Age' inevitably exposes us to aluminum in myriad ways. The majority of such exposures are benign in the shorter term while potentially harmful over decades of living. However, the injection of an aluminum adjuvant in a vaccine preparation is an acute exposure to a high concentration of aluminum, with cell death at the injection site the immediate consequence. Harvesting of aluminum adjuvant by immune-reactive cells at

injection sites transports this toxicity well beyond this site and in susceptible individuals is responsible for serious adverse events, which
may span the lifetime of affected individuals. This is no longer a
'dirty little secret' to those of us who understand the toxicity of aluminum. This is a serious book about a very serious subject, and it
demands to be taken seriously now." —Professor Christopher Exley,
PhD FRSB, Keele University

"'Should we give the HPV vaccine?' is an ethical question. Good
ethics starts with good facts. The authors of *The HPV Vaccine on
Trial* have conducted painstaking research, and their book is a rich
source of facts. Their book points to troubling conflicts of interest
of HPV vaccine researchers and those who have editorialized about
it. It makes a convincing case that the push for mandatory HPV vaccination should cease and that HPV vaccination of the individual
should only follow an informed consent process in which patients
are told of its benefits and risks." —Alvin H. Moss, MD, Center for
Health Ethics and Law, West Virginia University

"Like no other, this book provides thorough and sound scholarship on all that is known about the HPV vaccines, including the
junk science devised by the industry and its shameless promotion
by the government agencies that were created to regulate it. The
authors have left nothing out: *The HPV Vaccine on Trial* is a must-
read for every serious student." —Richard Moskowitz, MD, Author
of *Vaccines: A Reappraisal*

"What is happening to our young people? How is it that perfectly
healthy young women (and now men) suddenly lose energy, become
wheelchair-bound, or even die? Why are birth rates among teens
and young adults suddenly plummeting? Holland et al. provide
convincing evidence that these worldwide phenomena could be
linked to the HPV vaccine. Get informed!" —Gayle DeLong, PhD,
Associate Professor, Baruch College, City University of New York

"You may have heard that clinical trials of the HPV vaccine (which included thousands of children) did not include a saline placebo in the control arm. That's just the tip of the iceberg that the authors elucidate." —Shira Miller, MD, Founder and President, Physicians for Informed Consent

"This meticulously researched book deftly answers why wherever HPV vaccines have been introduced, young girls and boys have suffered unacceptably high rates of medically unexplained paralysis, autoimmune disease, syncope, infertility, severe chronic pain, and other devastating health problems, including deaths. Contrary to how the media and policy makers label and attack those who are raising questions about safety, the authors give clear and convincing evidence to support that the 'antiscience' label rests firmly on those who would dismiss these sudden or delayed onset symptoms as a 'coincidence.' The authors explain how vaccine manufacturers, policy makers, media, and NGOs have formed an unholy global alliance to hide the flawed science that formed the foundation for the HPV vaccine approval. These actors suppress science that raises safety concerns and market this neurotoxic vaccine to eleven- and twelve-year-olds, who are pressured by schools and their peers to get this vaccine, or else die of a disease when safer alternative preventative measures exist. This book will help you understand how to protect yourself from policies that put profit over health and safety—a must read." —Claire Dwoskin, Founder, Children's Medical Safety Research Institute

"No parent should make the decision to vaccinate their child until they have read and understood this book." —Jonathan Irwin, Founder, the Jack & Jill Foundation Ireland, former racetrack executive, parent of a child who reacted adversely to the HPV vaccine

"As a father who has witnessed debilitating side effects of 'Big Pharma' medications on his son, I am outraged to learn of thousands of injuries and even death suffered by girls and boys being given the unnecessary HPV vaccine to prevent cervical cancer. Once again, millions are being made by the same company (Merck) responsible for the Vioxx drug that killed more than 100,000 people before being withdrawn from the market. The meticulous research put forward in *The HPV Vaccine on Trial* should compel American lawmakers to follow the lead of Japan to withdraw its recommendation for the HPV vaccine." —Dick Russell, Author, *My Mysterious Son: A Life-Changing Passage Between Schizophrenia and Shamanism*

"As an oncology nurse of twenty-five years and a mother of four fully vaccinated children, I truly believe that *HPV on Trial* is a crucial and desperately needed exposé of the controversial HPV vaccine. The authors have done extensive research and reporting to uncover the devastating side effects that have long been dismissed as psychological, while also revealing the faulty clinical trials. With our children's lives in the balance, this remarkable and gripping story is essential reading for all parents and doctors concerned with the future of our youth." —Deborah Hall Sullivan, RN BSN OCN

"Finding a book that summarizes in a methodical, serious, and well-documented way the story of the great HPV vaccine fraud—described with the rigor of true connoisseurs—fills me with gratitude and respect. Few brave people have faced the power of two multinationals like Merck and GlaxoSmithKline. No one understands better than I the pain, frustration, and impotence of trying to prove the real injury for thousands of girls and women who lost their health and innocence because of this deception. History will smile on those who said and did the right thing, even if branded as fanatics, antivaccine activists, and crazy, merely for daring to do what every parent, ethical professional, and human being has a duty to do. Disguised as the greater good, the HPV vaccine is a farce that has harmed the lives of thousands of young people in the last decade. In the not-too-distant future, with the help of books like this, ethical scientists, the outcry of thousands of injured families, and courts that will not be fooled by the appearance of philanthropy and science, we will be able to declare in unison THE TRUTH HAS TRIUMPHED." —Monica Leon del Rio, Attorney for HPV vaccine-injured women in Colombia and mother of an HPV vaccine-affected daughter.

"If you care about your children's health and future, this book is a must-read. The book confirms the approval of the HPV vaccine without any adequate safety studies. US authorities' denial of the large number of harmed children is equivalent to what we experience in Europe. This book is scary reading. Unfortunately, it's not fiction. It is fact." —Karsten Viborg, Chairman, HPV Vaccine Victims, Denmark

"This is a forensic case against all involved with the development, marketing, and institutional defense of HPV vaccines, presented with formidable clarity. It is hard to believe that the proponents of these vaccines ever intended any good: either that they had any strong conviction in the long-term possibility of eradicating cervical cancer, or that they did not plan to cover up widespread harm to the recipients of the products from the earliest trials. In sum, it poses the most profound questions about the real purpose of public health programs in the twenty-first century." —John Stone, Author, UK Editor, Age of Autism blog

"Many new vaccines are being created and marketed to enrich corporations rather than improve our health. This important book exposes a corrupt system that no longer prioritizes safety and has been co-opted by profiteers. When we understand how HPV vaccine has managed to stay on the market despite its fatal flaws, we will understand how to fix a broken system." —J.B. Handley, Author, *How to End the Autism Epidemic* and Cofounder, Generation Rescue

"The authors have unmasked and exposed the clinical trials of the HPV vaccines, filtered out all the propaganda designed to mislead the public on the safety of this vaccine, and provided a clear and concise discussion of the effectiveness of the human papillomavirus vaccine. Too many women, girls, and boys are being harmed, only to be silenced by the medical community and treated as collateral damage." — Wayne Rohde, Author, *The Vaccine Court: The Dark Truth of America's Vaccine Injury Compensation Program*

"Parents, take heed—your child's health and life is at stake. Clinicians, here is the evidence on the risks of HPV vaccine—please take note. Regulators & legislators, the facts in this book are all you need to uphold the integrity of conflict of interest, account-ability, and honest reporting. The depth of research in this book is remarkable." —Sabeeha Rehman, Author, *Threading My Prayer Rug: One Woman's Journey From Pakistani Muslim to American Muslim*

THE
HPV
VACCINE
ON TRIAL

Seeking Justice for a Generation Betrayed

MARY HOLLAND, J.D.
KIM MACK ROSENBERG, J.D.
EILEEN IORIO

Preface by Dr. LUC MONTAGNIER, Nobel Prize Winner

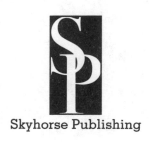

Skyhorse Publishing

Skyhorse Publishing books may be purchased in bulk at special discounts for sales promotion, corporate gifts, fund-raising, or educational purposes. Special editions can also be created to specifications. For details, contact the Special Sales Department, Skyhorse Publishing, 307 West 36th Street, 11th Floor, New York, NY 10018 or info@skyhorsepublishing.com.

Skyhorse® and Skyhorse Publishing® are registered trademarks of Skyhorse Publishing, Inc.®, a Delaware corporation.

Visit our website at www.skyhorsepublishing.com.

10 9 8 7 6

Library of Congress Cataloging-in-Publication Data has been applied for.

Cover design by Brian Peterson
Cover photo credit: iStock

Print ISBN: 978-1-5107-1080-1
Ebook ISBN: 978-1-5107-1081-8

Printed in the United States of America

DISCLAIMER

This book contains the opinions and ideas of its authors. It is a source of information only and does not constitute medical, legal, or other advice to the individual reader. Neither the authors nor the publisher are liable or responsible for any injury, loss, or damage allegedly arising from this book.

Contents

PREFACE

This book is not fiction. It is unfortunately the accurate description of facts occurring in our time: a promising vaccine against a virus involved in cervical cancer turns out to be the source of extremely grave side effects, even death, of young girls and boys.

This vaccine still has the support of official agencies—the WHO, FDA, CDC, EMA—and with the marketing and lobbying efforts of the manufacturers, it continues to be recommended in several countries, and even mandated in some US states!

The reader will see the truth: the side effects are underreported by medical personnel, while there is a growing number of parents suing manufacturers and governments for inducing lifelong handicaps, even death, of their loved ones.

In fact, this is the tragic example of various segments of our society, worldwide, placing economic interests before the health and protection of our younger generation.

I congratulate the authors of this book, who are showing the world this scandal.

What this vaccine is doing to thousands of our young worldwide is a crime.

Historically, vaccines have protected many people. Presently, over these last many years, too many vaccines, HPV and others, have harmed and killed so many people.

Let us mandate that ALL vaccines be safe for everyone. This is possible.

Our future depends on respect for medical ethics, according to the Hippocratic Oath:

FIRST DO NO HARM.

by Luc Montagnier, M.D.

Nobel Prize winner for the discovery of HIV

INTRODUCTION

Cancer strikes fear in people around the globe. So a vaccine to prevent cancer—as the human papillomavirus (HPV) vaccine is touted to do—seemed like a game changer. Since 2006, when the US approved the first HPV vaccine, over 125 countries have introduced it to prevent cervical and other HPV-related cancers. The three HPV vaccines bring in over $2.5 *billion* in annual sales for Merck (Gardasil, Gardasil 9) and GlaxoSmithKline (Cervarix). They have been pharmaceutical juggernauts, yet scandal has followed worldwide. The HPV vaccine is on trial—literally and figuratively—around the world in courts of law and public opinion.

No one disputes that cancer is a ravaging disease that leads to death, if uncontrolled. But the fact that cancer is a grave disease does not necessarily mean that a vaccine purporting to prevent it is safe and effective for everyone. The US Food and Drug Administration, the US Centers for Disease Control and Prevention, the European Medicines Agency, the World Health Organization, and many other public health agencies have embraced the HPV vaccine as a safe and effective way to prevent HPV-related cancers. Here are a few representative statements:

> **FDA:** Based on the review of available information by FDA and CDC, Gardasil continues to be safe and effective, and its benefits continue to outweigh its risks.

CDC: The HPV vaccine is very safe, and it is effective at preventing HPV. Vaccines, like any medicine, can have side effects. Many people who get the HPV vaccine have no side effects at all. Some people report having very mild side effects, like a sore arm, from the shot. The most common side effects are usually mild.

WHO: The WHO's Vaccine Safety Committee considers HPV vaccines to be extremely safe.

EMA: The benefits of HPV vaccines continue to outweigh the known side effects.

These official statements contrast starkly with the reports of devastating injuries and death that we recount in this book. You'll get to know these and other children and young adults.

Christina Tarsell, 21 years old.

Chris was an undergrad at Bard College, New York. A talented athlete, artist, and honor student, she received three Gardasil doses when she was twenty-one. Shortly after the third dose, she died in her sleep. After eight years of hard-fought litigation in the only judicial forum available, Chris's mom "won"—the Court of Federal Claims finally acknowledged that Gardasil more likely than not caused the heart attack that led to Chris's untimely death. You can see Chris, and a memorial to her, in the photo insert.

Alexis Wolf, 13 years old.

In 2007, when Alexis was in 7th grade, she began the Gardasil series. After the second dose, her health deteriorated. After the third, she could no longer focus, sleep, eat, or behave normally. She started to have many seizures every day. She was put in psychiatric hospitals. A year and a half after her symptoms began, Alexis tested at a 4th grade level. Today, at 25, Alexis still suffers from severe neurological injury, including daily seizures. You can see pictures of Alexis both before and after receiving the vaccine in the photo insert.

Joel Gomez, 14 years old.

Joel was an athletic, healthy teenager when he got two Gardasil doses in 2013. Without warning, Joel died in his sleep after the second dose. Joel's family sued for compensation in the Court of Federal Claims. The family's expert witness, Dr. Sin Hang Lee, testified that Gardasil likely caused his heart attack. The Department of Justice settled the case, awarding the family almost the full statutory death benefit.

Abbey Colohan, 12 years old.

In a small town in Western Ireland, Abbey received the first dose of Gardasil at school. Abbey fainted immediately and then had seizures for more than an hour. Two days later, she passed out again. Abbey started to have chronic pain, fatigue, and frequent fainting spells. Abbey's teen years have been consumed with illness and hardship. Ireland's health service denies that Abbey had an adverse vaccine reaction at school.

Colton Berrett, 13 years old.

Colton was an athletic, kind, helpful teenage boy. He loved all outdoor sports. Colton started the three-dose Gardasil series when he was thirteen. Shortly after the third dose, he became paralyzed from the neck down and had to use a ventilator. Through intensive physical therapy, Colton eventually recovered some mobility but remained on a round-the-clock ventilator. He committed suicide two months before his eighteenth birthday. In the photo insert, you can see pictures of Colton that convey far more than words ever can.

Lucy Hinks, 13 years old.

Lucy was a healthy English teenager when she began the Cervarix series in her school. Shortly after the third shot, Lucy's health plummeted. She could barely walk, slept 23 hours a day, and could not think straight. She could not attend school and had to be spoon-fed. Her parents described her as being in a "walking coma." Through many therapies and treatments, Lucy has substantially recovered but still suffers from chronic fatigue.

Maddie Moorman, 15 years old.

Maddie began the Gardasil series at the gynecologist's recommendation. After the second shot, Maddie became bedridden and ill. She had debilitating headaches every day and could no longer remember things. Her mom declined the third shot for her. Through conventional and holistic treatment, Maddie's health began to recover slowly, and she was able to complete high school and go to college. But some of Maddie's symptoms never abated, including a constant buzzing in her head and the inability to think the way she could before. She took her own life at twenty-one. You can see her pictures in the photo insert.

We show that the HPV vaccine clinical trials paved the way for such tragic results. Here are some of the little-known facts we'll explore:

HPV vaccines have never been proven to prevent cervical or any other cancer. Merck and GlaxoSmithKline, the manufacturers, did not have to prove that the vaccines prevent cancer. They were allowed to use precancerous lesions as "surrogate endpoints" in the clinical trials. Scientists do not know if the decline in cases of precancerous lesions will translate into fewer cases of cervical cancer in 20–30 years.

Even if they were 100 percent effective, which they are not, HPV vaccines do not prevent all cases of cervical cancer. The vaccines do not prevent infections from all HPV types associated with cancer, and not all cervical cancer is associated with HPV. HPV vaccines are *not* a replacement for cervical screening, yet evidence strongly suggests that young women are skipping screening in the mistaken belief that they no longer need it. HPV vaccine marketing hype appears to have contributed to a sharp drop-off in cervical screening among young women.

None of the participants in the clinical trials received a true saline placebo. None of the clinical trials included a straightforward comparison of the effects of the vaccine against a true control. We use the term "fauxcebo" to describe the aluminum-containing adjuvants, other vaccines, and chemical mixtures that control subjects received instead of true saline placebos. These fauxcebos masked the adverse effects of the vaccines, making them appear safer than they would have if compared to true placebos.

Merck told young female clinical trial subjects that the vaccine had already been proven safe and that the placebo was saline. Both claims were false. A key purpose of the clinical trials was to establish safety, and the placebo was not saline. Clinical trial subjects suffered because of these lies.

The manufacturers never tested HPV vaccines on human fertility. Although this vaccine is given to adolescents throughout the world, the manufacturers acknowledge in their package inserts that they never tested the vaccine for fertility effects in humans—only rats. We look at the substantial evidence of severe adverse effects on fertility, including miscarriage and premature ovarian failure in girls and young women.

Evidence shows that certain ingredients in HPV vaccines, including sodium borate (also known as borax, a cleaning agent), may have negative effects on fertility. The European Chemicals Agency requires sodium borate to carry the following warning: "DANGER! May damage fertility or the unborn child." In the US, borax is banned in food but allowed in vaccines.

The manufacturers never tested HPV vaccines to discover if they might cause cancer. The package inserts acknowledge that the vaccines have never been tested for "carcinogenicity." But clinical trial data suggest that if women have HPV infections when they get the vaccines (and prescreening is not recommended), then they may be at higher risk for precancerous cervical lesions or worse. Some clinical trial participants later developed cancer, including cervical cancer.

The Gardasil clinical trials used a new metric, "New Medical Conditions," as a way to claim that serious health problems after vaccination were unrelated to the vaccine or aluminum-containing fauxcebo. More than 50 percent of all clinical trial participants reported "new medical conditions," including infections, reproductive disorders, neurological syndromes, and autoimmune conditions. The FDA did not question this novel metric or whether the vaccine itself might be contributing to these conditions.

Although 11–12-year-olds are the target population for this vaccine (and it is approved for children as young as nine), the vast majority of clinical trial subjects were considerably older. Only a small percentage of participants were aged 12 or younger, and their age cohort, or group, lacked a true saline control placebo, as did the older age groups. Preteens, on the cusp of puberty, have significant biological differences from young adults, the primary age group in the clinical trials. Thus, the target population was insufficiently studied before the vaccine received approval.

Doctors and scientists have published peer-reviewed articles on the adverse effects that many young women reported after HPV vaccination. Here is a nonexhaustive list:

- Headache

- Orthostatic intolerance

- Syncope

- POTS

- Fatigue

- Cognitive dysfunction

- Disordered sleep

- Visual symptoms

- Blurring of vision

- Gastrointestinal symptoms

- Neuropathic pain

- Motor symptoms

- Skin disorders

- Voiding dysfunction

- Limb weakness

- Vascular abnormalities

- Irregular period

Despite US government assertions that the vaccine is safe,

the federal compensation program for vaccine injury has paid out millions of dollars in damages for HPV vaccine injuries. Families have received compensation for death, brain injury, multiple sclerosis, complex regional pain syndrome, Guillain-Barré syndrome, ulcerative colitis, and other severe, debilitating conditions. We delve into reported HPV vaccine injuries and the pursuit of justice.

All participants in the Gardasil clinical trials who received a "placebo" rather than the vaccine were encouraged to receive HPV vaccines at the end of the clinical trial period. By doing this, Merck destroyed any opportunity for large-scale, long-term safety and efficacy studies of vaccinated versus the original control subjects.

Lawsuits have been filed against Merck, GlaxoSmithKline, and government health agencies around world, including in the US, India, Colombia, Japan, Spain, and France. Families want treatment for their injured children and young adults. They also want to hold the manufacturers accountable and to prevent future injuries to other children.

National and international health agencies are working hand in glove with the HPV vaccine manufacturers to promote, advertise, finance, recommend, and even compel children to get HPV vaccines. We have included examples of CDC and UK National Health Service ads for HPV vaccines in the photo insert.

The US government earns royalties from Merck and GSK for licensing HPV vaccine technology. Scientists at the National Institutes of Health, with others, participated in the invention of HPV vaccines. While receiving millions of dollars in annual royalty income from these corporations, the US government ostensibly holds the upper hand in regulating them. The conflict of interest is obvious.

The HPV vaccine saga began just as Merck was trying to turn the page on its criminal conduct with Vioxx, its failed painkiller drug. Just as Vioxx was raking in $2.5 billion in annual revenue—almost the same amount Gardasil and Gardasil 9 are now bringing in—Merck withdrew it from the market because it was causing heart attacks, strokes, and death. Merck had not disclosed known heart attack risk in its clinical trial data. In 2005, Merck paid multimillion-dollar civil and criminal penalties and entered into a $4.85 billion settlement with injured plaintiffs. Congress, the Department of Justice, and the media investigated Merck for falsifying data, making false statements to regulators, making false marketing claims, failing to disclose material information to consumers, and more. In 2006, the FDA approved Gardasil, leading some to dub the HPV vaccine "Help Pay for Vioxx."

History repeats itself in the Merck Vioxx and Gardasil sagas.

In researching and writing this book, we spoke with more than a hundred people who shared with us their time, expertise, and deeply personal stories. We also spoke with many injured young people and their parents, as well as with parents whose children died. We are humbled that they trusted us with their stories and have done our best to give them voice.

We also reached out to doctors, scientists, and medical researchers. We met with advocates fighting for those who have been injured. We met personally with women who were subjects in the clinical trials and spoke with doctors who were principal trial investigators. We also contacted HPV vaccine proponents, including the FDA, and are grateful for their assistance. We reached out to Merck with a long list of questions on two occasions but received no replies.

We bring legal and financial backgrounds to this task. While we are not doctors or scientists, we believe that our perspective is critical to this debate. For too long, those with real and potential conflicts of interest in industry and government have dominated public discourse about vaccine safety.

Part I examines the clinical trials and the race to develop the vaccine. It analyzes surprising data that have received little attention to date. We also provide a primer on cervical cancer to explain its real risk factors. While we focus on the Gardasil clinical trials, we also look at Cervarix, GlaxoSmithKline's version, and at Gardasil 9, the only currently available HPV vaccine in the US. (GSK took Cervarix off the US market, likely because of low sales. Merck replaced Gardasil with Gardasil 9, the new HPV vaccine against a broader range of HPV viruses.) We use official documents and the accounts of two young women injured in the clinical trials to examine their many flaws. We close Part I with a look at India, where clinical trials led to national outrage and a legal battle against the pharmaceutical industry and its partners.

Part II covers what happened after the vaccines hit the market. How do you sell a vaccine for an infection that clears almost all the time? We look at the marketing magic and "disease branding" that created a market out of thin air. We also share heartbreaking stories of injury and death. We follow several families' fights for justice. We look closely at the US and Australia, powerhouses in HPV vaccine development, whose governments are leading the charge toward universal HPV vaccine uptake.

Part III is a deeper dive into the latest research on aluminum-containing adjuvants and other ingredients of concern, including DNA fragments. We discuss HPV transmission, the potential threat of "type replacement," cervical screening in both high and low resource countries, and more. If you don't need the deep science dive, skip ahead.

Finally, Part IV takes readers around the world to Japan, Denmark, Ireland, the UK, and Colombia. Each of these countries is a unique case study regarding the HPV vaccine, and the role that governments, media, and the law play. You'll get a close look at the latest developments in each country yet also see the global threads in common.

We strongly advocate for informed consent and hope that this book will help people to make truly informed decisions about this vaccine. Only you can be the ultimate judge for yourself or your loved one.

This story is ever-evolving, so inevitably there will be new developments before and after this book goes to print. We anticipate future editions, but in the meanwhile, for additional information or to contact us, please go to www.hpvvaccineontrial.org.

We include a glossary below to help with the "alphabet soup" of agencies and organizations that this topic requires.

GLOSSARY OF TERMS

AAHS Amorphous Aluminum Hydroxyphosphate Sulphate, the adjuvant used in Merck's Gardasil and Gardasil 9 vaccines

ACIP Advisory Committee on Immunization Practices

ACOG American College of Obstetricians and Gynecologists

Adjuvant Immune stimulating vaccine ingredient, most often an aluminum compound

AE Adverse Event

AMA American Medical Association

Antibody An immunoglobulin, a specialized immune protein, produced because of the introduction of an antigen into the body

Antigen A toxin or other foreign substance that induces an immune response in the body

ASIA Autoimmune Syndrome Induced by Adjuvants

AS04 GlaxoSmithKline adjuvant system consisting of aluminum hydroxide and monophosphoryl lipid (MPL) used in the Cervarix vaccine

CBER Center for Biologics Evaluation and Research at the US FDA

CDC US Centers for Disease Control and Prevention

Cervarix™ GlaxoSmithKline's bivalent HPV vaccine

CIN 1, 2, 3 Cervical Intraepithelial Neoplasia (1, 2, or 3)

CRPS Complex Regional Pain Syndrome

DTC Direct-To-Consumer (marketing)

EDC Estimated Date of Conception

E6 and E7 Oncoproteins in human papillomavirus that are involved in cancer or tumor initiation and progression

EMA European Medicines Agency

FDA Food and Drug Administration (US)

FUTURE I/II Females United to Unilaterally Reduce Ecocervical Disease I/II, two of the Gardasil Phase III clinical trials

GACVS Global Advisory Committee on Vaccine Safety

Gardasil™ Merck's first generation quadrivalent HPV vaccine

Gardasil 9™ Merck's second generation 9-valent HPV vaccine

GAVI Global Alliance for Vaccines and Immunization

GSK GlaxoSmithKline, manufacturer of Cervarix HPV vaccine

HBV Hepatitis B vaccine

HHS Health and Human Services (US)

HPRA Health Products Regulatory Agency (Ireland)

HPV Human Papillomavirus

HSE Health Services Executive (Ireland)

IARC International Agency for Research on Cancer of the

World Health Organization

IND Investigational New Drug Application with the FDA

L1 A major capsid protein of the human papillomavirus used to make the virus-like particles (VLPs) used in HPV vaccines

L2 A major capsid protein of the human papillomavirus considered but ultimately not used to make the virus-like particles (VLPs) used in HPV vaccines

MHRA Medicines and Healthcare Products Regulatory Agency (UK)

MITT Modified Intent To Treat (study population)

MPL Monophosphoryl lipid A, a lipopolysaccharide extracted bacterium Salmonellas Minnesota strain R595 and used as part of GSK's AS04 adjuvant system in Cervarix

NCI National Cancer Institute

NCVIA National Childhood Vaccine Injury Act

NHS National Health Service (UK)

NIH National Institutes of Health (US)

NMC New Medical Condition

NSAE Non-Serious Adverse Event

NVIC National Vaccine Information Center

OTT Office of Technology Transfer (US)

PATH Program for Appropriate Technology in Health

PATRICIA Papilloma Trial against Cancer in Young Adults, part of the Cervarix clinical trials

PCR negative A result indicating the absence of the DNA

sequence targeted by a specific test (for example, a specific strain of HPV), here obtained from cell samples

PCR positive A result indicating the presence of the DNA sequence targeted by a specific test

POF Premature Ovarian Failure

POTS Postural Orthostatic Tachycardia Syndrome

SAE Serious Adverse Event

Seronegative No active infection and no antibody titers at a determined measurable level

Seropositive Antibodies present above a determined measurable level, likely indicative of past exposure or infection

TGA Therapeutic Goods Association (Australia)

VAERS Vaccine Adverse Event Reporting System

VFC Vaccines For Children

VICP Vaccine Injury Compensation Program

VLP Virus-Like Particle

VRBPAC Vaccines and Related Biological Products Advisory Committee of the FDA

WHO World Health Organization

WIG Women In Government

PART I
CLINICAL TRIALS

1.

REWARDING THE INVENTORS

In September 2017, luminaries in the healthcare field gathered at the New York Plaza Hotel to celebrate an extraordinary achievement: a vaccine to prevent cancer. Two scientists at the National Institutes of Health had created the human papillomavirus, or HPV vaccine. By 2017, it had been on the market just over ten years, although scientists had been working on it for decades. The Lasker Foundation gives awards to key leaders in the medical field.

At the ceremony, Drs. Douglas R. Lowy and John T. Schiller received Lasker Awards for their groundbreaking innovation. The Foundation celebrates scientists, clinicians, and public servants for advances in research and health. Albert and Mary Lasker, the Foundation's namesakes, created the Awards in 1945, drawing on Albert's advertising fortune, which he amassed through selling cigarettes and other products. These prestigious awards, sometimes called "American Nobel" prizes, carry not just acclaim, but $250,000 for each winner.

Drs. Lowy and Schiller, cancer biologists at the National Cancer Institute, had attained a dream—a vaccine to prevent cervical cancer, a killer for women, particularly in the developing world. In 1950, cervical cancer had also been the Lasker Foundation's theme: Dr. George Papanicolaou won a prize for his Pap test, which could identify abnormal cervical cell growth. Pap tests have saved countless lives over the past 70 years. But Drs. Lowy and Schiller's work promised something even better: to prevent cancer in the first place. This is what the Lasker Foundation sought to honor.

Dr. Craig Thompson, head of the world-renowned Memorial Sloan-Kettering Cancer Center, presided at the gala. He called the HPV clinical trials "stunningly successful." Because of Lowy and Schiller's pioneering work, the FDA approved the HPV vaccine for females in 2006 and for males in 2011. By 2015, nearly 60 million people around the globe, mostly children, had received at least one dose. Dr. Thompson proclaimed that HPV vaccines had already prevented 400,000 cases of cervical cancer.[1] A Lasker Award video went further, saying that over the next 50–60 years, the vaccine would prevent 19 million cases of cervical cancer and 10 million deaths: "The HPV vaccine is like an immunological grand slam. It prevents most cervical cancer as well as other HPV-linked cancers."[2]

In his acceptance remarks, Dr. Lowy acknowledged that he and Dr. Schiller would not have been able to develop the vaccine without public investment. For the pharmaceutical industry, the incentives to prevent disease are not as great as those to treat it. Publically financed NIH research had been essential. He also thanked the key manufacturers, Merck and GlaxoSmithKline, for taking big risks. The vaccines have "exceeded even our most optimistic expectations, while also highlighting the value of public-private partnerships in health and disease. Amazingly, eliminating cervical cancer and other HPV-associated cancers as a major public health problem is now a realistic goal."[3]

The HPV vaccine sounded miraculous, promising to safely prevent cancer with only a few shots. It sounded almost too good to be true.

2.

INJURED IN THE TRIALS: TESTIMONY FROM DENMARK

"I didn't want it to be the vaccine." Kesia Lyng, Denmark

In December 2017, the online magazine *Slate* published "What the Gardasil Testing May Have Missed." With its publication, the article sparked renewed debate over HPV vaccine clinical trials.[1] The story focused on Kesia Lyng, a young Danish woman who participated in one of Merck's Gardasil trials in 2002.[2] The article's description of the clinical trials surprised many but brought a sense of relief to other young people who, like Kesia, had experienced ill health after the vaccine. They could recognize their experience in hers.

When she was eighteen and still in high school, Kesia received a brochure in the mail about an exciting clinical trial for a vaccine that would prevent cervical cancer. She didn't know it was possible to vaccinate against cancer. She had heard that getting regular Pap tests was the best way to prevent cancer because most problems could be caught early and treated. The brochure said that the vaccine had no side effects, as it had already been thoroughly tested. It read, "FUTURE 2 er IKKE et bivirkningsstudie," which translates to "the FUTURE 2 study is NOT a side effect study" (original emphasis on "NOT"). This piqued her interest, particularly because the vaccine had already been proven safe.

Only six months before Kesia received this brochure, her grandmother had died at 68 of cervical cancer. Kesia adored her grandmother; she was Kesia's world. Her grandmother was the glue that
held the family together. Kesia has the fondest memories of her entire
family celebrating holidays in her grandmother's home. She missed
her terribly. She wanted to do something, and getting the brochure
seemed serendipitous.

The brochure said that half the clinical trial subjects would receive the vaccine and half would receive saline, which seemed like
standard practice. When she inquired further, she found out that
the clinical trials would take place at her local hospital in Hvidovre,
just outside Copenhagen. It seemed like an easy way to do something positive and help the fight against cervical cancer. She signed
up.

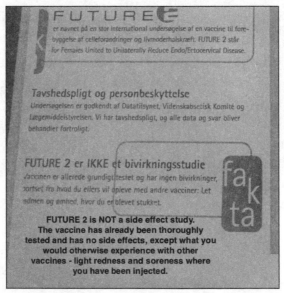

*Source: Excerpt from "Future 2" study recruitment brochure sent to all female
18–23 year-olds in Denmark, 2002.[3]*

Kesia's parents were skeptical, although they appreciated her
desire to do something constructive. They didn't want her to take
unnecessary risks. They discouraged her from participating in the
trials, but Kesia was resolute. She was proud to take part so that

she could help others avert a similar, painful loss. She had never heard of HPV before the study, but it sounded like a breakthrough. She learned that the study name, FUTURE 2, stood for "Females United To Unilaterally Reduce Endo/Ectocervical Disease." She couldn't wait to get started. And not least, she would earn around $500. That was a lot of money for an 18-year-old!

THE TRIAL BEGINS

Kesia enlisted in Study Protocol 015, a clinical trial, and received her first shot in September 2002. At this appointment, the clinicians examined her and took blood and urine samples. They told her she would either get the 3-shot Gardasil vaccine series, or three shots of saline placebo, which would have no effect. Since the study was double-blind, neither she nor the investigators would know which shots she got until the trial was over. Kesia was nervous. Part of her wanted to get the saline placebo, but part wanted to get the vaccine so that she would be protected against HPV. The nurse reassured her that if she did get the vaccine, it was perfectly safe; her mind was put at ease.

The first injection really hurt. Later that day, she felt tired, and her arm was weak. She was overcome by an unusual feeling all over her body; not dizzy, but strange, and disconnected. She had a weird sensation in her arm for weeks after the shot. But, in the end, she rationalized that she was doing something that might one day help women all over the world. She thought it was just a normal vaccine reaction.

Two months later, Kesia returned for her second shot. It was at this visit that she talked more with the clinicians. They asked her how things went after the first injection. The nurse read from a checklist of possible symptoms related to the injection site and other minor symptoms. Kesia hadn't received any information from the clinical staff when she received her first shot on how to record unusual reactions; they did not ask her to keep track. She didn't keep a journal and couldn't quite remember every ache or pain she had had the previous month. She was told that headaches and fevers were normal, so she took the second shot without hesitation. It was more painful than the first, but she put it out of mind. She had the same reaction as before—she was very tired, and her arm was weak. Her body felt very strange, but those feelings gradually subsided.

Shortly after this second appointment, though, Kesia developed flu-like symptoms, muscle pains, and a strange headache. At times, Kesia felt like her head was in a vice. She began having trouble sleeping for the first time in her life. She felt exhausted, but it would take hours to fall asleep, and she rarely stayed asleep for long, waking every hour. She tried everything, but nothing helped. Lack of sleep was the worst part of Kesia's illness. It was so stressful and upsetting to be this exhausted and not able to find relief. Kesia didn't realize it, but this was to be her new nightly experience for the next fourteen years.

Kesia's flu-like symptoms and sleep problems persisted that winter. There was no requirement for her to report back to the hospital. She missed a lot of school because of fatigue and constant pain but tried to catch up. She had to retake a few exams. As it got close to the third shot, and she still hadn't fully recovered, she thought perhaps she should not proceed with the trial. Her parents agreed and tried to dissuade her from continuing. But there was something about being part of this amazing trial that excited Kesia, so she continued.

To this day, Kesia remembers her third appointment vividly. She remembers the long corridor down which she walked to the room where she would get the shot. Looking back, there was something about it that stayed in her mind: the smells, the noise, the feeling of being wary, though she couldn't quite put her finger on why. At her appointment, she told the clinician she wasn't feeling well and was frequently tired and in pain. She asked if she should perhaps delay the shot. The nurse reassured her that what she was feeling had nothing to do with the vaccine and that she could get the third dose without problem. The nurse asked if Kesia had had any reactions after her second dose. Outside of the headaches, the fatigue, and muscle aches from her ongoing illness, Kesia couldn't remember the exact details from the last six months. She told the nurse about the headaches, which she got four or five times a week, lasting all day. The nurse told her not to worry and that some headaches were normal. She completed the paperwork and gave Kesia her third and final injection.

After this appointment, Kesia felt dizzy for the first time. She felt nauseated, and her arm hurt more than ever. During the following weeks, however, her health took a sharp turn for the worse. She went to her doctor, and when she told him she had participated in a clinical trial for a new vaccine, he was worried. He made a note in her file, and Kesia saw him put two exclamation points next to it. He asked her to talk to the trial staff again about her symptoms because all her blood tests were fine. Kesia returned to the hospital for a follow-up visit a month after her final shot. She tried to talk to the trial staff again about her symptoms based on her doctor's concerns, and they listened more intently this time. She told them that she was struggling to keep a normal, everyday life and that this was not something she had ever experienced before. But they told her once again that her symptoms were not the kind they would expect to see with the vaccine, and she should continue to see her regular doctor. Kesia accepted this explanation; after all, they were the experts, and she knew the vaccine had already been tested for safety. She tried to put it out of her mind, as she had a 50 percent chance she'd received the saline placebo and not the vaccine at all.

"I Didn't Want It to Be The Vaccine."

As months passed, Kesia became so ill that all she could think about was her next doctor's appointment. She missed so many exams in her last year of high school that she couldn't graduate alongside her classmates. She had to put her dreams and plans on hold until she could feel well enough to get through the day without a headache or pain in her joints and muscles. It was a daily struggle to get out of bed, let alone to attend school or university.

Kesia loved her high school, which focused on practical skills and crafts such as sewing, art, and design. She wanted to go to university to become an interior designer or glamorous window dresser for a fancy store in Copenhagen. Or perhaps she could be a journalist; she loved writing. She also had dreams of one day owning a coffee shop with her best friend. She had always been excited about the endless possibilities for her future, but now her whole life was on hold. She disliked having to rely on the government for financial and medical expenses. She lost count of the doctor's visits. She vowed one day to finish her exams and graduate from the high school she loved. She never thought months would turn into years, and years would turn into more than a decade.

When the trial investigators unblinded the trial in 2007, a year after the FDA approved Gardasil, Kesia learned that she had received the vaccine after all. She was relieved that the trial was over. If she had had the saline injection, she would have been strongly urged to go back to the hospital for the three vaccines, which would have been tough now that she was so ill. She heard no more from the clinical trial staff, although she agreed to be part of follow-up studies.

Some close friends and family began to ask Kesia questions about a possible link to the clinical trials, but she wouldn't listen. She was so convinced that she had made a positive contribution to cervical cancer research that she got upset when anyone suggested it. She wanted the vaccine to be a success so that other women did not die of cervical cancer like her grandmother had. She was very proud of her contribution to help find a way to prevent cancer. Gradually she began to forget about the clinical trials. She didn't want it to be the vaccine.

PIECING TOGETHER THE PUZZLE

Despite her illness, Kesia managed to keep her life going. The many doctors she saw could never find a reason for her incessant pain and fatigue. Resigned to thinking that this was how life would be, she found a way to tolerate the symptoms. She found love, married, and had two beautiful children. She worked part-time outside the home when her health permitted, but sometimes she could not. She loved being a mother and thought her most important job was at home, taking care of her children.

Kesia doesn't have a television and doesn't keep up with social media. In March 2015, Denmark was abuzz after the release of a controversial Danish documentary about the HPV vaccine, *The Vaccinated Girls*.[4] The film chronicled girls who suffered many neurological and physical symptoms following Gardasil vaccination. Two Danish physicians, Drs. Brinth and Mehlsen, gave interviews and explained why they were concerned that the vaccine may be contributing to unusual diseases, including Postural Orthostatic Tachycardia Syndrome (POTS) and other autoimmune conditions. People told Kesia about it, but she didn't watch. More than a year later, when she was sitting with her husband, watching an online news channel, things clicked. She heard a woman talk about getting the vaccine shortly after it was approved. As the woman described her reaction to each shot, Kesia's heart stopped. It was like listening to her own story—the same timeline, the same symptoms. At that moment, Kesia felt like the rug had been pulled out from under her. After all these years of wondering why she was so sick, here was another woman telling the exact same story.

She couldn't believe it. How could this happen if the vaccine had been "proven" safe? Every time she told the trial nurse about her symptoms, the nurse assured her that they weren't related. On the one hand, she was angry and upset; on the other, she was relieved to find someone else who could understand what she was going through and might even be able to help.

She barely slept that night. The next day, she went online to start looking for answers. She contacted Denmark's vaccine victim support group and spoke with Sara, who eventually became her dear friend. They talked for a long time, and Sara understood. She had heard it before. For Kesia, though, it was the first time she didn't feel crazy. It had been thirteen years of living with pain and hearing doctors deny that her condition was real.

In April 2016, she finally sat down with her husband to watch *The Vaccinated Girls*. She wasn't quite prepared to see Danish teenagers suffering from precisely what she had been living through for more than a decade. She cried for what she had suffered, but even more for what was happening to all the other girls since the clinical trials. If clinicians in the trials denied any connection between her

symptoms and the vaccine, it made sense that doctors today continue to deny them. She was determined to share her story.

SESILJE

Only a few miles away in Copenhagen, another young woman was
going through a similar awakening. Sesilje (pronounced Cecelia)
had also been in the FUTURE 2 study, and like Kesia, her health
too has suffered ever since. The two young women met through the
victim support group in July 2016. Sesilje's story is remarkably similar to Kesia's, with one significant difference: Sesilje received the
placebo. What could have made Sesilje so sick if she had received
saline? It didn't add up.

Sesilje had received the same brochure as Kesia about a clinical
trial at her local hospital in Frederiksberg, Copenhagen. Like Kesia,
Sesilje thought it would be exciting to contribute to an important
medical effort to protect women from cancer. Sesilje, a 21-year-old
undergraduate at the time, could do with the extra money, as well.
She read that the trial used saline as the placebo. Sesilje hoped
she would get the placebo because she was studying for exams and
didn't want to take any undue risks. But she had no way of knowing
if she would be in the vaccine or saline group, since the study was
double-blind. Thinking about all the good the trials might do, and
the money, she decided to participate, since the brochure said the
vaccine was safe.

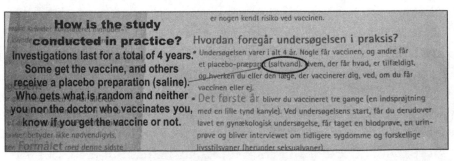

Source: Excerpt from "FUTURE 2" study recruitment brochure sent to
18–23-year-old women in Denmark, 2002.[5]

Sesilje didn't notice any strong reactions after the first shot, although it was quite painful. She had an unusual menstrual period the month following the vaccine but did not think it was related. The clinicians did not give her any booklet or form for recording symptoms. They did mention that she would feel injection site reactions and maybe a headache. The bleeding was just a coincidence, she thought.

A month later, Sesilje went back to the hospital for her second shot. And just like with Kesia, the clinicians asked about a checklist of reactions. Sesilje felt comfortable proceeding, as her reactions had been mild. They told her that she should see her personal doctor about the menstrual period, as it was unrelated. She would not return for another six months until she was due for the third shot. They told her to call with any questions but again did not give her any way to record reactions she might have.

It was after this shot that she noticed unusual symptoms, not just the heavy menstrual period. Her skin hurt, she had headaches, and she felt as if she had the flu. Her stomach really hurt, and she lost twelve pounds in a matter of weeks. She went to her doctor, but he could not figure out her symptoms. Sesilje couldn't understand; she had always been healthy.

When Sesilje returned for her third shot, the trial staff told her again that her recent health issues were unrelated. She should continue to see her own doctors and follow their advice. They assured her it was safe to proceed.

Finishing the series in 2003, Sesilje was told she had to wait until 2007 to find out if she had received the saline placebo or the vaccine. Her symptoms persisted, but no doctor could figure out why. She developed an allergy to her deodorant and various skin creams. She went to a dermatologist, who told her to switch brands, which didn't help. As part of her studies in medical research, Sesilje was around healthcare professionals, but no one could explain why she was so ill. Like Kesia, she learned to cope.

In 2007, when the clinical trial was unblinded, Sesilje learned that she had received the saline placebo. This silenced the voice in the back of her mind that the vaccine was somehow connected to her illness. Since she had received an inactive placebo, something else must have been the cause. At a follow-up visit with the clinical trial staff, she told them that her gynecologist had recently found that she had abnormal cervical cell growth. She asked the trial clinicians for information about whether she had had an HPV infection at the beginning of the trial in 2002. She thought they might know this information because she had had a gynecological exam before her first injection. She worried this might have something to do with her current diagnosis. The clinical staff told her they were not allowed to disclose her exam results and that her records belonged to Merck.

Sesilje was upset by this response because she had to decide about her treatment options for cervical dysplasia and didn't have enough information. Nevertheless, the staff strongly recommended that she get the vaccine because she could be at increased risk of cancer. Even though she had qualms, she felt enormous pressure from the staff to get the three Gardasil shots. Because she was more afraid of cancer than the vaccine, she did.

Then Sesilje's health plummeted. In the fall of 2007, she found out that she had a tumor on her pituitary gland. Could this be the reason for all her health problems? While she was scared, she was slightly reassured to know that she might have found the cause. She was still struggling with daily life, but now it seemed a little easier to understand.

Sesilje had played soccer in her spare time, but she was forced to stop because she was losing her balance; it was not safe to be on the field. She really missed being active, but her health had to come first. Her periods continued to be abnormal; something was not right.

Still, Sesilje was able to work in a job she loved, and she got married. Things were good when she could manage the pain and fatigue. She was worried about her pituitary tumor, but there was nothing doctors could do except monitor it. Despite menstrual problems, she conceived her first child in 2012. She experienced excruciating headaches during pregnancy, but doctors told her it was just migraines. Soon after her son was born, Sesilje found out that the tumor had unexpectedly ruptured. She was worried, but it slowly disappeared as if by magic and never returned. Her doctors were amazed. Her little baby may have saved her life, she thought.

Sesilje settled into life as a new mother and expected her pain and fatigue to go away, assuming the tumor had been the cause. But the symptoms worsened. She was confused and afraid. Luckily, her baby kept her busy. She tried not to complain. She returned to work and managed as best she could.

In 2015, everything changed. She read online that the Gardasil clinical trials had used an aluminum solution as the control, not saline, as she had been told. Sesilje worked in clinical research, so she knew that this should not have been permissible. She was certain that she had been told that the control was saline—it was even printed in the brochure she received years ago.

She was determined to research this, if only to prove the online information wrong. She expected to confirm that the placebo was "saltvand"—Danish for "saline." Instead, she found that there was no saline placebo group at all. What she had read online was correct: the control contained aluminum. Her heart sank. She knew what this meant: because the vaccine also had the same solution as the control, she had received six injections containing aluminum, three as the "placebo" and later three as the vaccine.

She knew aluminum was an active ingredient. She knew it has a measurable effect on individuals. She had read studies but wasn't sure how toxic it was. In that moment, Sesilje *knew* that the aluminum had been toxic to her. Her mind cast back over the last twelve years of ill health that started right after her first shot. She knew saline alone could not have caused her symptoms. It all began to make sense.

How could Danish authorities have approved FUTURE 2 with an aluminum-based adjuvant as a control group, and how could they have allowed trial participants to be told that the control was saline? How could this happen in Denmark, where health authorities rigorously scrutinize clinical trials? She didn't understand how the clinicians, assuming they knew the control was aluminum, could have dismissed her symptoms. She was healthy before the trial and terribly sick after it began. Wasn't the purpose of a trial to observe clinical symptoms?

Sesilje didn't yet know what to do, but her life had changed. She began to find out all she could about the clinical trials and Merck's proprietary aluminum adjuvant—the substance that boosted the immune system to make the vaccine work. She couldn't find safety information anywhere. She wondered if women in the vaccine group were experiencing the same problems.

Thanks to connections she made on social media, Sesilje found that there were many women like her, except that they had received the vaccine after it was officially on the market. Like Kesia, Sesilje got in touch with the victims' support group, and in July 2016, Sesilje and Kesia met.

Both felt duped into taking something without proper consent and now were suffering the consequences. They were distressed that no one had believed their symptoms were related to the vaccine trial. If they had only been able to make the trial staff see the connections, perhaps they could have helped spare countless people from suffering. Kesia and Sesilje share a sense of survivors' guilt.

BRINGING THE STORY TO LIGHT

When journalist Frederik Joelving began researching the *Slate* article, he sought to interview women who had taken part in the clinical trials. Kesia heard about Joelving's work and jumped at the chance to share her story. Even though Kesia didn't have documentation from that time, she and Joelving pieced together information from her medical records and Freedom Of Information Act (FOIA) requests. Journalists and the public alike use FOIA requests to access data from government agencies. Joelving took eight months to complete his comprehensive investigation.

Kesia and Sesilje learned from these documents and others that the clinical trial investigators knew, or should have known, that the placebo was not saline. They read the original study protocol for "V501-015" or FUTURE 2 that explained precisely that the placebo was Merck's proprietary adjuvant amorphous aluminum hydroxyphosphate sulfate, or AAHS, not saline.[6] Further, the clinical trial Protocol, although precise on many things, omitted from the vaccine and placebo descriptions the other ingredients contained in the approved vaccine: polysorbate 80, sodium borate, and L-histidine.[7] If the trial investigators didn't even know these ingredients were there, how could the participants have known?

The Protocol said that safety testing was the clinical trial's number one objective. Yet Merck had assured potential trial volunteers in the brochure they'd received that the control was saline and that FUTURE 2 was not a "side effect trial," because the vaccine had already been proven safe. Was this why their side effects were not taken seriously, because even the trial administrators didn't know exactly what they were injecting into participants? The clinicians did not collect any medical records from Kesia's or Sesilje's doctors and didn't record any details to explain why they thought the symptoms were unrelated. The reason Kesia and Sesilje felt safe enlisting in the trial was that Gardasil had been proven safe.

As they met others who participated in the Danish trials, they realized that they were not alone. But what about trial sites in other countries? They knew that Merck had FUTURE 2 sites all over the world. Did clinicians follow the same protocol everywhere? The protocol states that 10 percent of participants received a "vaccination report card" to record adverse effects in the first fifteen days after each vaccination, but only in the US.[8] Why did Danish girls not receive a report card? They had many more questions.

Kesia and Sesilje have met many other injured women from the clinical trials. Together, these women are supporting one another, and many are starting to get better. They have found a few doctors who believe them and are trying to help. But as they continue their research, they see a pattern: scandal follows the vaccine wherever it is introduced.

3.

RACING TOWARD
THE VACCINE

The HPV vaccine story began long before Kesia and Sesilje were born. Scientists had been trying to find the cause of cervical cancer since the 1800s, putting forward all manner of theories. Once they discovered that viruses could potentially cause cancer, they honed their focus. In 1971, US President Nixon declared a "war on cancer" and signed the National Cancer Act into law. He announced significant federal funding for cancer research; a "cure for cancer" became the ultimate prize. Virus research took off in the 1970s. As research started to explore a connection between viruses and cancer, it was only a matter of time before the starting gun would fire in the race to develop an anticancer vaccine.

THE SCIENCE BEHIND HPV VACCINES

As exciting as the prospects were, HPV research was exceptionally challenging and expensive. The virus replicates only in epithelial cells, such as those that cover or line body surfaces.[1] In the 1980s, advances in DNA technology and molecular cloning were game changers.[2] Germany's University of Freiburg led the way. Harald zur Hausen, who chaired the Virology Institute there at the time, was the first to successfully isolate HPV types to investigate their connections with cervical cancer.[3] In isolating HPV-11, zur Hausen and his colleagues used its DNA sequence to find similar, but not identical, HPV types in cancer cells.[4] He later won the 2008 Nobel

Prize in medicine for his contribution. He shared his Prize with this book's preface author, Dr. Luc Montagnier, who, with Françoise Barré-Sinoussi, shared the other half of the Prize "for their discovery of human immunodeficiency virus."[5]

In the mid-1980s, zur Hausen's team made another breakthrough. They cloned low-risk HPV types, making it possible to identify and isolate high-risk HPV 16 and 18 DNA in cervical cancer biopsies and cell lines.[6] Among the cells in which they found HPV-18 was the HeLa line, a cervical cancer cell culture dating back to 1951.[7]

Even though the team had isolated HPV types that seemed associated with cancer, they could not easily replicate them in the lab.[8] Researchers would need further technological advances to realize the dream of a vaccine against cancer.

THE RACE FOR AN ANTICANCER VACCINE

Two key discoveries laid the groundwork for HPV vaccines: technology to genetically modify viruses to be noninfectious and epidemiological evidence that HPV appears to be cervical cancer's primary cause.[9] During the 1990s, even before the population-based evidence on the relationship between HPV and cervical cancer was in, teams were competing intensely. Fame, fortune, and the sheer joy of discovery were at stake.

Scientists believed that to make a safe HPV vaccine, they needed to ensure the HPV virus would not replicate or cause disease in the body after vaccination. One way to do this is to use a weakened or "attenuated" virus to stimulate the immune system. Since scientists had not been able to effectively cultivate the virus on a large scale in the lab, they ruled that out. Another option was to genetically modify the virus into a virus-like particle or "VLP" to mimic the real virus. This would still require some replication but not as much. A *New York Times* article described early HPV vaccine research as "science fiction."[10] Scientists had found it difficult to isolate HPV, a "stumbling block" for those in "hot pursuit" of a vaccine.[11] They used everything from giant cow warts, to rabbit warts, to circumcised human foreskins grafted onto mice, to replicate the virus. The latter method eventually provided enough virus for continued re-search.[12] Replicating HPV in the lab was the tiny nugget of gold on the riverbed.

Viruses, including HPVs, contain multiple proteins. Scientists learned that certain HPV proteins—called "major capsid" proteins—could be used to create VLPs. They elicit a response from the immune system but do not cause infection. Researchers discovered that of the various HPV proteins, the "L1" protein was best suited to create these VLPs to mimic the actual virus. In the same article discussing the challenges of VLP replication, the *New York Times* described the HPV vaccine's self-assembly of VLPs as "almost magical" and didn't miss a beat in telling readers that Cervarix, GSK's version, was produced "in an insect virus grown in a broth of caterpillar ovary cells."[13]

Several labs around the world were also investigating HPV L1 and L2, another major capsid protein, and VLP technology. Each team knew that timely filed patents were key to a stake in this multibillion-dollar juggernaut, a vaccine whose worldwide potential was astronomical. Even though there were other ways to mitigate the risks of cervical cancer, like regular cervical screening, a vaccine to prevent it would be a blockbuster. Surely whoever reached the finish line first would win a Nobel Prize.

In 1991, Professor Ian Frazer, a Scottish immunologist who had emigrated to Australia, and his colleague, Jian Zhou, a postdoctoral fellow and expert in gene technology, developed a way to genetically engineer noninfectious VLPs. With Australia's University of Queensland backing their research, Frazer and Zhou successfully engineered HPV L1 and L2 proteins into VLPs. While their contributions were significant, the particles failed to activate the immune system sufficiently.[14] Despite this, Frazer and Zhou filed an international patent in Australia on July 19, 1991, and in the United States on July 20, 1992.[15]

Thousands of miles away, a team at Georgetown University filed its patent on June 25, 1992.[16] Unlike the other researchers, the Georgetown team did not develop VLPs, but its work with the L1 protein provided critical background science to the development of the eventual vaccine.[17]

As teams were competing, the US government joined the race. Drs. Lowy and Schiller of the US National Cancer Institute began their research in 1991 and made significant advances.[18] They grew their VLPs in an insect cell culture. They filed their initial patent on September 3, 1992, only a few months after Georgetown and Queensland.

Finally, on March 9, 1993, a team at the University of Rochester filed its patent.[19] The Rochester team, using the creative research methods described by the *New York Times*, eventually isolated the virus by grafting "bits of foreskin collected from hospital circumcisions and infected with genital wart extract into mice."[20] As grotesque as it sounds, this is what it took to create the vaccine.

Simultaneously, during the 1990s, scientists were gathering epidemiological evidence to justify the high cost of developing the vaccine. Dr. Nubia Muñoz, a Colombian doctor who is an HPV expert, headed a working group at the International Agency for Research on Cancer (IARC), to prove that HPV caused cancer and was the primary risk factor in cervical cancer.[21] In 1995, the IARC team reached a consensus that there is sufficient evidence in humans for the carcinogenicity of human papillomavirus HPV 16 and 18.[22] This gave Merck and GSK what they needed to justify further vaccine development. In 1999, in a later article titled *Human papillomavirus is a necessary cause of invasive cervical cancer worldwide*,[23] Dr. Muñoz concluded that "HPV infection was not only the unequivocal central cause of cervical cancer but it should also be viewed as a necessary one."[24]

The teams racing to invent the vaccine endured endless hours, secrecy, trial-and-error experiments, and tedious meetings with patent lawyers, all without knowing whether they would be successful. Only after patents were filed, and the epidemiological evidence was in, could the long process of licensing begin. By the 1990s, the stage was set for manufacturers and inventors to earn vast royalties if the HPV vaccine made it to market. A tangled web of patent interference litigation, licensing agreements, and cross-licensing deals ensued between the four teams, Merck and GSK, and other interested parties.

THE PATENT WARS

Sorting out the patents was a sticky business. The four scientific teams and their lawyers jockeyed and fought to sort out who owned what technology. They could not agree on whose research was the most valuable or which patents were the most vital. Ultimately, the courts resolved the dispute.[25]

All parties had a vested interest in making sure that clinical trials proceeded despite their disagreements. Merck and GSK entered into cross-licensing agreements, which allowed them to move forward with vaccine development while the legal battle wore on. After almost ten years of litigation before the US Patent and Trademark Office, first priority went to Georgetown in 2005. Frazer and Zhou quickly appealed, and in 2007, the Federal Circuit overruled the Patent Office's decision and awarded top priority to the Queensland team based on its 1991 Australian patent.[26] In the end, Frazer and Zhou received credit, and substantial royalties, for the discovery that HPV vaccines can be made from VLPs. Competitors contested their contributions,[27] but Frazer and Zhou took home the patent prize, carrying potentially unlimited royalty revenue.

Frazer and Zhou were not the only winners, however. Each team profits by sharing the royalties, including the NIH Office of Technology Transfer (OTT), which receives undisclosed annual royalty payments from Merck and GSK. In essence, OTT serves as a conduit between government and industry, enabling industry to harness technology developed by government researchers. While this collaboration has often allowed scientific advances to get to the public sooner, it has also created potential conflicts of interest, with the government and its employees profiting directly.

So just how much does the US government make in royalties from HPV vaccines? The short answer is, we don't know. In November 2010, NIH refused to comply with a FOIA request to disclose its HPV vaccine royalties from Merck and GSK.[28] One can glean some insight, though, from OTT's publicly available information. While OTT does not disclose HPV-vaccine specific information, it does report the "Top 20 Commercially Successful Inventions"—a ranking based on annual product sale royalties.[29] Since 2008, HPV-related technologies have ranked first or second.[30] In 2012, authors Mark Blaxill and Dan Olmsted analyzed available data and estimated that the licensing fees to the US government for HPV vaccines were about $15–$20 million annually.[31] That number is likely even higher today. In addition, vaccine inventors Drs. Schiller and Lowy are eligible to receive royalties individually and likely do receive them.[32]

Universities, government institutions, prize committees, and newspapers have showered HPV vaccine developers with accolades. As previously mentioned, Harald zur Hausen reached the pinnacle of scientific achievement, when on December 10, 2008, he received a Nobel Prize for isolating HPV 16 and HPV 18 in cervical cancer. In his acceptance speech, he spoke eloquently of the vaccine's great promise.[33]

The NIH Director lauded Drs. Lowy and Schiller, saying, "It's a heroic story about the effort to fight cervical cancer, the second-most deadly cancer for women worldwide."[34] President Obama awarded them prizes for their technological achievement. And in September 2017, they won Lasker Awards.[35] All the inventors and investors won fame, glory, and a share in the multibillion-dollar revenues to come.

POTENTIAL CONFLICTS OF INTEREST

The US government's role in HPV vaccine development, as investor, patent holder, regulator, and safety monitor, suggests obvious conflicts of interest. The manufacturers also have conflicts, funding clinical trials that should be unbiased, although they have clear incentives to produce favorable results.[36] Clinicians too often have direct and indirect conflicts through their ties to industry. Even when manufacturers do not fund trials, potential conflicts arise. For example, the US government, with support from GSK, conducted a Cervarix trial in Costa Rica.[37] Because the NIH licensed

HPV vaccine technology to Merck and GSK, it had potential revenue on the line, potentially biasing results.[38]

Even pharmaceutical industry insiders criticize how pharmaceutical products get to market. Weak oversight by regulatory authorities coupled with conflicts of interest raise serious questions about the reliability of reported results. As noted by Dr. Michael Carome, of the advocacy group Public Citizen and a former HHS employee, "Instead of a regulator and a regulated industry, we now have a partnership. . . . That relationship has tilted [the FDA] away from a public health perspective to an industry friendly perspective."[39] The HPV vaccine trials underscore these problems.

Funding from outside the government also raises potential conflicts of interest. Pharmaceutical companies pay billions of dollars in fees to the FDA to approve new drugs. For example, between 2000 and 2010, pharmaceutical companies paid the FDA $3.4 billion to gain drug approvals.[40] These payments certainly could influence regulators to view manufacturers more as clients than as entities to regulate.[41] Former FDA employees note that the more fees paid by industry for drug reviews and the greater the FDA's reliance on that funding stream, the more the FDA has "an inclination toward approval."[42]

The revolving door between government agencies and industry is also a potent source of conflicts. Scientists and others leaving government jobs often go to lucrative jobs in the private sector. For example, after serving as the Director of the CDC and waiting for one year as required by law, Dr. Julie Gerberding became the head of Merck's vaccine division. Regulatory agencies and their employees at least have the temptation to spare the hand that feeds them.

In the past twenty years, conflicts of interest have come to permeate research institutions, universities, and physician offices. Dr. Marcia Angell, former editor-in-chief of *The New England Journal of Medicine*, explains:

It is simply no longer possible to believe much of the clinical research that is published, or to rely on the judgment of trusted physicians or authoritative medical guidelines. I take no pleasure in this conclusion, which I reached slowly and reluctantly over my two decades as an editor of *The New England Journal of Medicine*.[43]

Dr. Angell writes that we occupy a world where "[d]rug companies now finance most clinical research on prescription drugs, and there is mounting evidence that they often skew the research they sponsor to make their drugs look better and safer."[44] In addition to sponsoring clinical trials, pharmaceutical companies provide sponsorship for individual researchers, labs, endowed chairs, and more.[45] Similarly, authors and medical journals rely heavily on pharmaceutical advertising, creating further potential for bias.[46] With money and careers at stake, regulators and other stakeholders have incentives, and few disincentives, to align with industry.

Even when pharmaceutical corporations commit fraud or otherwise act illegally, fines are usually insignificant compared to the profits they reap.[47] Real punishments are few and far between.[48] One need only think of the opioid crisis today to get a glimpse of the scope of pharmaceutical industry malfeasance. For example, in the early 2000s, Purdue Pharmaceuticals, the manufacturer of the painkiller OxyContin, hired Merck Medco, a Merck subsidiary, as a pharmacy benefits manager to facilitate wider access to the addictive drug by strong-arming insurance companies not to require preauthorization and to charge only low copayments. Merck helped ensure easy access to the opiates, especially in West Virginia, thus contributing to the opioid epidemic.

While many herald vaccines as a cornerstone of public health, there is no well-founded reason to presume that vaccine research, and vaccine clinical trials in particular, are exempt from such conflicts of interests.

4.

WHO'S REALLY AT RISK FOR CERVICAL CANCER?

"Instead of promoting drugs to treat diseases, [drug companies] have begun to promote diseases to fit their drugs."[1] *Dr. Marcia Angell (2009)*

Selling a product to prevent an infection that almost always resolves without treatment is a herculean task. Selling a treatment to prevent cancer is a winning market strategy, however. Most people fear cancer, and with good reason. To sell the HPV vaccines, the story had to be about cancer. The marketing tactic to emphasize that almost all cervical cancers are related to HPV has worked. This tactic creates a fear of HPV infection, equating infection with cancer, and deflecting attention from the actual risk of developing cervical cancer. But does the science really support the marketing hype?

WHO'S REALLY AT RISK TO DEVELOP CERVICAL CANCER?

Human papillomavirus (HPV) infections are endemic throughout the world. Almost all sexually active people contract HPV, usually unknowingly, at some point in their lives. As Nobel laureate Harald zur Hausen noted, HPVs have likely been with the human species for millions of years.[2] According to CDC data, about 79 million Americans have HPV infections, and about 14 million people contract them each year.[3] The overwhelming majority of HPV infections are innocuous, and approximately 90 percent of them resolve on their own within two years.[4]

Globally, the WHO's International Agency for Research on Cancer estimates that 291 million women are infected with HPV at any given time. It estimates 528,000 cervical cancer diagnoses each year.[5] These figures suggest that approximately 0.18 percent of infections progress to cervical cancer overall. A number of other sources similarly state that 0.15 percent of HPV infections overall progress to cervical cancer.[6]

In high-resource countries, cervical cancer is rare. According to the National Cancer Institute, cervical cancer is the twentieth most common cancer in the US, with a median age at diagnosis of 50.[7] Cervical cancer accounts for only 0.8 percent of all new cancer cases in the US; 0.6 percent of US women will receive a cervical cancer diagnosis in their lifetimes.[8] For those who are diagnosed, cervical cancer is largely treatable, and the 5-year survival rate is over 90 percent when the cancer is caught early enough.[9]

Common Types of Cancer	Estimated New Cases 2018	Estimated Deaths 2018
1. Breast Cancer (Female)	266,120	40,920
2. Lung and Bronchus Cancer	234,030	154,050
3. Prostate Cancer	164,690	29,430
4. Colorectal Cancer	140,250	50,630
5. Melanoma of the Skin	91,270	9,320
6. Bladder Cancer	81,190	17,240
7. Non-Hodgkin Lymphoma	74,680	19,910
8. Kidney and Renal Pelvis Cancer	65,340	14,970
9. Uterine Cancer	63,230	11,350
10. Leukemia	60,300	24,370
-	-	-
20. Cervical Cancer	13,240	4,170

Cervical cancer represents 0.8% of all new cancer cases in the U.S.

0.8%

Source: National Cancer Institute, SEER Cancer Statistics Review[10]

In lower-resource countries, the situation is far more serious. Studies estimate that 85 percent of cervical cancer cases occur in lower-resource countries, where access to routine gynecological care is often lacking.[11] Worldwide, cervical cancer is the seventh most common cancer overall and the fourth most common cancer among women.[12] Eastern Africa has the highest incidence of cervical cancer in the world.[13]

Most researchers believe that persistent, long-term HPV infection—not short-term or transient infection—is a significant risk factor in developing cervical cancer; it seems to be associated in approximately 90 percent of cervical cancers.[14] Even persistent HPV infection alone, however, appears to be insufficient to lead to cervical cancer. Cervical cancer is a multifactor disease, with HPV likely playing a role, together with many other environmental and genetic factors, including:[15]

- Rarely or never having Pap tests or other HPV screening (often a function of economic status and access to healthcare);

- Immunosuppression—for example, if one has HIV or another immunosuppressive illness or is being treated with high-dose steroids;

- History of vaginal, vulvar, or anal neoplasia;

- Family history of cervical cancer;

- Increasing number of sexual partners (increased HPV risk);

- Early age of sexual activity (increased HPV risk);

- Infection with chlamydia and possibly herpes simplex virus;

- Tobacco smoking;

- Overweight;

- Nutrient-poor diet;

- Long-term (more than 10 years) use of oral contraceptives (possible slight increase after 5 years);

- DES daughter (mother took the medication Diethylstilbestrol when pregnant);

- More than three full-term pregnancies;

- First full-term pregnancy before age seventeen

A number of these risk factors—such as poor access to health-care, poor diet, and early and multiple pregnancies—highlight endemic problems among people living in poverty, whether they live in high-, middle-, or low-resource countries. While smoking is now less prevalent among women in high-resource nations, it is on the rise—including among children—in many lower-resource countries. In many very poor countries with high rates of cervical cancer, women continue to cook over open fires or stoves in homes without adequate ventilation, creating a different but potent form of toxic smoke exposure.[16] Hormones also appear to be significant. Risk factors such as weight, pregnancies, and oral contraceptive use all relate to hormones. Examining hormones, especially estrogen, in young women could yield important information. While the role of estrogen in cervical cancer progression is not well understood, research is continuing.[17] Several recent studies have pointed to the potential importance of bacterial microbiota in the vagina to determine whether HPV infections persist.[18] Further, scientists are looking at the potential role of other viruses and the synergies between viruses and bacteria.[19]

Research into the non-HPV risk factors is urgently needed. India, as we show in Chapter 12, reduced cervical cancer rates substantially over the past several decades without a national screening program by improving nutrition, providing cleaner water, and other sound public health changes. Even in low-resource countries, the best defense against cervical cancer remains cervical screening, regardless of whether a woman has had the HPV vaccine. Many people, especially in low-resource countries, argue that it would be wiser to put scarce funds toward reproductive healthcare and cervical screening than into HPV vaccines.

HPV VACCINES: THE BASICS

All three HPV vaccines are intended to protect against infection with two "high risk" HPV types—HPV 16 and 18.[20] Cervarix only has VLPs for these two HPV types. Gardasil additionally includes VLPs for "low-risk" HPV 6 and 11, which are thought to cause genital warts in males and females. Gardasil 9 includes VLPs for five additional "high-risk" HPV types 31, 33, 45, 52, and 58. The theory behind the vaccines is that they will prevent HPV infection, which in turn will prevent cervical tissue abnormalities, called cervical intraepithelial neoplasia—CIN for short—and eventually prevent cervical cancer. The same basic theory is behind vaginal, vulvar, and anal cancers, for which the FDA has also approved the vaccine.

These CINs, categorized as CIN 1 (least severe) to CIN 3 (most severe), usually resolve spontaneously. When CINs do not resolve, routine gynecologic healthcare and treatment can ordinarily resolve them. This is why screening is so important and why medium- and low-resource countries are coming up with creative screening solutions.

The low risk of cervical cancer for girls in high-resource countries contrasts sharply with potential risks from the vaccine. Based on data extrapolated from the Gardasil package insert, the rate of serious adverse reactions following vaccination in the Gardasil clinical trials was 81.49/10,000 (128/15,706 participants), and the death rate was 13.3/10,000 (21/15,706 participants).[21] To put these figures in perspective, the highest rates of cervical cancer disease and death in the world are in East Africa, where cervical cancer rates are 4.27/10,000, and death rates from cervical cancer are 2.76/10,000.[22] Even if only a small fraction of the reported serious adverse reactions and deaths are attributable to Gardasil, these data raise red flags about the benefits of vaccinating all preteens.

HPV SCREENING

HPV vaccines are not a replacement for screening. If women who receive these vaccines forego regular screening in the mistaken belief that the HPV vaccines have eliminated all risk, cervical cancer rates may increase.[23] The vaccines cover a limited number of HPV types; they do not target all high-risk types, and they may not cover types prevalent among certain ethnic or racial groups. Moreover, in reducing or eliminating only some HPV types, other types may fill the void. Thus, screening remains essential.

Doctors have been using the Pap test, a screening technique developed by Dr. George Papanicolaou, for over 60 years to detect abnormal cell changes before they develop into cancer.[24] Pap tests are relatively inexpensive and widely available in high-resource countries. In countries with established and widely available screening, cervical cancer has dropped by as much as 80 percent.[25] By the 2000s, those women in the US who were diagnosed with cervical cancer were frequently women who had not had Pap tests within at least the last five years.[26] In addition to Pap tests, women can receive more recently available HPV DNA and RNA testing, which also analyzes cervical cell samples.[27]

Screening has been successful because cervical cancer develops slowly, often over twenty to thirty years.[28] Regular screening gives time to detect, observe, and treat precancerous lesions.[29] As Planned Parenthood explains on its website, "the vast majority of HPV infections are temporary and not serious, so don't spend a ton of energy worrying about whether you have HPV. Just make sure you're not skipping your regular checkups, including Pap and/or HPV tests."[30]

Dr. Diane Harper was an investigator in both the Cervarix and Gardasil clinical trials. She is a practicing family physician specializing in women's health and has been a researcher at a number of medical schools. Dr. Harper has written that combining screening with vaccination "does not significantly lower the number of women getting cervical cancer every year, but does decrease the number of women with abnormal screening tests."[31] Without Pap tests, even assuming women are vaccinated and that the vaccine works indefinitely—neither of which is true—the rates of cervical cancer are likely to rise.[32]

Despite these warnings, Dr. Harper and her colleague Dr. Leslie DeMars report screening trends that "should cause alarm for cancer control officers."[33] In the US, the age of vaccination appears to play an important role in women getting regular Pap tests. Girls who received HPV vaccines before turning 21 are far less likely to get cervical cancer screening that those who received the vaccines after turning 21: 24 percent versus 84 percent went for regular screening.[34] The CDC recently reported that women under 30 and women with lower income, less education, lack of insurance, or access to healthcare are among those who often don't receive adequate screening. Rates have declined to worrisome levels at some federally funded clinics.[35] The US is not alone. Drs. Harper and DeMars reported similar trends in Australia and the UK, comparing older versus younger women's cervical screening.[36] Screening behaviors are an obvious area of inquiry. We look further at proposed changes to screening protocols in Chapter 23.

VACCINE EFFECTIVENESS: HOW LONG DO HPV VACCINES LAST?

When the FDA approved HPV vaccines, no one knew how long they would protect against HPV infection. If they didn't at least protect through young adulthood, then the vaccines would likely only delay cervical cancer, not prevent it.

Recent long-term studies suggest that the vaccines lower the risk of HPV infections from vaccine types and related cervical lesions.[37] How this translates to cervical cancer rates is unclear, though, in part because of other confounding factors, like declining screening rates.[38]

Scientists believe that persistent HPV infections are a risk factor for cervical cancer, as opposed to transient and self-limiting ones. Current empirical evidence suggests that Gardasil protects for five years and Cervarix for ten against persistent HPV 16 and 18 infections. Because preteens get the vaccine before they reach sexual maturity, waning protection against persistent infection in individuals' twenties and thirties, periods of peak sexual activity, is of concern.

HPV vaccine advocates often point to the low-resource world where women die from cervical cancer because Pap tests are largely unavailable. One has to wonder whether these vaccines will offer real protection there, where people often suffer from malnutrition and poor health. "Perfect" clinical trial participants like Kesia and Sesilje in Denmark do not really resemble women in low-resource countries. Gardasil's coinventor Ian Frazer made this point himself:

> [I]t will be necessary to evaluate field effectiveness of the vaccines in the developing world, particularly in view of the malnutrition, endemic malaria, and adolescent iron deficiency, each of which impact the development of new immune responses and are concerns in many countries with a high prevalence of HPV infection and cervical cancer.[39]

Long-term HPV vaccine effectiveness remains unknown. Screening programs substantially reduce cervical cancer rates, and many HPV infection risk factors are well known. Countries like India show us that addressing those risk factors reduces cancer rates and provides broad public health benefits.

5.

CLINICAL TRIALS:
THE FOUNDATION FOR
THE HPV VACCINE

To make HPV vaccines available to the world, Merck and GSK had to shepherd them through human subject trials and demonstrate their safety and effectiveness.

Vaccine proponents, including the WHO, the CDC, and industry spokespeople, trumpet the HPV vaccine clinical trial data, arguing that they unequivocally demonstrate safety and efficacy. In the 2011 film *The Greater Good*, Dr. Paul Offit stated: "[t]here is no evidence that HPV vaccine causes any of the serious side effects that it has been alleged to cause. It's a beautiful vaccine. It's safe, effective. It doesn't matter what people say. It really doesn't matter what people's opinions are. All you have to do is look at the data and the data, I think, will tell you, you know, how one should approach a problem."[1]

Vaccine promoters dismiss reports of serious injuries and deaths after licensure, downplaying these tragedies as "anecdotal." They criticize researchers who explore potential causal relationships between HPV vaccines and serious adverse outcomes. The public trusts these institutions and individuals that the HPV vaccine trials were well designed, well run, and well policed by powerful health regulators, like the FDA.

Is this true? We now know that the FDA and European Medicines Agency (EMA) did not even rely on all available data to approve

HPV vaccines. In January 2018, an independent study by Lars Jørgensen and Peter Gøtzsche of the Nordic Cochrane Centre and Tom Jefferson of the Centre for Evidence-Based Medicine indexed all known industry and nonindustry clinical trials, a daunting task, demonstrating how difficult it is even for savvy researchers to get information about clinical trials.[2] The authors found it "very disturbing" that the regulators assessed as little as half of all available clinical trial results when they approved each of the HPV vaccines.[3]

Despite the concerns that Jørgensen, Gøtzsche, and Jefferson raised only months earlier, the issue of limited analysis of clinical trials was brought into focus in May 2018, when the Cochrane Collaboration published a favorable review of HPV vaccine clinical trials.[4] Cochrane reached its conclusions relying on only twenty-six studies (twenty-five of which were funded by vaccine manufacturers), just over half the studies available, per the indexing study. Regardless of the circumscribed scope of the review, the Cochrane Collaboration concluded that HPV vaccines were safe and effective in preventing precancerous lesions. Interestingly, the BMJ had rejected a Nordic Cochrane Centre review that had included all the studies and apparently was more critical than the May 2018 review. Dr. David Healy reports that this review likely will be published elsewhere soon.[5]

In July 2018, things heated up further. Jørgensen, Gøtzsche, and Jefferson published an article in BMJ Evidence-Based Medicine highly critical of the Cochrane May 2018 review. They revealed that they sent their index to the Cochrane group working on the review, but the group nonetheless relied on just more than half the available studies, essentially ignoring half of all clinical trial participants.[6] In particular, Jørgensen, Gøtzsche, and Jefferson noted that none of the studies relied on in the May review used a saline placebo and that "[t]he use of active comparators probably increased the occurrence of harms in the comparator groups and thereby masked harms caused by the HPV vaccines."[7] As we discuss in detail in Chapter 7, this is an important shortcoming in assessing the true safety of these vaccines and provides false confidence in their safety. These scientists touch on many of the issues we discuss here, including surrogate endpoints, assessment of adverse events and safety signals, and conflicts of interest. They conclude: "Part of the Cochrane Collaboration's motto is 'Trusted evidence'. We do not find the Cochrane HPV vaccine review to be 'Trusted evidence', as it was influenced by reporting bias and biased trial designs."[8]

Only days later, on August 9, 2018, BMJ published a news article by Nigel Hawkes titled "HPV vaccine safety: Cochrane launches urgent investigation into review after criticisms."[9] The Cochrane team admitted that it had received the index late in their process; they dispute that they missed almost half the studies they should have considered. Yet David Tovey, Cochrane Library's editor-in-chief, states that Cochrane "understand[s] the severity and importance of the criticisms" and the potential wider-ranging implications. He stated that editors and the review's authors were "investigat[ing] the claims as a matter of urgency."[10]

More than a decade after the clinical trials concluded, they still pose many questions:

- What if the subjects had no opportunity to give informed consent?

- What if the protocols did not compare the vaccine to a true placebo?

- What if investigators dismissed reports of serious adverse events?

- What if they didn't collect adverse event data systematically?

- What if government regulators failed to provide rigorous oversight?

- What if investigators had wide discretion to decide what constituted an adverse event?

- What if they had wide discretion to select the trial participants?

- What if the protocols were designed to eliminate long-term data for safety analysis?

What if you learned that all of the above—and more—was true of the HPV vaccine clinical trials? In that case, then we should look at the clinical trial data in a completely different light. Human subjects like Kesia and Sesilje tell a profoundly different story about HPV vaccine clinical trials from the glowing claims from industry, government, and the media.

How Do Clinical Trials Work?

According to US law, the purpose of human subject clinical trials is to "distinguish the effect of a drug from other influences" to determine if a pharmaceutical product is safe and effective before licensing it.[11] In the case of vaccines, a manufacturer must assure the FDA of the safety, purity, and potency of the vaccine.[12] While the FDA reviews materials from trial sponsors, typically manufacturers, it does not conduct its own research or even require significant independent oversight.

When a sponsor wants to begin clinical trials in the hope of getting FDA approval for a new vaccine, the sponsor submits a new drug application to the FDA's Center for Biologics Evaluation and Research (CBER).[13] It usually includes detailed scientific[14] and manufacturing information, and a proposed protocol to study the vaccine in human subjects.[15]

Clinical trials generally have four phases, serving different but overlapping purposes:[16]

> **Phase I trials** are the first human trials. They are small—often only a few dozen or a few hundred participants. In this phase, investigators look for safe dose ranges, side effects, and immunogenicity, which means how well the immune system mounts the desired response. These studies may take place over several months or even a few years.

Phase II trials involve a larger group of people who receive the product to further evaluate safety, dosage, and efficacy, which means whether the product does a better job against the endpoints tested than the placebo or control. Phase II trials may include several hundred participants and last anywhere from a few months to a few years.

Phase III trials are the larger and longer trials most familiar to consumers. They typically enroll anywhere from a few hundred to several thousand participants and last from one to four years, though vaccine trials are often shorter. Phase III trials primarily monitor safety and efficacy.

Phase IV trials are studies the sponsor completes after FDA approval and are intended to provide additional safety and efficacy information after licensure.

In most cases, a sponsor can submit a Biologics License Application for the vaccine once the first three clinical trial phases are complete. The FDA reviews the application and may refer its findings to the Vaccines and Related Biological Products Advisory Committee (VRBPAC), made up of experts from within and outside the FDA for further review before licensing.[17]

THE GARDASIL TRIALS

While this book discusses all three HPV vaccines—Gardasil, Gardasil 9, and Cervarix—we primarily focus on the Gardasil clinical trials. In each phase, Merck conducted multiple studies, referred to as "protocols." Each protocol had an identifying number, linking it to the overall Gardasil clinical trials, which were code-named "V501." For example, Kesia and Sesilje took part in Protocol V501-015, also known as FUTURE II, which was the largest Phase III trial.

Merck and other manufacturers tend to closely guard documents describing study designs and changes they made while the trials were ongoing. Even when documents are available, manufacturers frequently block out or obscure key information, making analysis challenging.[18] We obtained unredacted FUTURE II documents, some of which are linked to the December 2017 *Slate* article. Generally, the public has to rely on limited information from the FDA and other regulators.

Merck began the Gardasil Phase I trials in 1997. However, instead of finishing one phase and assessing data before moving to the next, Merck overlapped Phase I with II, and Phase II with III.[19] Without waiting for all results from each phase, Merck ran concurrent trials on human volunteers, assuring young women like Kesia and Sesilje that the vaccine had been proven safe.

The Phase I and IIa trials tested single HPV-type vaccines, such as only HPV 16.[20] By design, these early trials could not capture information on how well a vaccine combining different HPV types would work or how safe it would be. In 2000, before completing Phase I studies, Merck began Phase IIb, for the first time testing vaccines with four HPV types.[21] The table below outlines the Phase IIb and III clinical trials.

PHASE	PROTOCOL	LOCA-TIONS	POPULATION(s)	FORMULATION(s)	VACCINE RECIPIENTS n=enrolled	CONTROL	CONTROL RECIPIENTS n=enrolled	Dates of Study
PHASE IIb	V501-007	23 sites 5 countries	16-23 yo women	20/40/40/20 & 225 mcg AAHS/0.5ml	290	AAHS: 225 mcg/0.5ml 450 mcg/0.5ml	146 146	5/26/00-5/10/04
				40/40/40/40 & 225 mcg AAHS/0.5ml	284			
				80/80/40/80 & 395 mcg AAHS/0.5ml	292			
PHASE III	V501-013* (FUTURE I)	62 sites 16 countries	16-23 yo women	20/40/40/20 & 225 mcg AAHS/0.5ml	2723	225 mcg AAHS/0/5ml	2732	12/28/01-7/15/05 (& follow up)
	V501-015 (FUTURE II)	90 sites 14 countries	16-23 yo women (26 yo in Singapore)	20/40/40/20 & 225 mcg AAHS/0.5ml	6087	225 mcg AAHS/0/5ml	6080	6/24/02-6/10/05 (& follow up)
	V501-016	61 sites 19 countries	9-15 yo boys and girls 16-23 yo women	20/40/40/20 & 225 mcg AAHS/0.5ml	506 (10-15 yo girls) 510 (10-15 yo boys) 513 (16+ women)	none	none	12/7/02-9/20/04
				12/24/24/12 & 225 mcg AAHS/0.5ml	252 (10-15 yo girls) 256 (16+ women)			
				8/16/16/8 & 225 mcg AAHS/0.5ml	255 (10-15 yo girls) 259 (16+ women)			
				4/8/8/4 & 225 mcg AAHS/0.5ml	252 (10-15 yo girls) 252 (16+ women)			
	V501-018	47 sites 10 countries	9-15 yo boys and girls	20/40/40/20 & 112.5 mcg AAHS/0.5ml	616 girls 568 boys	Carrier Solution/0.5ml	322 girls 275 boys	10/8/03-1/19/05 (& follow up)

Source: Authors, based on data cited in endnotes 19 and 21.

Long before Phase IIb was complete in 2004, Merck began Phase III trials, starting with Protocol 013 in late 2001, with the final Gardasil formulation.

Merck's initial Gardasil trial design favored extremely healthy young women, like Kesia and Sesilje, as human subjects. These young women had limited or no prior exposure to HPVs and few sexual partners. In addition, Merck recruited a small number of young children. The exclusion criteria for FUTURE II (V501-015) were lengthy and broad, but investigators still had wide discretion to exclude anyone simply based on "[a]ny condition which in the opinion of the investigator might interfere with the evaluation of the study objectives."[22]

This healthy user bias in the trials may lead to results that over-estimate effectiveness and underestimate risk.[23] The Gardasil trials were spread across multiple clinical sites in a number of countries, with 2,301 investigators.[24] While there are advantages to numerous sites in many countries, there are disadvantages, as well. Often only a relatively small number of trial participants was at any one site. It's easy to see how investigators might miss or discount safety signals, particularly rare ones, like menstrual changes, or migraines, or seizures.

Merck's Protocol had exclusion criteria for subjects with allergies to vaccine ingredients, including aluminum, yeast, and the enzyme Benzonase.[25] Ironically, Benzonase is not even listed as an ingredient in the final package insert for Gardasil.

> f. Individuals allergic to any vaccine component, including aluminum, yeast, or BENZONASE™ (nuclease, Nycomed [used to remove residual nucleic acids from this and other vaccines]).

Source: FUTURE II Protocol, V501-015, Protocol/Amendment No. 015-00, at 32.[26]

Oddly enough, though, the Protocol did not list other potential allergens in Gardasil: polysorbate 80, sodium borate, and L-histidine. Merck's failure to identify these components raises questions: Were these ingredients in the clinical trial vaccine formulations? If yes, without telling clinicians about this information, how could they accurately decide whom to exclude from the trials based on allergies? Without allergy testing, how could trial subjects know if they were allergic to these unfamiliar ingredients? How could they then give true informed consent?

THE DENIAL OF INFORMED CONSENT

The bedrock of any clinical trial is informed consent. The human volunteers in trials must receive accurate information and understand the potential risks and benefits before agreeing to participate. Merck, GSK, and the hospitals and clinicians who undertook HPV vaccine trials had legal and ethical obligations to be certain that each person gave true informed consent. The subjects had to sign consent forms, and shortcuts simply do not exist.

Strict observance of informed consent rules came out of the bitter lessons of World War II, when Nazi doctors, the foremost doctors in the world at the time, performed medical atrocities on human subjects in the name of science. Dr. Josef Mengele and others performed experiments that killed children for research purposes alone.

In the aftermath of these crimes, the court that sat in judgment prepared the Nuremburg Code, which has served as the blueprint for informed consent norms ever since. The global medical community has embraced the Code, and over time, it has become the basis for all medical experimentation and treatment.[27]

Nuremburg Code Article 1 states:

> The voluntary consent of the human subject is absolutely essential. . . . The duty and responsibility for ascertaining the quality of the consent rests upon each individual who initiates, directs or engages in the experiment. It is a personal duty and responsibility, which may not be delegated to another with impunity.[28]

A 2002 Danish informed consent form, shown below, for the FUTURE II trial states (in the circled area): "One half of the participants receive the active vaccine while the other half receives a so-called placebo vaccine (*i.e.* a vaccine without an active substance)." A September 2004 consent form goes further, clearly calling the placebo "saltvand," or saline. By all appearances, Kesia and Sesilje would have been required to sign these consent forms.

Hvad omfatter undersøgelsen?

Der forventes at deltage i alt 11500 kvinder i undersøgelsen, som foregår både i USA, Sydamerika og Europa, herunder i alle de nordiske lande.

I Danmark vil der deltage ca. 1750 kvinder i alderen 18-23 år. Den ene halvdel af deltagerne får den aktive vaccine, mens den anden halvdel får såkaldt placebo vaccine (dvs. en vaccine uden virksomt stof). Det afgøres ved lodtrækning, hvilken en gruppe den enkelte deltager kommer i. Undersøgelsen er "dobbelt-blind", dvs. at hverken du eller den læge der vaccinerer dig, vil vide om du modtager aktiv eller inaktiv vaccine.

Undersøgelsen varer i alt 4 år. I løbet af det første år vil du blive vaccineret 3 gange med enten den aktive eller den inaktive vaccine (ved undersøgelsens start, efter 2 måneder og efter 6 måneder). Udover dette skal du komme til undersøgelse 7 måneder efter forsøgets start og herefter 1 gang årligt. Ved alle besøg, bortset fra besøgene 2 og 6 måneder efter start, vil du få foretaget en gynækologisk undersøgelse samt få taget en blodprøve og en urinprøve. Urinprøverne vil blive undersøgt for bl.a. klamydia- og gonorré-infektion. Ved det første besøg vil du blive interviewet om livsstilsvaner og tidligere sygdom.

Side 2 af 8

V501/015-00, Informeret samtykke og fuldmagt, version 1, 22APR2002

Source: Danish Cancer Society.[29]

Nogle har oplevet følgende almindelige bivirkninger:
Feber, hovedpine, svimmelhed, kvalme og trætheds-/svaghedsfornemmelse.   Saline

Det vides endnu ikke om ovennævnte bivirkninger skyldes placebo (saltvand) eller aktiv behandling, da data endnu ikke er blevet afblindet.

Under behandling med aktiv vaccine eller placebo er der set følgende alvorlige bivirkninger: Et tilfælde af åndedrætsbesvær; et tilfælde af forringet ledbevægelse med smerter; et tilfælde hovedpine, feber og kulderystelser; et tilfælde af hovedpine og forhøjet blodtryk samt et tilfælde af en overfølsomhedsreaktion.

Source: Authors' files.

Based on these documents, Kesia, Sesilje, and the other Danish girls did not give informed consent. They were denied that basic human right. Was this just the tip of the iceberg?

6.

RUSHING RESULTS: SURROGATE ENDPOINTS AND FAST-TRACKING

The clinical trials did not test whether HPV vaccines prevent cervical or any other cancer. Instead, they tested the vaccines against the development of certain cervical lesions, i.e., abnormal tissue called CIN2 and CIN3 and similar lesions for other genital and anal cancers. These "surrogate endpoints" allowed Merck and GSK to shorten the clinical trials to a few years. Merck further took advantage of FDA fast-tracking and priority review to shrink both Gardasil's and Gardasil 9's approval times. Based on the FDA's own criteria, the wisdom of its decision to accelerate Gardasil's approval is debatable.

SURROGATE ENDPOINTS

Merck and FDA agreed that cancer as the clinical trial endpoint "disadvantages too many women."[1] Researchers also knew that because cervical cancer is rare and has a long latency period, clinical trials using it as the endpoint would need an impossibly large number of participants followed over a long period of time to measure efficacy.[2] So Merck looked for surrogate endpoints to "fill the gap" and overcome these otherwise insurmountable challenges.[3] While surrogate endpoints have become common in drug trials, trial designers and regulators must still analyze whether the proposed endpoints make sense.[4] The FDA has stated that "[i]t is believed that prevention of cervical precancerous lesions is highly likely to result in the prevention of those cancers."[5] But are CIN lesions good surrogates for cervical cancer? Understanding the progression of an HPV infection is key.

When Merck presented information to the FDA to approve Gardasil in April 2006,[6] it included the following graph, purporting to show HPV progression from infection to cancer:

MERCK'S SUBMISSION TO FDA ON HPV PROGRESSION

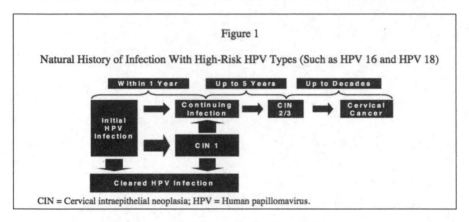

Figure 1

Natural History of Infection With High-Risk HPV Types (Such as HPV 16 and HPV 18)

CIN = Cervical intraepithelial neoplasia; HPV = Human papillomavirus.

Source: Merck April 19, 2006 VRBPAC final briefing document.[7]

Merck's graph potentially leaves the incorrect impression that once an HPV infection has progressed to a CIN2 lesion or worse, the march to cervical cancer is inevitable. In fact, the progression of an HPV infection is far more complex, and only a very small percentage, perhaps as low as 0.18 percent, progress to cervical cancer.

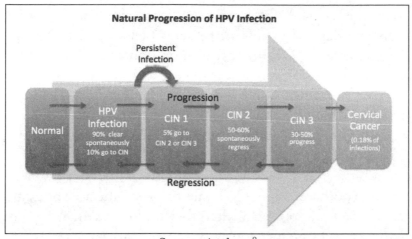

Source: Authors;[8]
see endnote 8 for details.

Keeping these graphics in mind, we can now look in more detail at CINs. CIN lesions are generally divided into three categories, from least to most severe: CIN1, CIN2, and CIN3. CIN1 lesions were not considered appropriate as surrogate endpoints for the clinical trials, and with good reason. They are not precancerous and are a poor predictor of cervical cancer.[9] While more prevalent than CIN2 or 3 lesions, the vast majority of CIN1 lesions resolve spontaneously. CIN1 typically progresses when the infection is persistent, and other risk factors, like smoking, play a role.[10] We address these risk factors in detail in Chapter 4.

What about CIN2? Is this a good surrogate endpoint for cervical cancer? Cancer experts like NCI's Dr. Mark Schiffman recognize that CIN2 may not be precancerous either, and it too may be a poor surrogate: "A large proportion of CIN2 lesions regress, suggesting that such lesions should be viewed as 'severe appearing' HPV infection rather than precancer."[11] In particular, as Dr. Schiffman, his colleague Dr. Philip Castle, and others point out: "[i]nclusion of CIN 2 . . . in the definition of an endpoint in clinical trials likely results in a high proportion of diagnoses with little or no invasive potential."[12] Because CIN2 is not necessarily precancerous and often resolves on its own,[13] perhaps there is a limitation in using this as a true endpoint for cervical cancer.

So we are left with CIN3. The NCI reports that 50 percent or less, and perhaps as low as 30 percent, of CIN3 lesions progress to cervical cancer.[14] Cochrane Collaboration recently assessed the probability of CIN3 progression to cervical cancer to be as low as 12 percent.[15] So while CIN3 lesions may be the most relevant endpoint, even Drs. Castle and Schiffman and their colleagues have recognized that CIN3 is an "imperfect" surrogate for cancer,[16] in part because the *majority* never progress. These experts raise the issue of whether HPV vaccine clinical trials are "underpowered" to test their hypotheses about CINs and cervical cancer.[17] For example, trials may be underpowered when they are not adequate in size or design, such as using inadequate surrogate markers.

At a minimum, Merck's chart above implies a stronger association between CIN2 and CIN3 lesions and cervical cancer than accepted science acknowledges. We won't know for years if these CIN2 and 3 endpoints used in the clinical trials were valid surrogates. In fact, because of confounding factors, like changing cervical screening recommendations, it may be impossible to ever determine whether the vaccines will prevent cervical cancer cases that would not have been prevented otherwise.

FAST-TRACKING AND PRIORITY REVIEW: WHY THE RUSH?

"Because Merck was so aggressive, it went too fast. I would have liked to see it go much slower."[18] *Dr. Diane Harper, Principal Investigator, Gardasil and Cervarix clinical trials*

In 2002, the FDA agreed to speed up the Gardasil approval process.[19] The FDA fast-tracked Gardasil, allowing Merck to submit data to support its licensing application on a rolling basis rather than all at once. In 2005, FDA also granted Merck priority review—a process that shortened the review period from ten months to six.[20] Fast-tracking is coveted in the industry. It streamlines the clinical trial process and means that FDA is working closely with the manu-facturer to ensure any problems can be resolved in a timely fashion.

The FDA explained in a letter to the authors that fast-tracking is justified when the new drug or biologic treats "serious or life-threatening conditions" and "addresses unmet medical needs." The FDA asserted that a vaccine against cervical cancer met these criteria, whereas a vaccine to prevent genital warts alone did not.[21] According to the FDA, whether a condition is "serious" is a matter of judgment but depends on such factors as "survival, day-to-day functioning, or the likelihood that the condition, if left untreated, will progress from a less severe condition to a more serious one."[22] The FDA defines "filling an unmet need" as providing a drug or therapy where none exists or where the proposed therapy is poten-tially superior to the existing one.[23]

In 2002, the FDA fast-tracked Gardasil, deciding that Merck met the "serious condition" and "unmet needs" criteria. However, a year later, in a press release discussing HPV DNA tests, FDA admitted that most HPV infections are neither serious nor life-threatening but rather are "short-lived and not associated with cervical cancer."[24] In that same press release, it advised that if women get regular cervical screening, they could avoid cancer or get treatment to potentially cure it. This undermines the assertion that HPV vaccines will fill an unmet medical need.[25] There is a clear disconnect in the FDA's positions.

When there is an effective existing intervention, the FDA has es-tablished five additional criteria to determine if fast-tracking is appro-priate.[26] The FDA did not apply these criteria, because Pap tests (and now HPV DNA tests) are diagnostic tools, not preventive ther-apies.[27] Because it was not obliged to consider Pap tests as an "avail-able therapy" to prevent cervical cancer, the FDA was able to dis-regard that Gardasil would not have met the additional criteria for fast-tracking. If the goal is to prevent cancer, then Pap tests should have been considered, and Gardasil should have been required to meet these additional criteria. Let's look at each criterion in turn.

(1) Superior effectiveness to the existing treatment? NO.

While Pap tests are diagnostic and not therapeutic, they have proven to be effective at preventing cervical cancer, particularly in high-resource countries like the US. In the absence of cervical screening, Gardasil and Cervarix will likely be less effective than Pap tests.[28] Even when combined with screening, Dr. Diane Harper has said that the vaccines likely will not substantially reduce cervical cancer cases.[29]

(2) New therapy avoids serious side effects of existing therapy: NO.

Side effects from Pap tests are rare and minor. They include false positives and anxiety from abnormal results. While interventions following an abnormal Pap test may have some negative health consequences, like thinning of the cervix and premature birth, they are rare.[30]

(3) Improves "the diagnosis of a serious condition where early diagnosis results in an improved outcome." NO.

Even assuming the vaccine can prevent cervical cancer, Gardasil fails to meet this criterion. When combined with Pap tests, HPV vaccines are unlikely to reduce cervical cancer rates in high-resource nations.[31] Pap tests have been highly effective in identifying CIN lesions and reducing cervical cancer, regardless of HPV type. The fact that almost all HPV infections and lesions never progress to cervical cancer should have made fast-tracking unavailable.

(4) Decreases "a clinical significant toxicity of an available therapy that is common and causes discontinuation of treatment." NO.

There is no "clinical significant toxicity" related to Pap tests or to the HPV DNA and RNA testing now available. In contrast, Gardasil contains substances with known toxicity and also substances for which the toxicity is not well understood.

(5) Addresses "an emerging or anticipated public health need." NO.

Before Merck's aggressive marketing campaign, there was no HPV public health emergency in high-resource countries. HPV was considered a benign infection that most people cleared without ever knowing they had it. Pap tests protected women from cervical cancer, which is rare in the US.[32]

Merck and FDA faced a conundrum. The only conceivable surrogate markers available to them, CIN 2 and CIN 3, were not well suited to stand in the place of cervical cancer. However, with no other choice, the FDA accepted these markers and allowed the Gardasil trials to proceed. Then, as the trials progressed, by relying on the distinction between prevention and diagnosis of cervical cancer, the FDA did not require Merck to fulfill all the criteria discussed above, which made it easier for the FDA to justify fast-tracking. Somehow, Merck convinced the FDA to green-light a vaccine that, even more than a decade out, has been shown to, at best, prevent conditions that would have resolved in most cases without any intervention.

7.

"FAUXCEBOS" AND PLACEBOS

"The goal of a clinical trial is to establish the truth about an intervention designed to alter the natural history of disease. The trial may concern prevention, diagnosis or therapy, and the specific questions may focus on effectiveness, relative effectiveness, or on benefits, risks and costs. The subject and society as a whole have a stake in the outcome. The subject and society are both mistreated if the trial has no chance of establishing the truth because of flaws in design or interpretation."[1] James F. Holland, MD

WHAT MAKES A PLACEBO?

When we think about clinical trials, we imagine that neither the investigators nor the volunteers know who receives the treatment or vaccine and who gets the benign substance, like saline.[2] This classic "gold standard" trial is called a "randomized double-blind place-bo-controlled trial." Comparing a new product against an inactive control provides an accurate picture of the product's effects—both good and bad. Further, when participants and investigators don't know who receives what, the results and reporting are thought to be more reliable and unbiased. Unlike trials for drugs to treat illnesses or conditions, vaccine trials don't have to worry about the "placebo effect"—where people appear to get better even when they receive an inactive substance.

The WHO and FDA endorse saline placebos in vaccine trials. The WHO notes that they are particularly valuable for evaluating the safety and efficacy of *new* vaccines.[3] But in most vaccine clinical trials, saline placebos are the exception, not the rule. Instead, designers typically test new vaccines against existing ones as controls. They claim it would be unethical to deprive the control group of vaccine benefits.[4] Even with this justification, though, the WHO recognizes that using another vaccine as a control creates a "methodological disadvantage." It states that "[i]t may be difficult or impossible to assess fully the safety" of a vaccine when there is no true placebo.[5]

Gardasil and Cervarix are just the kind of new vaccines that Merck and GSK should have compared to saline placebos. They did not. No HPV vaccine clinical trial had a true saline placebo control. Instead, Merck and GSK used a variety of adjuvants, other vaccines, and chemical solutions as the so-called placebos.

NOTHING TO SEE: THE FAUXCEBO EFFECT

Merck used "fauxcebos"—or false placebos—as controls in the Gardasil trials, with the FDA's blessing. These fauxcebos appear to have masked Gardasil's ill effects. For all but a few hundred clinical trial participants, Merck used AAHS, Gardasil's aluminum-containing adjuvant, as the primary control. AAHS is an active ingredient that boosts the immune system to enhance the vaccine's effect. Only one small group of approximately six hundred 9-to-15-year-olds in Protocol 018 received something other than AAHS. But they didn't receive saline, either.

What did they receive? It looks like they got an active "carrier solution" fauxcebo, which contained everything in the vaccine except the VLPs and AAHS. It's confusing, though. When the FDA approved Gardasil, it described the Protocol 018 control as a "true saline placebo."[6] The FDA even said that this supposed "saline placebo-controlled" trial was "of particular interest," because this group allegedly used a true placebo compared to the AAHS control.[7] Was the FDA wrong? It certainly seems that way.[8]

In 2007, several Merck scientists and others published a study on Protocol 018. They described the control as a solution containing "identical components to those in the vaccine with the exception of HPV L1 VLPs and the aluminum adjuvant."[9] In other words, the carrier solution contained a number of potentially toxic components: Polysorbate 80, sodium borate (Borax), genetically modified yeast, and L-histidine.[10] Even while allowing Merck to add it to Gardasil, the FDA has banned sodium borate in food products because of its risks.[11] Polysorbate 80 crosses the blood-brain barrier and is associated with many health problems, including infertility and cardiac risk.[12] Scant research supports the safety of these ingredients.

The Australian drug approval agency, the Therapeutic Goods Administration (TGA), acknowledged that the Protocol 018 control group did not receive saline. In 2015, Dr. Deirdre Little, an Australian gynecologist, brought Merck's inaccurate description of the study 018 control to the TGA's attention. In a letter, the TGA advised Dr. Little that they investigated and found that "the current information is a misrepresentation of the situation. That is, that the current reference to the placebo being 'saline' misrepresents the actual placebo in Protocol 018."[13] They assured her that they asked Merck to change its package insert to reflect that the placebo was *not* saline. As of the time of writing, in July 2018, however, the Australian package insert still refers to saline as the placebo.[14]

Like Merck, GSK had no saline placebos in its clinical trials. GSK's Cervarix vaccine used a novel and proprietary adjuvant called "Adjuvant System 04," or "AS04" for short. This adjuvant system includes aluminum hydroxide and a substance that has a potent immune system effect called MPL (see Chapter 20). In the clinical trials, GSK used fauxcebos, including unlicensed vaccines, and different adjuvants as "controls" to assess Cervarix's safety.[15]

Did anyone in any of the HPV clinical trials receive a true saline placebo, as the WHO recommends? Out of the tens of thousands of children, women, and men who participated in the Merck and GSK trials that the FDA reviewed, it appears that only a few hundred in one Gardasil 9 trial group *may* have received a saline placebo. Even these young women and girls were not true controls, though, because they had already received three doses of Gardasil before the Gardasil 9 trial.[16] In short, it appears that *no one* in the HPV vaccine trials ever received only a true saline placebo as a control.

MASKING SAFETY SIGNALS AND CAUSING HARM?

Many experts believe that aluminum-based adjuvants should never be used as controls in vaccine clinical trials because they pose substantial health risks and obscure safety results.[17] World-class aluminum expert Dr. Christopher Exley has stated that one must "make a very strong scientific case for using a placebo which is itself known to result in side effects and I have not found any scientific vindication for such in the recent human vaccination literature."[18] He is far from alone in the scientific community.[19] For those concerned about aluminum, Chapter 20 is a deep dive on the subject.

According to federal regulations, a manufacturer should not add an adjuvant to a vaccine if it poses safety risks.[20] When the authors asked the FDA for clinical safety data in humans for AAHS, the FDA did not supply any. Despite mounting evidence of aluminum's health risks and lack of any known benefits, the FDA continues to presume its safety. The FDA bases this on longtime use of aluminum-based adjuvants generally.[21] The bottom line is that no definitive studies show that these adjuvants are safe.[22]

How does the FDA justify allowing Merck to use AAHS in vaccines, let alone as a control? The FDA's surprising answer has nothing to do with safety. In a letter to the authors, it stated that using AAHS as a control was necessary to ensure "blinding the study," explaining that AAHS "looked similar" to the vaccine, so neither investigators nor participants knew who received what.[23]

Of course, blinding is a critical aspect of rigorous placebo-controlled studies, but the FDA's claim that AAHS was necessary is preposterous. In Protocol 018, the control group received the carrier solution, which did not look like the vaccine. That study had a work-around, using staff who did not otherwise work with trial

participants to prepare and administer injections.[24] Investigators in
the Gardasil 9 "saline placebo" group also used this method.[25]

Is there any rationale to include an adjuvant control group in a
vaccine clinical trial? Maybe. Scientists could argue that an adjuvant
control might signal whether the vaccine/adjuvant combination
has unexpected safety results. This reasoning might support an aluminum-based control as a secondary control group, but not the primary one. To see a true safety signal, a saline placebo is preferable,
as the WHO had made clear.

Merck and FDA concluded that because the vaccine and AAHS
control had similar safety profiles, the vaccine must be safe. This is
a bit like saying that because cigarettes and cigars have similar risk
profiles, they both must be safe. Given aluminum's known toxicity,
assuming its safety is mind-boggling.

In an apparent attempt to obfuscate things, Merck frequently
combined safety data from the AAHS controls with the group that
received the carrier solution. This data pooling creates the false impression that adverse events occurred at similar rates across both
groups:

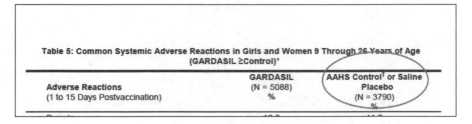

Table 5: Common Systemic Adverse Reactions in Girls and Women 9 Through 26 Years of Age (GARDASIL ≥Control)*		
Adverse Reactions (1 to 15 Days Postvaccination)	GARDASIL (N = 5088) %	AAHS Control† or Saline Placebo (N = 3790) %

Source: *Gardasil Package Insert, at 6 (Table 5).*[26]

A bit of sleuthing, however, demonstrates that the AAHS and
carrier solution results were starkly different. Locating separate safety data for the two groups is challenging because the FDA provided insufficient information. Occasionally, though, one can cross-
reference tables. FDA's Table 229, below, shows that *none* of the
9-to-15-year-olds in the Protocol 018 carrier solution group had any
serious adverse events, or SAEs, in days 1 to 15 after vaccination:[27]

TABLE 229		
Protocol 018: Clinical Adverse Experience Summary Days 1-15 Postvaccination – Protocol 018 (Overall)		
	HPV vaccine group N=1179	Placebo group N=594
Subjects with follow-up	1165	584
N (%) with 1+ AE	963 (82.7%)	392 (67.1%)
N (%) with IS AE	877 (75.3%)	292 (50.0%)
N (%) with systemic AE	541 (46.4%)	260 (44.5%)
N (%) with SAE	5 (0.4%)	0 (0.0%)
Deaths	0	0
D/C due to AE	3 (0.3%)	0(0.0%)
D/C due to SAE	1 (0.1%)	0 (0.0%)
Source: From Table 8-1, CSR 018v1, p. 140		

Source: FDA 2006 Gardasil Clinical Review, at 316 (Table 229)
(emphasis added).[28]

By contrast, FDA's Table 295 below *combines* data from AAHS and carrier solution groups and collectively labels them the "placebo."[29] The Table below shows 43 SAEs in this combined group. We know from Table 229 above that all 43 SAEs occurred in the AAHS controls, and not in the carrier solution group, which had zero SAEs.[30] Unless one delves into this opaque data, though, one would assume that the SAEs occurred across both control groups.

TABLE 295		
Protocols 007, 013, 015, 016, and 018 Clinical Adverse Experience Summary (Days 1 to 15 after any Vaccination Visit) - Safety Population (Cumulative Data)		
	Gardasil N=11778	Placebo N=9686
Subjects with Follow-up	11641	9578
	N/%	N/%
Subjects with ≥ 1 AE	5729 (49.2%)	3659 (38.2%)
Injection Site AEs	5195 (44.6%)	3049 (31.8%)
Systemic AEs	3750 (32.2%)	2571 (26.8%)
Subjects with SAEs	59 (0.5%)	43 (0.4%)
Deaths	3 (0.03%)	1 (0.01%)
Discontinued due to AE	15 (0.1%)	10 (0.1%)
Discontinued due to SAE	4 (0.03%)	3 (0.03%)
Source: Source: Summary of Clinical Safety, Table 2.7.4:4, p. 29 (3/8/06)		

Source: FDA 2006 Gardasil Clinical Review, at 378 (Table 295)
(emphasis added).[31]

In Protocol 018, the carrier solution group was small, with only 594 children. Unlike every other protocol, where vaccine recipients and controls were matched roughly 1:1, here the ratio was 2:1, with twice as many vaccine recipients as controls.[32] Because of this, Protocol 018 lacked statistical "power" or significance. In addition, it has the only non-AAHS control group and the only trial group with children aged 9 to 15, the ultimate target population for the product. Merck should have published separate and consistent data for the two distinct groups, the AAHS and carrier solution controls. The FDA should have required it. Unfortunately, it did not.

When the trials ended, HPV vaccines superficially appeared to be as safe as their controls because of fauxcebos. When Kesia and Sesilje found out that there had been no saline groups, they were outraged. Not only had they been duped and put at risk, but the science on which the vaccines now rest is fatally flawed. The public, including most medical professionals, remain in the dark about these faux clinical trials. Yet this was not the worst of the HPV vaccine data manipulation.

8.

PROTOCOL 018: HIDING IN
PLAIN SIGHT?

In the last chapter, we shone a light on fauxcebos, including the carrier solution Merck used in the Protocol 018 Gardasil trial. In this chapter, we shift our focus to that study's vaccine formulation, given to 9-to-15-year-olds. Hidden in plain sight in an FDA document is evidence that the vaccinated children in Protocol 018 received just *half* the AAHS adjuvant than in the licensed vaccine.[1] It is possible, although not likely, that this is a typographical error. But, if proven true through full disclosure, the implications are enormous.

The FDA's 2006 Clinical Review shows evidence of this dose anomaly.[2] Table 210 below describes the vaccine formulation as "per mL" (milliliter), but Gardasil is dosed by the half-milliliter. Simple division shows that the 0.5 mL dose administered in the 018 study contained only **112.5 mcgs** (micrograms) of AAHS, as well as the standard ratio of the four HPV L1 VLPs:

Clinical Material	Formulation Number	Dosage	Package and Storage	225 mcg of AAHS per mL = 112.5 mcg per 0.5 mL
		TABLE 210 Protocol 018: Vaccine Products Used		
Quadrivalent HPV (Types 6, 11, 16, 18) L1 VLP Vaccine	V501 VAI025T004	40/80/80/40 mcg plus 225 mcg aluminum adjuvant /mL 0.5 mL	0.75-mL single dose vial	
Placebo for Quadrivalent HPV (Types 6, 11, 16, 18) L1 VLP Vaccine	PV501 VAI036P001	Carrier Solution Only /0.5 mL	0.75-mL single dose vial	
HPV = Human papillomavirus; VLP = Virus-like particles.				

Source: FDA 2006 Gardasil Clinical Review, at 301 (Table 210) (emphasis and text box added).[3]

No other clinical trial described the vaccine formulation this way. For example, the table below shows the standard *per 0.5 mL* dose description used in Protocol 015:

Products Mandated by Protocol			
TABLE 26			
Protocol 015: Clinical Products Used			
Clinical Material	Formulation Lot Information	Dosage	Package
Initial Enrollment Period			
Quadrivalent HPV 6, 11, 16, 18 L1 VLP Vaccines	V501 VAI018I001, V501 VAI025T001, V501 VAI025T002.	HPV 6, 11, 16, 18 L1 VLP 20/40/40/20 mcg with 225 mcg aluminum adjuvant/0.5 mL	0.75 mL single dose vial
Placebo	PV501 VAI019A001	225 mcg aluminum adjuvant/0.5 mL	"

Source: Excerpted from Table 26, 2006 FDA Gardasil Clinical Review, at 50. (Emphasis added by authors.)[4]

The way Merck presented the formulation is unnecessarily confusing and obfuscates the true formulation used in the study. Nothing in the title of the study or the FDA's discussion in the Clinical Review hints at a substantially different AAHS dose. Other studies with nonstandard AAHS and VLP doses clearly disclose that information.[5] Why would Merck give the children in study 018 a vaccine with only half the standard AAHS amount?[6]

Protocol 018 is unique. The FDA considered it important because it is the only study in the preteen target population comparing Gardasil to a non-aluminum-containing control (the carrier solution).[7] A lot was at stake, as it would provide the *only* long-term study cohort for this age group. We can only speculate as to why Merck would want this group to receive only a half AAHS dose. Perhaps Merck was testing different adjuvant levels in various studies to find the "sweet spot" for the ratio of AAHS to VLPs. Or perhaps giving the children a lower AAHS dose might avoid a larger disparity in reactions between the vaccine and carrier solution groups. Whatever the reason, illuminating the dosing discrepancy would likely have meant more questions from the FDA and more costly clinical trials, possibly delaying Gardasil's much-awaited launch.

MISSING A RED FLAG?

Was the AAHS half dose sufficient to elicit an antibody response that would satisfy the FDA that the vaccine produced a strong enough immune reaction? The data suggest that it was. Children in Protocol 018 had similar antibody levels to another small group of 10-to-15-year-old children, in Protocol 016, who got the full 225 microgram AAHS dose.[8] *Both groups* of children had much higher antibody responses than the young women in the trials, whose levels Merck and the FDA considered acceptable.[9]

This should have raised a red flag to study whether preteens needed the full AAHS dose. But it appears that the FDA missed this signal and approved the vaccine with the higher AAHS dose without question.

DOES THE DOSE MAKE THE POISON?

If the higher AAHS dose was not needed to provoke a strong enough immune response in preteens, what does it imply for safety? No Gardasil clinical trial, regardless of age group, tested the vaccine against a true saline placebo. Assuming Table 210 is correct, there is also no trial study comparing standard Gardasil to a nonaluminum placebo of any kind. Given that the vaccine is administered to healthy preteens with essentially zero immediate risk of cervical or other HPV-related cancers, the highest safety standards should apply. To minimize the risk of harm, these children should receive the lowest possible dose of AAHS.

The idea that aluminum is safe at any dose and in any form is not supported by any scientific research. A growing body of research demonstrates its harmful effects, which we examine further in Chapter 20. Some vaccine experts explain that if a vaccine contains too much aluminum, the excess may bind to nonvaccine proteins, including the host's own proteins or latent viruses, and may trigger autoimmune and other serious conditions.

Unfortunately, we can't compare long-term health outcomes between the two groups of children in Protocols 016 and 018 because the FDA chose not to publish safety data on Protocol 016 past day

15.[10] We can compare some long-term health effects, however, in the Protocol 018 children against pooled results from several trial protocols. Using data from "new medical conditions" (see Chapter 11), we see that 29 percent of children in Protocol 018 reported new illnesses compared to 49.6 percent in the pooled group.[11] It's difficult to draw a conclusion from these data, as the time periods don't match and the pooled data include Protocol 018 itself. Still, one must wonder if the pooled results would have been even worse if the 018 results had not been included. Furthermore, Merck and the FDA do not consider that "new medical conditions" may be vaccine-related. These data, however, are all we have to examine to try to uncover the true risk of HPV vaccines in the preteen target population.

TABLE 245 Protocol 018: New Medical Conditions Day 1 through Month 12		
Subjects in analysis population	Gardasil N=1128	Placebo N=562
Subjects with new medical history	327 (29.0%)	174 (31.0%)

Source: Excerpted from Table 245, 2006 FDA Gardasil Clinical Review, at 329 (emphasis added).[12]

TABLE 302 Protocols 007, 013, 015, 016 and 018: New Medical Conditions Day 1 through Month 7 in the Safety Population		
Subjects in analysis population	Gardasil N=11778	Placebo N=9686
Subjects with new medical history	5842 (49.6%)	4750 (49%)

Source: Excerpted from Table 302, 2006 FDA Gardasil Clinical Review, at 393 (emphasis added).[13]

The FDA could have required Merck to conduct larger trials on children to see if the antibody data from the small, underpowered studies held up, and more important, to further explore safety signals. The FDA also could have asked Merck to include a true saline placebo group in a larger study of preteens. But it failed to do so.

THE PROTOCOL 018 FOLLOW-UP STUDIES

The CDC and American Academy of Pediatrics proclaim Gardasil both safe and effective based on follow-up studies of Protocol 018. None of the three published articles[14] on Protocol 018 addresses the AAHS dose anomaly, yet surely some of the authors must have been aware of it. Several Merck experts, including Dr. Eliav Barr, are co-authors on key Protocol 018 studies.[15] Dr. Barr is now a senior vice president of Merck Global Medical Affairs but from 1998 to 2008, led the Gardasil clinical research and regulatory program.[16] He testified before the FDA's vaccine advisory committee to win Gardasil's approval.[17] Did Dr. Barr or others involved in the trial design know about the AAHS anomaly?

Perhaps Merck and the FDA will claim that the formulation information is an error and that Protocol 018 used the standard formulation. If that's the case, why didn't anyone at Merck or the FDA correct this mistake over the course of twelve years, since Gardasil first came on the market?

WHAT HAPPENS NEXT?

A 2017 follow-up study based on Protocol 018 in *Pediatrics* confidently asserts that it "should help to dismiss any lingering doubts about the safety and durability of HPV vaccine-induced protection."[18] The authors clearly hope that the article will hammer the final nail into the coffin of HPV vaccine skeptics. Clinicians around the world rely on it to dismiss a connection between the vaccine and injuries. *Pediatrics* carries a lot of weight with pediatricians. But if the Protocol 018 data are based on a different vaccine formulation, *Pediatrics* should immediately retract both the 2014 and 2017 follow-up studies. If Merck used a half AAHS dose, the data from that Protocol do *not* support safety of the standard Gardasil formulation.

In fact, journals should retract *any* articles relying on Protocol 018 for the same reason.

Physicians need accurate information so that their patients can make well-informed decisions. Any revised and republished articles should also clarify that the placebo group in Protocol 018 received the carrier solution, not saline.

If we are correct in our reading of the FDA Clinical Review text, this may go a long way toward explaining the disconnect between what the follow-up data purportedly show and the very serious re-actions that families report. The AAHS dose anomaly demands urgent attention.

But is this anomaly the tip of the iceberg? Just before this book went to press, the authors obtained evidence that the AAHS dosing anomaly may not be an isolated incident; there are serious addition-al questions about the ingredients in both the vaccine and control formulations for Protocol 018 as well as the vaccine formulation for Protocol 015.[19] Further investigation into precisely what injections the clinical trial participants received is imperative. The discrep-ancies that have come to light raise questions not only about trial safety and integrity, but also about the informed consent of clinical subjects.

9.

ENHANCING RISK: "NEGATIVE EFFICACY"

When people say a vaccine is "effective," they mean that it works in the real world to protect against a specific disease. "Efficacy," on the other hand, is a narrower, technical term in a clinical trial to compare a test group to a control group. Here, it compares the reduction in disease incidence between a vaccine group and a control group. The HPV clinical trial data raise a troubling question of "negative efficacy." Negative efficacy means that the vaccine might *cause or contribute* to the very condition it is meant to prevent. In both the Gardasil and Cervarix clinical trials, data show that there is a frightening possibility that some vaccinated girls who had an HPV infection or HPV antibodies when they were vaccinated are more likely to develop CIN2 or CIN3 lesions, or even cancer. Can HPV vaccines enhance the risk of cervical cancer? We don't know for sure, but the "negative efficacy" findings in the clinical trials certainly suggest that they may.

"NEGATIVE EFFICACY": COULD THE VACCINE CAUSE CERVICAL CANCER?

Merck and GSK state that the vaccine may not protect women who have been exposed to HPV before. What they do not say, however, is that women who have been exposed to HPV before may have enhanced risk for cervical disease.

The clinical trial results show this risk, which should have prompted Merck and GSK to strongly consider screening before vaccination, or prescreening. Instead, by recommending the vaccine for children who are sexually naive, this appeared to avoid the problem of so-called "negative efficacy."

In the trials, Merck reported that women who had a current HPV 16 or 18 infection *and* evidence of prior exposure to those types on day 1 were 44.6 *percent* more likely to develop CIN2 or CIN3 lesions or worse compared to the fauxcebo group, even within a few years of receiving the vaccine:[1]

	Gardasil™ N=2717				Placebo N=2725					
Endpoint	N (subgroup)	Number of cases	PY at risk	Incidence Rate per 100 person years at risk	N (subgroup)	Number of cases	PY at risk	Incidence Rate per 100 person years at risk	Observed Efficacy	95% CI
HPV 6/11/16/18 CIN 2/3 or worse	156	31	278.9	11.1	137	19	247.1	7.7	-44.6%	<0.0, 8.5%

Table 17. Study 013: Applicant's analysis of efficacy against vaccine-relevant HPV types CIN 2/3 or worse among subjects who were PCR positive _and_ seropositive for relevant HPV types at day 1. [From original BLA, study 013 CSR, Table 11-88, p. 636]

Negative Efficacy: Gardasil
Source May 2006 VRBPAC Background Document, at 13 (Table 17)
(emphasis added).[2]
(nb: PCR positive means a positive HPV DNA test result, suggesting current infection; seropositive means testing positive for HPV antibodies in the blood, suggesting a prior exposure.)

Similarly, women who either had a current infection and/or a prior exposure for relevant types showed negative efficacy of -33.7 *percent* compared to the controls:[3]

	Gardasil™ N=2717				Placebo N=2725					
Endpoint	N (subgroup)	Number of cases	PY at risk	Incidence Rate per 100 person years at risk	N (subgroup)	Number of cases	PY at risk	Incidence Rate per 100 person years at risk	Observed Efficacy	95% CI
HPV 6/11/16/18 CIN 2/3 or worse	685	48	1385.6	3.5	664	35	1350.3	2.6	-33.7%	<0.0, 15.3%

Table 19. Study 013: Analysis of efficacy against vaccine-relevant HPV types CIN 2/3 or worse among subjects who were PCR positive _and/or_ seropositive for the relevant HPV type at day 1.
[From additional efficacy analyses requested by CBER and submitted March 15, 2006, table 1e-2, p. 13.]

May 2006 VRBPAC Background Document, at 14 (Table 19)
(emphasis added).[4]

The FDA asserts that these women had "enhanced risk factors" for CIN 2 or worse, including smoking or a history of sexually transmitted infections. These enhanced risk factors reflect real-world cervical cancer risk, though. The FDA minimized these risk factors, suggesting that the data merely showed that the vaccine "lacks therapeutic efficacy among women who have had prior exposure to HPV and have not cleared a previous infection." In its 2006 clinical review of Gardasil, however, the FDA "concluded that there was *no clear evidence* of vaccine related disease enhancement." (Emphasis added.)[5] The FDA did not deny, however, that there was *some* evidence of risk enhancement.

In several clinical trial subgroups, risks seem to have outweighed benefits. And not just with Gardasil. The signal appears in Cervarix data, as well:[6]

Negative Efficacy: Cervarix

Table 136-Study HPV-008: Incidence rates and vaccine efficacy against CIN2+ associated with HPV-16 and/or HPV-18 (by PCR) in HPV DNA positive and seropositive subjects at baseline with normal or low-grade cytology at baseline, using conditional exact method (Subset of TVC-1)						
					Person-year rate	VE
Event Type	Group	N	n	T (yesr)	(n/T) per 100 [96.1% CI]	% [96.1% CI]
HPV 16/18	HPV	315	43	821.95	5.23 [3.72, 7.15]	-32.5% [-123.1, 20.4%]
	HAV	290	31	784.99	3.95 [2.63, 5.70]	-
HPV 16	HPV	244	39	630.50	6.19 [4.32, 8.58]	-31.2% [-127.8, 23.1%]
	HAV	218	28	594.97	4.71 [3.06, 6.92]	-
HPV 18	HPV	82	4	222.49	1.80 [0.45, 4.77]	-48.1 [-1019.1, 77.0%]
	HAV	91	3	247.10	1.21 [0.23, 3.69]	

2009 FDA Cervarix Clinical Review, at 218 (Table 136) (emphasis added).[7]

The chart above shows enhanced risk for those who received Cervarix compared to controls, ranging from negative 31.2 percent for women positive for HPV 16 alone to negative 48.1 percent for those positive for HPV 18 alone. The FDA did not consider these results statistically significant or flag them for further scrutiny. Notably, in the Cervarix trial of women aged 26 and over ("VIVIANE"), the investigators reported as serious adverse events two cases of cervical cancer among women who received the vaccine.[8]

To this day, the FDA and CDC do not recommend prescreening before vaccination.

The American College of Obstetricians and Gynecologists, a leading US professional association, goes even further. It recommends that physicians *not* prescreen patients. In a 2017 opinion, it stated:

> Testing for HPV DNA is not recommended before vaccination. Vaccination is recommended even if the patient is tested for HPV DNA and the results are positive. Even if a patient previously has had an abnormal Pap test or history of genital warts, vaccination is still recommended.[9]

Given what we know about the trial data, it's hard to understand why this association would counsel its members to intentionally remain ignorant about their patients' HPV status. One must at least consider that this recommendation concerns legal liability. If it turns out that those with positive HPV DNA results have enhanced risk, then gynecologists might be more vulnerable to successful malpractice lawsuits if they test.

In June 2018, Merck filed an application with the FDA for priority review to approve Gardasil 9 to 27-to-45-year-old men and women.[10] If Merck succeeds, then potentially more adults with enhanced risk factors may receive these vaccines.

The target population of preteens seemed to sidestep the problem of enhanced risk. But that may not be the case, as we know that some young children in the clinical trials had positive markers for HPV, even though their exposures were not sexual. We simply don't know if children or adults who have enhanced risk factors will be at higher risk for cancer. Logically, though, if positive efficacy means enhanced protection, then negative efficacy must mean enhanced risk.

10.

FERTILITY EFFECTS—TRIAL SIGNALS MISSED?

The vaccine manufacturers state in their package inserts that they have not tested the vaccines' effect on human fertility. One would expect that a vaccine targeting a sexually transmitted virus would at least have some studies on fertility. This is not the case. While they did some studies on rats, they did not do any in humans. Some women did become pregnant during the trials, however, and Merck and GSK collected and reported findings. A closer look at these data provides some insight into fertility signals, although the FDA did not flag them as such.

PREGNANCY IN THE TRIALS—EARLY MISCARRIAGE SIGNAL?

Young women have far fewer miscarriages than older women. Miscarriage is the spontaneous loss of a pregnancy before 20 weeks. Merck used the term "spontaneous abortion" to describe miscarriage throughout the trials. Even though women couldn't be pregnant on day 1 as a clinical trial condition, some women became pregnant during the study period. Trial investigators recorded pregnancy outcomes, specifically miscarriages and congenital birth defects.[1] When Merck combined all clinical trial data, the average miscarriage rate was similar in both the Gardasil and AAHS control groups at around 25 percent.[2] The FDA accepted that overall, because the groups had similar rates, there was no cause for concern. It did not look to a background miscarriage rate in the US or any other country for comparison.

Rates vary, but in women under 30, the miscarriage rate in the US is around 10–15 percent.[3] A large study in Denmark looked at over 1.2 million pregnancy outcomes from 1978 to 1992 and found that the miscarriage rate in women aged 20 to 24 years old was 8.9 percent.[4] The clinical trials took place only 10 years after researchers collected these data. While we don't have a direct comparison to every country that took part in the trials, we do know that the miscarriage rate in healthy young women is relatively low and much lower than the 25 percent rate in the Gardasil trials. The miscarriage rate in the Gardasil 9 trials was even higher at 27.4 percent,[5] which we'll examine below.

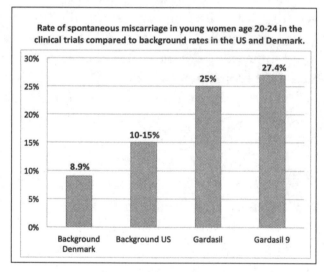

Source: Authors–see details in endnote and text above.[6]

Data from the Cervarix clinical trial review show higher early miscarriage rates in those who received the vaccine versus the controls, at 13.5 percent versus 8.3 percent.[7] The FDA was concerned enough about this "imbalance" between the vaccine and control groups to conclude that it was a "safety signal" and recommended that GSK study this further postapproval.[8] Researchers later reanalyzed the clinical trial data, showing higher miscarriage rates in the vaccinated women who became pregnant within 30 and 60 days of receiving Cervarix.[9] In that time frame, the Cervarix miscarriage rate was double that of controls. Remarkably, while investigators concluded that there were no long-term effects of the vaccine on pregnancy, they could "not completely rule out" an increased risk of miscarriage in the first trimester.[10] This risk was the exact safety signal that the FDA asked GSK to study, but no warning was issued to the public.

GARDASIL 9 AND MISCARRIAGE

The same 30-day window signal appears in the Gardasil 9 trials. Since Gardasil and Cervarix are no longer available on the US market, it is especially important to review Gardasil 9's data. The rate of miscarriage in those who received Gardasil 9 within 30 days of conception was 28.4 percent and only 12.7 percent in those who received the Gardasil control.[11] The FDA did not explain this large difference. There was also a higher rate of 40 percent in women aged 23 to 26, compared to 18.9 percent in 16-to-22-year-olds.[12] There was something amiss with these data, but the FDA posed no questions. Once Merck submitted all the Gardasil 9 trial data, the package insert was able to report a slightly lower miscarriage rate of 27.4 percent in the vaccine group and 12.7 percent in the control group, without referring to the 30-day window.[13] Even though the Gardasil 9 miscarriage rate was more than double the Gardasil control rate, the FDA failed to recognize this as a safety signal and instead referred to it as an "imbalance."[14]

Unlike the FDA, the European Medicines Agency did raise this miscarriage signal as a concern in its preapproval process.[15] The agency remarked on the unusual disparity between those who became pregnant before and after the 30-day vaccination window. Merck's response was in follow-up documents, saying that the miscarriage rates in the trials were similar to background rates.[16] Accepting Merck's explanation at face value, the EMA approved Gardasil 9, failing even to mention the 30-day anomaly in its approval.[17]

CONGENITAL ABNORMALITIES

Before approving original Gardasil, the FDA did highlight a safety signal for birth defects in babies conceived in the 30-day window.[18] The vaccine group had 5 babies with congenital abnormalities versus *zero* in the AAHS group. This risk of birth defects is consistent with the miscarriage risk in the 30-day window. While the FDA considered a possible birth defect warning on the package insert, it ultimately rejected one for unstated reasons.[19]

Table 35. Distribution of congenital anomaly cases. [From March 8, 2006 safety update submitted to BLA, table 2.7.4:26.]		
	Gardasil™	Placebo
Congenital anomaly infant or fetus	15	16
EDC within 30 days	5	0
EDC beyond 30 days	10	16

Source: May 2006 VRBPAC Background Document, at 24 (Table 35).[20]

Could regulatory complacency, at least in part, be because the target preteen population removes pregnancy risk? If so, this is a weak reason, since the vaccine is already indicated for 9-to-26-year-olds and may soon be approved for women up to 45 in the US, as in Canada, Europe, and Australia. While the vaccine is generally not recommended for pregnant women, the US package insert does not warn that it is unsafe. Instead, it says that "there are no adequate and well-controlled studies of GARDASIL 9 in pregnant women. Available human data do not demonstrate vaccine-associated increase in risk of major birth defects and miscarriages when GARDASIL 9 is administered during pregnancy."[21]

Perhaps the clinical trial data should have received more attention, and regulators should have required an explicit warning. It appears that only the Canadian package insert contains a clear warning: "It is not known whether the vaccine is harmful to an unborn baby when administered to a pregnant woman. The use of the vaccine is not recommended during pregnancy."[22] The public again does not have all the information and therefore cannot adequately assess the risk.

FERTILITY AND PREMATURE OVARIAN FAILURE

Manufacturers only tested the vaccine on rats as a way to assess fertility safety in humans. Australian gynecologist Dr. Deirdre Little sought Merck's clinical data on the rodent fertility studies through a freedom of information request to Australia's Therapeutic Goods Association. She published her observations in 2014 in the *Journal of Investigative Medicine*.[23] She found that Merck had not conducted toxicology studies on the female rats' reproductive system, and it destroyed the male rats after a short period. There was no long-term observation of the rats' fertility. Dr. Little believes that had Merck studied the female rats' ovaries for a longer period, it might have clarified the vaccine's possible role in premature ovarian failure (POF) and other reproductive disorders.

Dr. Little also examined the other ingredients in the vaccine, including polysorbate 80, which has either "a suggested association with autoimmune ovarian damage, or known direct ovarian toxicity."[24] She forcefully concluded, "it is known that safety research before and after licensing has inadequate capacity to determine ovarian safety."[25] In 2012, she published a case study in the *British Medical Journal Case Reports* on POF in an otherwise healthy teenager following Gardasil vaccination.[26] She published three case studies in 2014, including the previously published 2012 case, examining why the vaccine might be related to this condition in teens and young women that is extremely rare.[27]

A peer-reviewed article from Poland, citing Dr. Little, reiterated the need for more research into the possible vaccine effects on ovarian failure.[28] In 2013, another article in the *American Journal of Reproductive Immunology* described three cases of POF associated with other autoimmune symptoms after HPV vaccination.[29]

POF in adolescents in the US is so rare that when researchers at Stanford University School of Medicine learned about just one case, they checked their database for others. They published their findings in

2015 in the *International Journal of Pediatric Endocrinology*.[30] They looked at the rates of idiopathic, or unexplained, POF from 1998 to 2013 and found 15 cases in total, with 13 occurring after 2008. The timing of these cases matches Gardasil's introduction into the mass market in 2007. The Stanford researchers could not explain the reason for this sudden appearance of idiopathic POF cases. They concluded that if other institutions found similar numbers of cases, future research should focus on environmental causes and genetic predispositions. These researchers did not explore any connection to HPV vaccines.

In looking at VAERS data, the US vaccine adverse event reporting system, we see that POF was never reported as an adverse event to vaccination until 2006.[31] Since then, the data show many cases of POF that relate to HPV vaccines. In a 2016 press release, the American College of Pediatricians, a small pediatric group, also raised a concern about Gardasil's association with "ovarian failure, premature menopause, and/or amenorrhea."[32] The WHO conducted its own review of VAERS and other European safety databases in 2017 and found no causal link between the vaccines and POF.[33] It may be too early to see the full impact of HPV vaccines on fertility when administered to 12-year-olds beginning in 2007, but many experts agree a large follow-up study on POF should be an urgent priority. For example, in 2018, *The Journal of Toxicology and Environmental Health* published an article by Gayle DeLong, exploring declining birth rates in young women in the US, and a possible association with the HPV vaccine. DeLong suggests that there may be a link, which demands further research.[34]

DECLINING TEEN PREGNANCY RATES: A POTENTIAL SIGNAL?

Since the 1970s, when birth control and abortion became available, teen pregnancies in high-resource countries have been falling steadily. Most teen pregnancies are unplanned, so governments generally welcome falling rates. Since 2007–08, however, there has been a sharp decline in teen pregnancies in many countries where HPV vaccine uptake is high.

In the UK, where uptake has consistently been around 90 percent, the government has reported that teen pregnancies have almost halved since 2008, when the vaccine was introduced, with
no increase in abortion rates.[35] In 2017, the UK's *The Independent*
reported that teen pregnancy rates are at their lowest recorded level
ever.[36] The reason the newspaper gave was increased sex education
and access to birth control, but it gave no reason why the decline
would begin in 2008. Rates of conception for under-18-year-olds
fell by 44 percent since 2007, while rates in those over 40 years old
increased.[37] The Office for National Statistics stated, "the decline
was most notable among women aged under 16 years."[38] Scotland
and Wales have similar statistics, both of which have the same
school-based programs ensuring high uptake. Rates in under-16s in
Scotland decreased by over 60 percent from 2007 to 2015.[39]

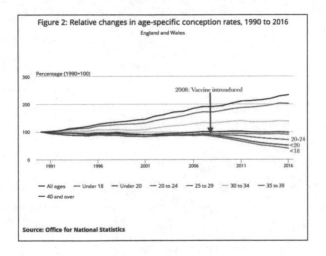

Source: Office for National Statistics UK Conception Statistics 2016
Authors inserted vertical line and labels.[40]

The United States has also seen a 50 percent drop in the teen
pregnancy rate since 2007, after a period where rates had leveled off
(see next graph).[41] According to the CDC, US teen pregnancy rates
are now at the lowest recorded level ever.[42] A 2016 Congressional
Research Service report noted that teen pregnancies fell in all racial and ethnic groups from 2007 to 2015. Experts are at a loss to

agree on the reasons for the dramatic drop, citing factors such as reality TV shows, social media, and the 2008 recession.[43] Economic
factors likely do not play a role in unplanned teen pregnancy rates,
however, so the 2008 recession cannot explain this phenomenon.
Over-the-counter access to the morning-after pill became available
to those under 17 in the US in 2013, so that access may account
for some of the drop.

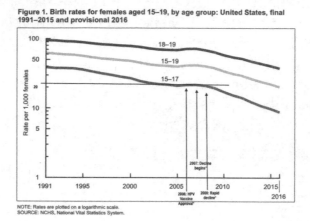

Figure 1. Birth rates for females aged 15–19, by age group: United States, final 1991–2015 and provisional 2016

NOTE: Rates are plotted on a logarithmic scale.
SOURCE: NCHS, National Vital Statistics System.

*Source: NCHS, National Vital Statistics System, Natality Brief No. 002,
June 2017 *Authors inserted vertical lines and labels.[44]*

What if pregnancy rates have dropped at least in part because
of an environmental factor? Many countries besides the UK and
US are reporting similar headlines. Canada, Ireland, Denmark,
Norway, and Australia all reached record low teen pregnancy rates
in the last decade. It is impossible to know whether miscarriages
or infertility have increased, or whether teens simply have better
access to contraception, are more abstinent, or some combination
of these or environmental factors. Given that the clinical trial data
for all three HPV vaccines show unusually high miscarriage rates,
especially within the 30-day window of conception, it is reasonable
to speculate that the vaccines may be playing some role. While there
is no hard evidence of a causal link between falling teen pregnancy
rates and the vaccine, this possible association requires more study.

By making 9-to-12-year-old girls the target population for the vaccine, the risks of miscarriage and birth defects essentially disappeared. Yet the risk of reproductive harm remains and may be masked because of the girls' prepubescent age. Young girls have minimal, if any, menstrual history, thus making causation almost impossible to establish. With declining teen pregnancy rates making headlines around the world, experts are scratching their heads as to why. While any link to the vaccine would be difficult to establish because of many confounding factors, it surely deserves serious scientific inquiry.

11.

CLINICAL TRIAL
MALFEASANCE?

After reviewing thousands of pages of clinical trial data, the FDA and EMA ultimately concluded that HPV vaccines are safe. They acknowledged that known side effects are largely limited to issues like short-term injection site reactions, fainting, and headaches. In previous chapters, we looked at dangerous flaws in the clinical trials' design and execution. Here, we enter a labyrinth of reported side effects, which clinical trial investigators seem to have labeled "new medical conditions." Looking at these data may give pause when deciding that there are no long-term safety risks.

SAFETY AND MONITORING: WHO'S WATCHING OUT?

Vaccine safety depends on having good placebos and unbiased monitoring; there are no substitutes for these requirements. In FUTURE II, the trial in which Kesia and Sesilje took part, Merck identified safety as the study's primary goal. Merck vaguely defined "safety" as three doses of Gardasil being "generally well tolerated."[1] We are unable to know how Merck assessed whether Gardasil was "generally well tolerated" in analyzing the data.

Within the trial guidelines, investigators seemed to have broad discretion to determine what constituted a reportable adverse event.[2] And Merck was under no obligation to review a participant's medical records, even if a participant developed a "serious medical condition that meets the criteria for serious adverse experiences" as defined in

81

the Protocol.[3] Based on Kesia's and Sesilje's experience in Denmark, it appears that trial staff asked subjects at each visit if they had experienced any side effects since the previous visit. We know from Kesia's and Sesilje's accounts that this subjective data collection method was subpar, relying on the participant's recollection and the potentially biased viewpoint of the trial investigator. In Kesia's case, the clinicians did not report the onset of her illness as potentially vaccine-related, and they made no attempt to look further into her concerns.[4]

Some trial participants did receive Vaccination Report Cards. These cards provided a simple way for participants to record data concerning adverse experiences following each shot, both serious and nonserious, such as temperature, injection site reactions, and headaches.[5] In FUTURE II, only 10 percent of participants, all in the US, got cards. Even then, Merck instructed those participants to record information for only 14 days after each injection.[6] These cards, designed to capture straightforward, immediate reactions, are not well suited to capture chronic conditions like autoimmune or menstrual cycle problems.

We have spoken with several clinical trial investigators who shared the challenges they face. These doctors want to do good work, but the clinical trial system is sometimes stacked against them. They criticize the time, significant duties, and low compensation for clinical trials. Many drop out after only one trial. The paperwork, especially reporting requirements for adverse events, can be time-consuming and onerous. Investigators, who don't receive additional compensation to fill out more paperwork, may lose income if they complete that work rather than see patients. One has to ask whether these same barriers may have influenced the behavior of some of the clinical trial investigators in the HPV vaccine trials, either consciously or subconsciously, especially because they had broad discretion to decide what constituted reportable events.[7]

New Medical Conditions

The *Slate* article that featured Kesia brought to light the safety gaps in the Gardasil trials, and in particular in reporting "new medical conditions."[8] Based on documents *Slate* author Joelving uncovered, it appears that trial staff recorded one-word descriptions on the form to record "new medical history." The trial staff appeared to believe that her new and worsening symptoms couldn't be related to the vaccine.

When did Merck add this "new medical condition"category to the trial protocol? According to the 2002 Gardasil trial design, it was not part of the study protocol. A 2006 peer-reviewed article reviewing the Gardasil trials in the *New England Journal of Medicine* did not report data on "new medical conditions."[9] Likewise, a 2006 EMA prelicensure scientific discussion made no reference to the term.[10] The first place we find reported data is in the FDA's 2006 Clinical Review immediately before it approved the vaccine. The document does not define this category and lists it as "new medical history" in the table of contents. It uses the terms "new medical history" and "new medical condition" interchangeably. Buried near the end of the FDA review document, tables 302 and 303 (below) reveal that almost *half* of all trial participants, regardless of whether they received the vaccine or a fauxcebo, reported "new medical conditions."[11]

Because the overwhelming majority in the fauxcebo group received the AAHS control, could this explain the comparable results in both groups? A true saline control group of a similar size would shed light on this, but unfortunately, Merck didn't do such a study.

TABLE 302
Protocols 007, 013, 015, 016 and 018:
New Medical Conditions <u>Day 1 through Month 7</u> in the Safety Population

Subjects in analysis population	Gardasil N=11778	Placebo N=9686
Subjects with new medical history	5842 (49.6%)	4750 (49%)

Source: Excerpted from Table 302, 2006 FDA Gardasil Clinical Review, at 393 (emphasis added).[12]

(Authors' Note: "Placebo" = AAHS adjuvant, sodium borate, polysorbate 80, and L-histidine. A small portion of the "placebo" group was from Protocol 018 and received a nonaluminum placebo, which included sodium borate, polysorbate 80, and L-histidine.)

Table 303 below shows that approximately half of participants in both groups continued to report new medical conditions after the initial study period, including chronic medical conditions such as thyroiditis, arthritis, or multiple sclerosis.[13]

TABLE 303 Protocols 007, 013, 015, 016 and 018: New Medical Conditions after Month 7 in the Safety Population		
Subjects in analysis population	Gardasil N=10452	Placebo N=9385
Subjects with new medical history	5178 (49.5%)	4883 (52.0%)

Source: Excerpted from Table 303, 2006 FDA Gardasil Clinical Review, at
395 (emphasis added).[14]
(Authors' Note: "Placebo" = AAHS adjuvant, sodium borate, polysorbate 80,
and L-histidine. A small portion of the "placebo"
group was from Protocol 018 and received a nonaluminum placebo, which
included sodium borate, polysorbate 80, and L-histidine.)

All subjects in Protocol 018 show remarkably lower "new medical conditions" compared to the other clinical trial protocols in the clinical trials. Recall from Chapter 8 that the subjects in Protocol 018 were aged 9 to 15, the vaccine group likely received half the regular AAHS dose, and the control group received only the carrier solution. We can only imagine what the "new medical conditions" would have been in the placebo group had this been a true saline controlled trial.

TABLE 245 Protocol 018: New Medical Conditions Day 1 through Month 12		
Subjects in analysis population	Gardasil N=1128	Placebo N=562
Subjects with new medical history	327 (29.0%)	174 (31.0%)

Excerpted from Table 245, 2006 FDA Gardasil Clinical Review, at 329
(emphasis added).[15]
Gardasil= possible nonapproved formulation with half AAHS per Chapter 8.
Placebo = Saline plus sodium borate, polysorbate 80, and L-histidine.

Despite the high overall rate of new conditions reported, Merck only disclosed a small subset of these data on the package insert. On Table 9 (below), Merck disclosed that 2.3 percent of participants in both groups reported "new medical conditions potentially indicative of a systemic autoimmune disorder,"[16] although it did not define the term:

Table 9: Summary of Girls and Women 9 Through 26 Years of Age Who Reported an Incident Condition Potentially Indicative of a Systemic Autoimmune Disorder After Enrollment in Clinical Trials of GARDASIL, Regardless of Causality		
Conditions	GARDASIL (N = 10,706)	AAHS Control* or Saline Placebo (N = 9412)
	n (%)	n (%)
Arthralgia/Arthritis/Arthropathy[†]	120 (1.1)	98 (1.0)
Autoimmune Thyroiditis	4 (0.0)	1 (0.0)
Celiac Disease	10 (0.1)	6 (0.1)
Diabetes Mellitus Insulin-dependent	2 (0.0)	2 (0.0)
Erythema Nodosum	2 (0.0)	4 (0.0)
Hyperthyroidism[‡]	27 (0.3)	21 (0.2)
Hypothyroidism[§]	35 (0.3)	38 (0.4)
Inflammatory Bowel Disease[¶]	7 (0.1)	10 (0.1)
Multiple Sclerosis	2 (0.0)	4 (0.0)
Nephritis[#]	2 (0.0)	5 (0.1)
Optic Neuritis	2 (0.0)	0 (0.0)
Pigmentation Disorder[Þ]	4 (0.0)	3 (0.0)
Psoriasis[à]	13 (0.1)	15 (0.2)
Raynaud's Phenomenon	3 (0.0)	4 (0.0)
Rheumatoid Arthritis[è]	6 (0.1)	2 (0.0)
Scleroderma/Morphea	2 (0.0)	1 (0.0)
Stevens-Johnson Syndrome	1 (0.0)	0 (0.0)
Systemic Lupus Erythematosus	1 (0.0)	3 (0.0)
Uveitis	3 (0.0)	1 (0.0)
All Conditions	245 (2.3)	218 (2.3)
*AAHS Control = Amorphous Aluminum Hydroxyphosphate Sulfate		

Source: *Gardasil package insert (emphasis added).*[17]

Why did Merck single out only 2.3 percent of the "new medical condition" data, particularly when 49 percent of participants reported other new conditions indicating all kinds of serious illnesses, including blood, lymphatic, cardiac, gastrointestinal, immune, musculoskeletal (arthritis), reproductive, neurological, and psychological ones, and even conditions requiring surgery, such as appendectomies? Even with the autoimmune subset data disclosed on the insert, Merck could justify them by noting that the Gardasil and control groups had virtually the same results. Merck and the FDA apparently interpreted these similar data as support for safety rather than as signals for alarm.

At some point before 2006, the FDA permitted Merck to use "new medical conditions" as a metric, but the details of when and why are unknown. How is a "new medical condition" different from a vaccine reaction, a suspected reaction, or a serious adverse event? Why was it not described or detailed in the 2002 clinical trial design? Why is the term not part of the FDA or WHO guidelines on clinical trials?

New Medical Conditions and Gardasil 9

It is curious, therefore, that it wasn't until 2014 when a regulatory agency questioned Merck on this metric. When the EMA evaluated Gardasil 9, it raised this study method as one of its "major objections," which made the vaccine "not approvable."[18] It referred to "new medical conditions" as "an unconventional and suboptimal study procedure."[19] Almost 52 percent of participants in the Gardasil 9 trials reported new medical conditions, a slightly higher rate than for original Gardasil. The EMA was also concerned that Merck had not supplied information on serious conditions appearing in less than 1 percent of the total trial population.[20] In other words, out of 20,000 people in the Gardasil 9 trials, 200 people would have to report a serious condition before the EMA would even receive the data. The EMA specifically asked Merck to report further on illnesses of great concern, such as multiple sclerosis and narcolepsy.[21]

Merck's November 2014 response explained away rare conditions occurring in less than 1 percent of participants as having no real pattern and thus as unrelated.[22] Merck offered the explanation that there was a similar number of subjects with illnesses in the Gardasil 9 and Gardasil control groups. But they considered all of these conditions unrelated to the vaccine.

The EMA did not address that over half of the trial participants reported new illnesses. The EMA reviewers were concerned, however, that there was "only specific, short, AE reporting periods," and any new symptoms were considered "new medical conditions."[23] The EMA reviewers criticized the data collection method as suboptimal in cases where side effects could appear long after vaccination.[24]

The EMA eventually approved Gardasil 9, so the reviewers must have ultimately been satisfied with the data. The EMA's final report made no reference to "new medical conditions," though.[25] Again, the public, and even doctors, have no idea about the "new medical conditions" data and regulators' concerns.

GARDASIL 9 AND LEUKEMIA

Before it approved Gardasil 9, the EMA also asked Merck in 2014 for more data on acute leukemia cases.[26] (The December 2017 *Slate* article provided links to these documents.)[27] Of the five cases Merck reported, four were in the Gardasil 9 group, including three in Colombia, and one in the Gardasil control group. Merck disputed that the cases were cause for concern because the time to disease onset was prolonged (482 to 1,285 days) in all cases but one, when a trial subject received a diagnosis within a month after the third dose.[28]

Vaccine group	Allocation Number	Country	Race	Diagnosis	Age at Enrollment	Time of Onset	Age at Diagnosis
Listing of Cases of Acute Leukemia (V503 – P001 and P002 Studies)							
Protocol V503-001							
9vHPV	▓▓▓	Colombia	Multi-racial	Acute promyelocytic leukemia	▓	1285 days post-dose 3	▓
9vHPV	▓▓▓	Colombia	Multi-racial	Acute lymphoblastic leukemia	▓	27 days post-dose 3	▓
qHPV	▓▓▓	Canada	White	Acute lymphocytic leukemia	▓	1279 days post-dose 3	▓
Protocol V503-002							
9vHPV	▓▓▓	Colombia	Multi-racial	Acute leukemia	▓	482 days post-dose 3	▓
9vHPV	▓▓▓	United States	White	Acute myeloid leukemia	▓	705 days post-dose 3	▓

Source: Table–Assessment of the responses to the CHMP list of questions, Nov 25, 2014.[29]

The EMA expressed concern and commented that the number of cases in the trials was greater than what they would expect in the general population at this age, although ages were redacted in the report (see above table). It asked Merck to take a closer look at each case to see if there was a connection to the vaccine. The EMA asked

Merck to provide an analysis of "expected" versus "observed" numbers of leukemia cases in subjects under 20 years old. We do not know Merck's response, but since the EMA approved the vaccine shortly thereafter, we infer that the EMA was content with Merck's response.[30]

Despite Gardasil 9's eventual approval, publicly available documents could mislead the public into assuming a higher level of safety than actually exists. Since passive surveillance systems do not generally capture illnesses with long latency periods, it is at least possible that an illness, such as leukemia, could occur long after vaccination and yet be vaccine-related. Yet again, the public and doctors are in the dark that there was ever a question about this serious health outcome.

DEATHS IN THE TRIALS

When the FDA approved Gardasil in 2006, Merck reported 10 deaths in the vaccine group and 7 in the AAHS group, out of 21,458 participants.[31] Reasons for deaths varied, but one cause stood out—motor vehicle accidents.[32] There were four in the vaccine group and three in the AAHS group. In postmarket surveillance studies, we now know that syncope, or fainting, is a recognized side effect of the vaccine that had not yet been identified at that time. In the FDA's Gardasil 9 statistical review, four subjects in the trial died because of motor vehicle accidents.[33]

Since each trial investigator had the discretion to determine whether a serious event was vaccine-related, an investigator might choose not to report a car accident as related. Intuitively, there appears to be no connection between a vaccine and a car accident weeks or months later. But since syncope is one of the recognized side effects of Gardasil, perhaps it shouldn't be dismissed out of hand.

The background death rate in young women in the US is low. Based on data from the CDC from 2002, the average death rate in girls and young women in the general population was 4.37 per 10,000.[34] When the vaccine was approved in 2006, the trial data showed that the rate of death in the Gardasil groups was 8.5 per 10,000 (10 deaths out of 11,778), or almost double the background rate in the US. The rate in the fauxcebo groups was 7.2 per 10,000 (7 deaths out of 9,680).[35] The FDA Clinical Review dismissed all deaths as coincidences and failed to compare the clinical trial death rate to any background death rates.[36] Two more deaths were reported after approval, one in the vaccine group and one in the carrier solution group of Protocol 018.[37]

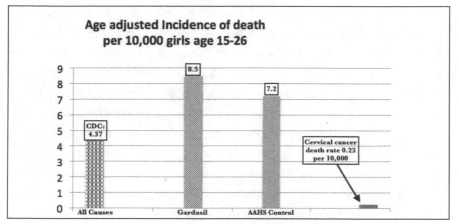

Background CDC rate 4.37, source: National Vital Statistics Report Vol. 53 2002 page 24.[38]
Gardasil rate 8.5: 10/11,778. AAHS control rate 7.2: 7/9,680[39]
Cervical cancer mortality: 2.3 per 100,000, source: National Cancer Institute SEER Cancer Statistics Review 2015[40]

In seeking approval to recommend the vaccine to older women, boys, and men, Merck reported results from two additional trials. One trial was on older women aged 26–45 (Protocol 019) and the other on men aged 16–26 (Protocol 020). Both trials reported results after Merck had already received FDA approval and the vaccine was already on the market.

Protocol 019 had seven deaths in the Gardasil group and one in the AAHS group.[41] The Gardasil group's rate of death was over *four times* that of previous studies in younger girls. According to an FDA clinical review of Protocol 019, seven of the eight deaths were in Asian women, although they made up only 31 percent of the trial population.[42] Experts should reexamine these deaths in light of the high number of postvaccination reactions in Japan to explore a potential susceptibility. Again, the FDA was satisfied that there was no signal in these data and that none of the reported deaths were associated with the vaccine. The FDA, however, did not approve the vaccine for older women following this study, allegedly because of poor efficacy.

Protocol 020, an all-male trial of 16-to-26-year-olds, had thirteen deaths out of 4,065 study participants.[43] Uniquely in this trial, there were three deaths in the Gardasil group and ten in the fauxcebo group. The rate of death was *seven times higher* than in the other fauxcebo groups. In all other trials, the fauxcebo group deaths never exceeded those in the vaccine group. Two of the deaths in the vaccine group were due to traffic accidents, and one from a gunshot wound. In the fauxcebo group, three were due to gunshot wounds, two to drug overdoses, two to suicides, one to a traffic accident, one to chemical poisoning, and one to a heart attack.[44] Once again, the FDA did not note any unusual remarks in their review of the data and accepted Merck's assertions that no deaths were due to the vaccine. The FDA approved the vaccine for boys and men based on these data.

Once Merck added in these belated clinical trial death results from Protocol 019 and 020 to the original 2006 data set, the death rate jumped significantly to 13.3 per 10,000 (21 deaths out of 15,706) in the Gardasil groups and 14.5 per 10,000 (19 deaths out of 13,617) in the AAHS groups.[45] The table below captures the different rates of death in all reported Protocols. The FDA did not note any of these rates as unusual:

Deaths in the Clinical Trials				
	N	Gardasil Deaths	N	AAHS Control Deaths
2006 Approval Data (Protocols 007, 013, 015, 016, 018)	11778	10 (0.08%)	9680	7 (0.07%)
Additional deaths reported*		1		1
Protocol 019	1908	7 (0.37%)	1907	1 (0.05%)
Protocol 020	2020	3 (0.15%)	2030	10 (0.49%)
All Protocols	**15706**	**21 (0.13%)**	**13617**	**19 (0.14%)**

* Miller, et al., 2008 Table 43: One death in Gardasil group (Protocol 013) and one death in non-alum control (Protocol 018).

Source: Authors, see endnotes.[46]

Clinical trial investigators did not observe this relatively high death rate in Gardasil 9. Only 10 deaths were reported, five in each group. Even though numbers were lower, the package insert reports that there was one death due to a motor vehicle accident and one due to acute leukemia in the vaccine groups.[47] Investigators asserted that all deaths were unrelated to the vaccine.

When investigating exciting new medical innovations, it's perhaps understandable why some investigators might disassociate adverse events from what they are testing. Rather than looking at how the vaccine could have contributed to an adverse event, like a car accident or heart attack, investigators may instead try to rule out any causal connection, consciously or unconsciously. Here, because the death rates in the control and vaccine groups were essentially identical, it might be easy to dismiss the deaths as unrelated at first blush. But given aluminum's toxicity and the higher-than-normal death rates in both the vaccine and control groups of otherwise healthy teens and young adults, investigators and regulators should have scrutinized these deaths more rigorously.

12.

INDIA: A CLINICAL TRIAL SCANDAL

India's experience with the HPV vaccine hinges on so-called "demonstration projects" with Merck and GSK HPV vaccines. The Indian Parliament alleges they were unauthorized and unethical; the manufacturers and their allies strongly disagree. Here's the background.

Over 25 percent of all newly diagnosed cases of cervical cancer in the world occur in India. It is the second-leading cause of cancer death in women, claiming approximately 74,000 lives a year. Despite this large and unfortunate number, cervical cancer deaths by 2005 had dropped almost 50 percent.[1]

Shortly after the FDA approved Gardasil in June 2006, a US nongovernmental organization, Program for Appropriate Technology in Health (PATH), started a five-year so-called "demonstration project" with "the main objective . . . to generate and disseminate evidence for informed public sector introduction of HPV vaccines" in India, Uganda, Peru, and Vietnam.[2] These four countries, with different ethnic populations, could potentially be useful sites to monitor the safety and efficacy of the newly approved vaccines. In addition, and perhaps more important, these four countries have state-funded national immunization programs. If any of these countries, but especially India, adopted HPV vaccines into their universal vaccine programs, major financial gains would result.[3]

The "demonstration projects" involved many agencies, policy makers, special interest groups, and the public at large. India became one of four global sites to participate in these Gardasil and Cervarix trials. The trials took place in two remote provinces, Andhra Pradesh and Gujarat. Seven girls allegedly died in the trials in 2009–10.[4] The subsequent investigation, while initially focusing on the girls' deaths, uncovered systemic failures in government agencies' oversight of the trials. Ultimately, this inquiry led to a Parliamentary investigation, rebukes against India's highest medical agencies, reform of clinical trial laws, and ongoing human rights litigation in the Indian Supreme Court. As a result, a national Indian HPV vaccine program has to date failed to materialize.

PARLIAMENTARY REPORT ON THE HPV STUDY

According to a 2013 detailed report of an Indian Parliamentary Committee, PATH entered into a memorandum of understanding with the Indian Council of Medical Research, the highest medical research body in India, to study HPV vaccination.[5] To obtain approval, PATH described the project to vaccinate approximately 23,000 girls between ages 10 and 14 as an "observational study," since "it did not conform to the definition of clinical trial."[6] Merck and GSK supplied the vaccines to PATH at no cost. PATH then distributed the vaccines to local medical agencies for free. The Bill and Melinda Gates Foundation funded the other costs of the study, as part of its global public health activity.[7]

The Parliamentary Committee dismissed PATH's explanations that these studies were not clinical trials. It opined:

> The choice of countries and population groups; the monopolistic nature . . . of the product being pushed; the unlimited market potential and opportunities in the universal immunization programmes of the respective countries are all pointers to a well-planned scheme to commercially exploit a situation. [8]

The report alleges that PATH resorted to subterfuge. In the process, PATH jeopardized the health and wellbeing of thousands of vulnerable Indian girls.[9] The Parliamentary report makes clear that these de facto clinical trials could not have occurred without corruption within India's leading health organizations. The Committee noted "serious dereliction of duty by many of the institutions and individuals involved" and accused some of having "undisclosed conflicts of interest with the vaccine manufacturers."[10] The report criticizes an earlier inquiry into these irregularities, noting that it failed to pursue an investigation to its logical end, providing full details of exactly who was culpable and how.[11]

PATH engaged in extraordinary practices to obtain "informed consent" from minors in economically vulnerable areas. Indian law requires that parents or guardians consent on behalf of minors to participate in clinical trials. For uneducated subjects, an independent person must be present to explain and witness the consent process. The Committee reviewed thousands of consent forms from the two provinces signed by dormitory supervisors in schools where the girls lived without their parents. These supervisors were not the girls' legal guardians. They found forms with no witness signatures and signatures by thumb impression of those who could not write. Many forms had no dates.[12] Direct interviews revealed that trial participants had received grossly inadequate information about potential risks and benefits while being offered financial inducements to participate.[13]

A different 2014 fact-finding report carried out by physicians details several interviews with subjects and their family members.[14] These authors learned that families were told that the vaccine would protect the subjects from all cancers; they were not told about any side effects; and they were not provided any medical insurance in the event of injury or death. Moreover, they learned that several of the girls suffered adverse events, including loss of menstrual cycles and psychological changes such as depression and anxiety.[15] The report concluded that "the safety and rights of the children in this vaccination project were highly compromised and violated."[16]

The Parliamentary Committee harshly criticized PATH's treatment of adverse events. The Committee noted that there were clear situations when a vaccination should not have been given to a girl, but those conducting the study ignored such contraindications. The Committee observed that this was "clearly an act of willful negligence."[17] They noted that the project design failed to account for the possibility of serious adverse events and failed to provide for an independent monitoring agency. "[I]nvestigations into causes of deaths took an unacceptably long time," and there were critical discrepancies in the investigation.[18]

The report notes PATH's wrongful use of governmental logos to make it appear as if the project were part of the Indian Universal Immunization Program.[19] The Committee found governmental responses "very casual, bureaucratic and lack[ing] any sense of urgency."[20] The report concludes that "PATH has exploited with impunity the loopholes in our system" and "has violated all laws and regulations laid down for clinical trials by the Government."[21]

> [PATH's] sole aim has been to promote the commercial interests of HPV vaccine manufacturers who would have reaped windfall profits had PATH been successful in getting the HPV vaccine included in the UIP [universal immunization program] of the country. . . . This act of PATH is a clear cut violation of the human rights of these girl children and adolescents . . . [and] an established case of child abuse.[22]

The report stopped short of finding the deaths directly related to the vaccine trials and failed to call for prosecution of those responsible. But it laid the groundwork for petitions to the Indian Supreme Court about the HPV clinical trials.

HPV Vaccine Litigation in the Supreme Court

In October 2012, activists on behalf of the girls in the trials filed a petition in the Indian Supreme Court against the Drug Controller General, the Indian Council of Medical Research, the State of

Andhra Pradesh, the State of Gujarat, PATH, GSK, Merck, and others. The petition alleged that the clinical trials for Gardasil and Cervarix were unethical, that the vaccine use was illegal, and that various actors enlisted girls in an experiment and then abandoned them without follow-up, treatment, or adequate information.[23]

The complaint states that "adverse events were grossly under reported and hidden. Records were falsified. Deaths that took place were stated as having nothing to do with administering of the vaccines and were described as deaths due to suicides, insecticide poisoning, and snake bites." Kalpana Mehta, an attorney for the activists, stated that there had been "gross anomalies in the death-related documentation."[24] Deaths were reported without dates or signatures. The petitioners asked that the Court rescind the Gardasil and Cervarix product licenses in India and withdraw both vaccines from the market until their safety and efficacy was proven.[25] At the time of this writing, the case is still pending.

IS MASS HPV VACCINATION APPROPRIATE FOR INDIA?

A 2012 article in the *Journal of the Royal Society of Medicine* raises fundamental questions about the appropriateness of data collection methods in the PATH study in Gujarat and Andhra Pradesh.[26] The Indian scientists who published the article found that cancer surveillance, registration, and monitoring in India in general, and in Gujarat and Andhra Pradesh in particular, were incomplete, "meaning that it would be impossible to tell whether the vaccine would be successful in preventing the disease."[27] The dramatic drop in cervical cancer rates occurred without the vaccine and without widely accessible screening. They attributed this drop to several factors, including better hygiene, cleaner water supply, improved nutrition, and changing reproductive patterns, among others.[28]

The scientists concluded, "neither epidemiological evidence nor current cancer surveillance systems justify the general rollout of an HPV vaccination programme in India or in the two states where PATH was conducting its research."[29] Effective surveillance requires baseline incidence, prevalence, and mortality rates. "The effectiveness of an intervention cannot be measured if there is no monitoring or follow-up on epidemiological data."[30] They argue that better uses for primary care medical resources in India include malaria, maternal anemia, and malnutrition. The HPV vaccine, as the most expensive vaccine on the market, is not justifiable without strong epidemiological evidence of disease and adequate surveillance and monitoring.[31]

A 2013 article in the *South Asian Journal of Cancer* also concludes that the HPV vaccination program is unjustifiable.[32] It argues that "it would be far more productive to understand and strengthen the reasons behind this trend [of decreasing cervical cancer rates] than to expose an entire population to an uncertain intervention that has not been proven to prevent a single cervical cancer or cervical cancer death to date."[33] The authors of the 2013 article conclude that it is "grossly premature to judge the efficacy of these vaccines from a public health perspective."[34]

The article also questions the vaccine's fundamental safety. Because vaccines are administered to healthy individuals, "the highest standards of safety are (rightly) expected of them."[35]

> [A] healthy 16-year-old is at zero immediate risk of dying from cervical cancer but is faced with a small but real risk of death or serious disability from a vaccine that has yet to prevent a single case of cervical cancer. . . . [T]here is genuine cause for concerns regarding mass vaccination in this country.[36]

In addition to efficacy and safety, the authors of the 2013 article also address cost. They argue that HPV vaccination does not remove the need for cervical screening and that the infrastructure for screening does not exist in India. Based on empirical cost-effectiveness data, they argue that cervical screening is more cost-effective than either vaccination alone or vaccination with screening.[37] In conclusion, they ask a series of reasonable questions that everyone should wonder about:

• How, "with zero evidence," can these products be promoted as "cervical cancer" vaccines?

- Should regulators rely solely on data provided by manufacturers for public health decisions?

- With low or declining cervical cancer incidence, how is mass vaccination to prevent it in 30 years justified?

- Shouldn't there be a mandatory requirement to fully convey the small but real and serious risks of vaccination to potential recipients?

- Shouldn't cervical screening programs be a much higher public health priority in India than mass HPV vaccination?[38]

THE CURRENT SITUATION

Largely because of the HPV vaccine scandal, the Indian government restricted clinical trials in 2013 and forced an end to the Merck and GSK "demonstration projects."[39] That same year, the Supreme Court suspended 162 drug approvals pending the creation of a better monitoring system.[40] In 2014, the government published new guidelines for audiovisual recording of informed consent in clinical trials.[41] Since 2015, though, provinces obtained the right to approve some drugs without national approval, bypassing federal regulators.[42] The Delhi government launched a school-based HPV vaccination program in November 2016, and the Punjab government followed suit in early 2017.

Dr. Mark Feinberg, then a Merck senior executive, maintained that "[d]emonstration projects, such as those suspended in India, are not clinical trials; rather, they help accelerate access by providing local experience on the most regionally appropriate immunization strategies."[43] He maintains that the projects were not "industry studies," but were "collaborations between the Indian Council of Medical Research, state health departments, and the international non-profit organization PATH."[44]

Similarly, PATH vehemently denies any wrongdoing and "strongly disagree[s] with the findings, conclusions, and tone of the released

[Parliamentary] report and its disregard of the evidence and facts."[45] PATH points to what it says is the "voluminous evidence on the safety and efficacy of HPV vaccines," and it claims that the report "falsely suggests that deaths may be causally linked to the vaccines."[46] PATH suggests that this is inaccurate and "may have tragic consequences for delivering these and other lifesaving vaccines to those who need them most." Because PATH is a nonprofit, it states that it receives no industry funding and has no financial stake in the vaccine.

PATH also contests any notion that there may have been conflicts of interest in India: "Any suggestion that inappropriate collusion existed in this project is baseless, wholly inaccurate, and defies the very spirit of our cross-sector partnerships, which are essential in India and around the world."[47] PATH sees itself as an international nonprofit organization that "transforms global health through innovation," taking "an entrepreneurial approach to developing and delivering high-impact, low-cost solutions, from lifesaving vaccines, drugs, diagnostics, and devices to collaborative programs with communities."[48]

The Bill and Melinda Gates Foundation funded the PATH demonstration projects and has invested heavily in India's vaccine program. The Foundation has funded two organizations that have influenced vaccine policy since 2002: the Global Alliance for Vaccines and Immunization (GAVI) and the Public Health Foundation of India (PHFI). Pharmaceutical executives sit on GAVI's board, which has a public-private partnership with the Indian government, providing hundreds of millions of dollars to fund vaccine programs.[49] PHFI is India's largest public health nonprofit organization. Although the Indian government set up PHFI, the Gates Foundation largely funds it. Critics, such as the right-leaning Swadeshi Jagran Manch organization, argue that the Indian government has conflicts of interest because of these public-private partnerships with the GAVI, PHFI, and PATH. It argues that through these partnerships, the pharmaceutical industry wields undue influence over the Indian immunization program.

In April 2017, the Indian government blocked the Gates Foundation and other foreign entities from further funding PHFI and other nongovernmental organizations. The Foundation maintains that it has no conflicts of interest and works only to ensure "the adequate production and affordability of vital and safe vaccines for the world's poorest populations. . . ."[50]

In 2018, the debate about a national HPV vaccination program resumed, but so far it is just talk.[51] The HPV controversy seems contained for now, at least until the Supreme Court issues a judgment on the demonstration projects. The vaccines' unintended effect, though, was to spur the country to adopt new laws to better ensure informed consent in clinical trials. That result may yield long-lasting benefits.

PART II

THE HPV VACCINE HITS THE MARKET

13.

A Market out of Thin Air

Looking solely at financials, Merck's and GSK's HPV vaccines have been glittering successes. In 2017, Merck made $2.3 billion in revenue worldwide from Gardasil and Gardasil 9, up from $2.2 billion in 2016.[1] GSK earned 134 million pounds (roughly $186 million) globally in the same year,[2] although down from a pinnacle of 506 million pounds (roughly $708 million) in 2011. To date, these pharmaceutical giants have distributed over 270 million doses of HPV vaccines around the world.[3]

Gardasil is critical to Merck's overall financial health. Merck identifies Gardasil as one of its "Key Company Products," meaning that any change in Gardasil's cash flow affects the corporation as a whole. Merck's 10-K financial reports note that discovery of previously unknown side effects or removal of Gardasil from the market would hurt Merck's bottom line.[4] GSK similarly notes that Cervarix is one of its leading products and that its revenue is material to the corporation as a whole.[5]

How is it that these corporations, some of the world's largest, now depend for their survival on HPV vaccines?[6] How did Merck and GSK create a market out of thin air?

THE HPV VACCINE: HELPING PAY FOR VIOXX

By the early 2000s, scientists, corporations, and governments had been working for years to promote the possibility of HPV vaccines.

But Merck's sense of urgency to market Gardasil is hard to understand without some historical context. Merck had just suffered a fiasco from its drug Vioxx. Some critics have dubbed the HPV vaccine the "Help to Pay for Vioxx" vaccine. Vioxx is the brand name for the drug rofecoxib, a nonsteroidal anti-inflammatory drug (NSAID) to treat chronic and acute pain from arthritis and other conditions. The FDA approved Vioxx in May 1999. Because of safety concerns, Merck voluntarily withdrew it from the market in September 2004, just five years later.

While on the market, 80 million people worldwide took Vioxx, and, in 2003 alone, it generated $2.5 billion in revenue.[7] Merck's abrupt "voluntary" withdrawal of Vioxx preceded possible FDA action to remove it from the market. The drug carried significant, undisclosed cardiovascular risks. FDA analysts estimated that in the five years Vioxx was on the market, it likely caused between 88,000 and 139,000 heart attacks and 26–42,000 deaths.[8] Dr. Peter Gøtzsche of the Nordic Cochrane Centre puts the estimate of deaths much higher, at about 120,000 people.[9]

The FDA had serious concerns about Vioxx before its approval. When it approved Vioxx, the FDA stated that it lacked "complete certainty" that the drug increased cardiovascular risk.[10] As Peter Gøtzsche points out, this is as if a doctor told his patient, "I'm not completely sure this drug will kill you, but please take it."[11] Federal agency officials and physicians dominate FDA advisory committees with few, if any, representatives of the public. Dr. Gøtzsche believes that if patient representatives had participated in the FDA advisory committee for Vioxx, they would have rejected Merck's application, as it was clear that the drug posed heart risks.[12]

Not only do Merck and the FDA bear responsibility for this disaster, Gøtzsche also points to the *New England Journal of Medicine*. The *NEJM* published inaccurate data from the Merck clinical trial called VIGOR, omitting heart attack information, although that information was on the FDA's website. After five years of silence, the journal became concerned about litigation exposure and published an "expression of concern" about its role in the Vioxx scandal.[13]

Had the *NEJM* acted earlier, it might have spared lives; it also would have lost between $697,000 and $836,000 in reprint sales.[14]

Emails made public through litigation showed that high-level Merck scientists Dr. Edward M. Scolnick and Dr. Alise Reicin asked researchers to recharacterize deaths from Vioxx as the result of "unknown" causes.[15] Dr. Scolnick urged a researcher to change the description "so that we don't raise concerns" to the FDA. Another email said that if they attributed a particular woman's death to the drug in the clinical trial data—they ultimately did not—it would have "put us in a terrible situation."[16]

Merck also published a fake journal, the *Australasian Journal of Bone and Joint Medicine*, which looked like a peer-reviewed medical journal, to include articles favoring Merck products, including Vioxx, without disclosing sponsorship.[17] In Australian litigation, emails showed that Merck made a "hit list" of doctors who criticized Vioxx, indicating after their names the words: "neutralize," "neutralized," or "discredit." According to an Australian newspaper, Merck emails from 1999 showed company executives complaining about doctors who disliked Vioxx. One mob-style email read, "We may need to seek them out and destroy them where they live. . . ."[18]

Even once the FDA was fully aware of the cardiac risk, it procrastinated for nearly two more years before putting a warning on Vioxx. In the meantime, Merck continued to aggressively market Vioxx, even after the FDA asked it to inform doctors of the risk in February 2001. Instead, in May 2001, Merck issued a press release, stating, "Merck reconfirms favorable cardiovascular safety of Vioxx."[19] And the marketing for Vioxx was prodigious—Merck promoted it for at least 30 different conditions, ranging from schizophrenia, to seven types of cancer, to premenstrual acne.[20]

Merck's preapproval clinical trial studies showed the heart attack risk, but Merck downplayed the risk in marketing to doctors and the public.[21] Dr. Gurkirpal Singh, a doctor who reviewed Merck documents for a Congressional hearing, noted that Merck scientists were concerned about heart attack risk as early as 1997. He characterized Merck's failure to investigate as a "marketing decision" designed to minimize the possibility of finding cardiovascular adverse events.[22]

Merck's Vioxx clinical trials were small, had short treatment periods, enrolled people at low risk for heart problems, and did not have a procedure to collect and review cardiac problems that arose. All these aspects have analogues in the HPV vaccine trials: short observation periods, certain studies without statistical power, clinical trial subjects with "perfect" profiles, and no standard adverse event reporting procedures. For both Vioxx and Gardasil, these techniques permitted conscious avoidance or willful blindness of risks.[23] Dr. Gøtzsche contrasts the low-risk participants in Merck's Vioxx clinical trials with the typical patients prescribed Vioxx, who often had eight times higher cardiac risk than those in the trials.[24]

At a US Senate hearing in 2004, Dr. David Graham, formerly the associate director in the FDA's Office of Drug Safety, called FDA's approval of Vioxx the "single greatest drug safety catastrophe in the history of this country or the history of the world."[25] Dr. Graham argued that the victims from this unwarranted approval far outnumbered those from previous FDA blunders, including the 5,000 to 10,000 infants born with birth defects from thalidomide and the 100 who died from sulfanilamide in the 1930s. Senator Grassley, chair of the Senate Committee hearing, suggested that the problem was that the FDA's relationship with drug companies was too cozy. Dr. Graham pointed out that the FDA had an inherent conflict of interest because the same group that approved the drug was also responsible for taking regulatory action against it once it was on the market.[26]

Shortly after Merck withdrew Vioxx from the market in 2004, the FDA, in a 2007 report, concluded that it "is in a precarious position: the Agency suffers from serious scientific deficiencies and is not positioned to meet current or emerging regulatory responsibilities."[27] The FDA's scientific base had eroded, and its organizational structure was weak. American lives were at risk, and the FDA's inability to perform jeopardized the public.

In 2005, in the first of many lawsuits, Merck paid $253 million in damages. In subsequent cases, though, Merck won a string of victories. Still, Merck faced 27,000 lawsuits on behalf of 47,000 plaintiffs. In November 2007, Merck garnered agreement from over

85 percent of the Vioxx plaintiffs for a global settlement for $4.85 billion.[28] The average plaintiff would receive about $100,000 less 30-50 percent to cover legal fees and other expenses. As a *New York Times* correspondent put it, "While eye-popping, the settlement payment represents less than one year's profits for the company." The settlement "put to rest any fears that the Vioxx lawsuit might bankrupt the company, or even have a significant financial impact."[29]

In 2012, almost eight years after Merck withdrew Vioxx from the market, it pleaded guilty to one criminal violation of the Food, Drug and Cosmetic Act for introducing a misbranded drug into interstate commerce.[30] Merck also entered into a civil settlement under which it paid fines to resolve additional allegations of off-label marketing and false statements about Vioxx's cardiovascular safety. The $322 million criminal fine and $628 million civil settlement concluded long-running investigations.[31] Merck also entered into a corporate integrity agreement with the Office of Inspector General of HHS, whose intent was to strengthen oversight procedures and to deter similar conduct in the future.[32]

Merck, the FDA, and others deprived more than 80 million Vioxx users of informed consent to accurately weigh the drug's risks and benefits. Thousands died needlessly.[33] Despite clear errors in corporate and regulatory judgment and ethics, the Vioxx fiasco did not trigger widespread outrage, nor did Merck pay any price other than the financial one. No officers went to prison, and in fact several key players in the Vioxx scandal remain at the highest levels of the corporation today.[34]

So with this troubling track record at Merck, the FDA, and the *New England Journal of Medicine*, the HPV vaccine marketing saga began.

"DISEASE BRANDING" OR SELLING CERVICAL CANCER

Although the FDA approved Gardasil in June 2006, less than two years after Vioxx came off the market, Merck's aggressive direct-to-consumer marketing started in September 2005, seven months ahead of FDA approval. In a marketing effort that CEO

Richard Clark dubbed "flawlessly" executed, Merck sold fear of cervical cancer, not the vaccine itself, to consumers. Scholar Carl Elliott explains that "disease branding" is the marketing buzzword for promoting a disease that a new drug can treat.[35] Merck has perfected this reverse engineering over decades. As far back as the 1960s, Merck's strategy for marketing a new antidepressant drug, amitriptyline, was to "sell clinical depression."[36]

While Merck could sell clinical depression—and thus amitriptyline—only to doctors at the time, since the mid-1990s, the FDA has allowed direct-to-consumer (DTC) pharmaceutical marketing.[37] The United States is an outlier on this.[38] New Zealand, with only four million people, is the only other country allowing DTC prescription drug advertising. The overwhelming majority of countries do not accept that advertising prescription medical products to consumers is in the public interest. Even the American Medical Association, the US voice of mainstream medicine, has called for a halt to DTC marketing for prescription drugs and medical devices.[39] It expressed concern in 2015 that commercial drug promotion drives demand for expensive treatments when less expensive and more effective alternatives exist. Overall, DTC advertising contributes substantially to the ultimate cost for drugs and medical care, with advertising at $4.5 billion per year.[40] With billions invested in consumer outreach, you can bet Merck and other pharmaceutical giants are factoring that expenditure into their pricing models.

Recognizing that most girls and women were ignorant of any relationship between HPV and cervical cancer, Merck first drew attention to the issue in two widespread ad campaigns that did not even mention "Gardasil." Following Edward Bernays's advice in the classic 1928 book *Propaganda*, Merck understood that "it is not enough to sell a product. Instead, you need to sell the vision that will lead to desire for the product, with the consumer believing that it is their [sic] own idea."[41]

First, Merck funded a group called Cancer Research and Prevention Foundation, "a drug industry funded group wrapped in non-profit clothing," to run a campaign called "Make the Connection."[42] Merck urged women to link HPV with cervical cancer; a bracelet-making component of the campaign symbolized making a connection. Then it launched the "Tell Someone" ad campaign, urging women to tell their loved ones about the connection between the virus and cancer.

Finally, having primed the market, Merck launched an advertising blitz aimed at preteen girls urging each to "Be One Less" victim of cervical cancer in her lifetime. Merck saturated print and broadcast media with ads for Gardasil as the only solution to the omnipresent threat of cervical cancer. Such an ad campaign would have been illegal in almost every other country in the world, but not the US.

SELLING GARDASIL: "BE ONE LESS"

The FDA's approval of Gardasil in June 2006 was only the first step. Step two was to have the Advisory Committee on Immunization Practices of the CDC approve Gardasil. The Committee reviewed data from the clinical trials, held regular meetings from 2004 to 2006, and ultimately approved the vaccine for the US recommended childhood vaccine schedule. With ACIP's approval only a few weeks later, the ad campaign began in earnest.

Merck's DTC advertising was unprecedented in the vaccine market. In the past, manufacturers named vaccines after the diseases they prevented, like measles or mumps, or after their inventors, like Salk or Sabin. Never before had any company marketed a vaccine so aggressively under a trade name like Gardasil, evoking images of protection or a guard. Nor had any vaccine ever come on the market at such great expense, costing approximately $360 for its three doses, excluding doctor costs. Two doses of Gardasil 9 now cost about $410, plus the cost of two office visits, at the private sector price.[43] Contrast that with a polio vaccine at $32 a dose or a Diphtheria-Tetanus-Acellular Pertussis vaccine at $24 per dose.[44]

Merck's sales efforts employed sophisticated marketing messages to girls and their moms, playing on a kind of consumption feminism to suggest that smart, independent girls and women choose to vaccinate with Gardasil. Ironically, Merck at the same time aggressively lobbied state legislators to mandate Gardasil to all sixth-grade girls, thus taking away the very choice it was pitching.

Merck's "One Less" ad campaign featured athletic girls and young women skateboarding, playing basketball, surfing, dancing, and swimming; and their mothers, showering them with affection. The ads said nothing about sex, how women might acquire the virus, or how they might protect against it. Nor did the ads say anything about potential side effects from the vaccine.[45]

The ads also conveyed that "good mothers vaccinate." The only responsible option for good mothers would be to protect daughters from cervical cancer with Gardasil as soon as possible. As Dr. Diane Harper, principal investigator for Gardasil, said, "[Merck] created a sense of panic that says you have to have this vaccine now."[46]

The ads also framed the choice as "get the vaccine" or "risk cervical cancer."[47] Of course, the HPV infection does not equate to cervical cancer; and there were many other choices, including regular Pap tests and practicing safe sex, that could have a decisive impact on getting infected with HPV as well as on developing malignant cervical lesions or cancer later.[48] (We discuss cervical cancer risk factors in Chapter 4.) Merck's hard-sell marketing was only possible because of US laws allowing pharmaceutical ads to target children.

Although the ads mentioned that the vaccine was not a substitute for cervical screening, that message was lost in the hype to "be one less." The FDA regulations that apply to drugs, requiring corporations to note in DTC ads important risks and side effects, do not apply to vaccines.[49]

Merck emphasized the importance of "third-party credibility" in marketing Gardasil and went to great lengths to get a variety of endorsements: it enlisted professional medical associations, women's health groups, and government organizations. Merck gave generous donations to these nonprofit groups, and the groups in turn educated their members. Merck also reached out to individual doctors, offering them the opportunity to give lectures about Gardasil for $4,500 per lecture.[50]

The public relations genius behind Merck's Gardasil campaign was Edelman, a leading global public relations firm that has represented many corporate behemoths.[51] Edelman has strong connections to the pharmaceutical industry and emphasizes the importance of working with third-party actors to enhance credibility.

Accolades for Merck's savvy Gardasil ad campaign poured in. The journal *Pharmaceutical Executive* named Merck the first annual "Brand of the Year" in February 2007.[52] The author of the article gushed that "Gardasil is Merck at its best." She called Gardasil a "pharmaceutical breakthrough" and described it as "empowerment for a generation of girls and young women." She also accurately pronounced that Merck had "made a market out of thin air."

THE CDC's ADVISORY COMMITTEE ON IMMUNIZATION PRACTICES (ACIP)

The Advisory Committee on Immunization Practices (ACIP), the CDC expert committee that makes all federal vaccine recommendations in the US, approved Gardasil in June 2006, fast on the heels of FDA approval.[53] The ACIP has institutional and corporate insiders with long and deep connections to industry. A Congressional Committee once found that the CDC routinely grants conflicts of interest waivers to ACIP members; members own stock in vaccine makers under review; and those not allowed to vote because of financial conflicts are nonetheless allowed to participate in deliberations.[54] While on rare occasions ACIP has not recommended a vaccine, in general it recommends almost all proposed vaccines, and its recommendations dramatically affect uptake and revenues.

Medical associations, like the American Academy of Pediatrics, generally follow ACIP recommendations, and individual states over time usually mandate ACIP-recommended vaccines. Furthermore, once ACIP recommends a vaccine, that vaccine becomes eligible for tort liability protection under the 1986 National Childhood Vaccine Injury Act. This means that those injured by the vaccine no longer have the right to sue the manufacturer directly in the first instance. The injured party must sue the US Department of Health and Human Services to receive any compensation. Most compensation program cases are extremely acrimonious and take many years to resolve, most often in a loss for the injured party. There are many problems with the program, including a short time window within which to file, no right to discovery, and no formal rules of civil procedure.[55] Although in theory, injury victims preserve the right to sue for damages in civil court after filing in the compensation program, in reality, the grounds for doing so are exceptionally limited. Approximately 0.5 percent of victims go on to sue for vaccine injury in a state or federal court.[56]

The ACIP recommendation for an HPV vaccine set a new standard for pediatric medical care. Because this recommendation came with funding for about 40 percent of US girls through the Vaccines For Children Program, Merck could be sure that pediatricians and gynecologists would purchase, recommend, and administer the vaccine routinely. The ACIP decision not only made the vaccine free to girls aged 9 to 18 who were uninsured or on Medicaid, but led the private sector to follow suit, with 95 percent of insurance plans adding Gardasil immediately to keep up with this new standard of care.[57]

As one journalist wrote in 2009, Merck "really captured lightning in a bottle—to perfection! Hats off to Merck and their agency teams . . . for creating a campaign that is positive, upbeat, educational, empowering and relevant . . . Oh and did I mention the resulting $1.4 billion in Gardasil sales in 2007? A very effective campaign indeed."[58]

In part, Merck was simply applying lessons it had learned from its hepatitis B vaccine years earlier. In the late 1980s, ACIP had initially recommended the hepatitis B vaccine only for high-risk groups: men having sex with men, IV drug users, and hepatitis B-positive pregnant women. Merck did not initially propose the vaccine for universal use. But allegedly because high-risk groups were not vaccinating against hepatitis B, ACIP recommended the vaccine in 1991 for all infants on the first day of life. When Congress enacted the Vaccines for Children Program in 1994, making ACIP-recommended vaccines free to uninsured and Medicaid-eligible children, sales of the hepatitis B vaccine skyrocketed. By 2002, 90 percent of children under age three were receiving hepatitis B vaccines.[59]

Merck knew to avoid the hepatitis B launch pitfalls. This time, it immediately promoted a universal recommendation and state mandates. Although only a few groups of American women—such as African American women in the South, Latina women on the Mexican border, and white women in Appalachia—were at high risk for cervical cancer because of inadequate Pap screening, Merck did not target these women to get the HPV vaccine.

Merck targeted and funded professional medical associations, providing them "slide kits" for lectures. The kits asked lecturers to lobby state and federal agencies for mandates and insurance coverage. They instructed doctors to "downplay the sexually transmitted infection issues surrounding HPV"[60] and left out any broader context of women's sexual health.

This omission was dangerous because the HPV vaccine alone does not fully protect against cervical cancer. Gardasil at best protects against the HPV types thought to be associated with 70 percent of cervical cancers, and the additional types in Gardasil 9 bump that figure to, at most, 90 percent.[61] Thus, absent any overall emphasis on women's reproductive health, Gardasil might even have a negative impact, leading women to skip cervical screening.

While the vaccine would generate incredible revenue for Merck, it was unclear that it would actually improve women's health. The notion that any teenage girl would be "one less" if she receives a Gardasil vaccine was dangerously misleading. Young American girls in the target population are at almost zero immediate risk of cervical cancer. If a woman gets routine screening throughout her life, even her lifetime risk is exceedingly low. As Dr. Diane Harper said, "Being 'one less' means nothing because you weren't going to be one in the first place."[62]

Merck's "Be One Less" slogan and its rhetoric implied that the vaccine would protect for life. Yet the reality was starkly different: proven efficacy at the time of the campaign for Gardasil was just 4.5 years—hardly a lifetime for preteen girls.[63] The "Be One Less" slogan still appears on Gardasil 9's website and remains part of Merck's marketing strategy.[64]

Evidence already suggests that young women who received HPV vaccines are less likely to get Pap tests and thus may be at higher risk for cervical cancer.[65] Yet "[w]ithout regular Pap tests and follow-up, Gardasil and Cervarix will be at best expensive Band-Aids."[66]

Merck's ads had other problems, as well. To say that the vaccine is "anticancer" is misleading. To date, research shows only that it prevents precancerous lesions and genital warts, not cancer itself. Furthermore, HPV infections alone do not appear to lead to cervical cancer; other cofactors, such as persistent HPV infection, poor nutrition, and toxic exposures, seem necessary. Worse yet, the data do not yet rule out that HPV vaccines themselves could lead to cervical and other cancers in some women.[67] (See Chapter 9.) Until HPV vaccines have been on the market for decades, and scientists have proved that they reduce HPV-related cancers that otherwise would not have been prevented, it is misleading to assert that HPV vaccines prevent cancer. But that has not stopped Merck and GSK from making these expansive claims.

SELLING A CERVICAL CANCER VACCINE TO BOYS

Just how does one go about selling a product to prevent cervical cancer to someone who doesn't have a cervix? Having targeted teenage girls so intensely and having branded Gardasil as a feminist product, it might seem a stretch to rebrand the vaccine as "masculine" and good for boys and men. But that is precisely what Merck has done. In 2011, Merck secured ACIP's recommendation to administer Gardasil to 11-to-12-year-old boys, and in 2015 it got ACIP to recommend Gardasil 9 to all boys and girls. By 2015, the uptake of the vaccine among US boys was 42 percent for a first dose, compared to 60 percent of the same-aged girls.[68]

Initially, the marketing emphasized ending male-to-female sexual transmission of HPV. Over time, though, Merck adopted a broader "cancer prevention" message. In August 2016, Merck stopped distributing Gardasil in the US. At the same time, GSK stopped selling Cervarix in the US as its market share had continued to dwindle. Gardasil 9 is now the sole HPV vaccine on the US market.

The current pitch is that the vaccine can prevent many HPV-related cancers—penile, anal, oral, throat, and head and neck cancers, as well as vaginal, vulvar, and cervical cancers. There's only one problem: there are no clinical trials that show the vaccine is effective for throat, penile, head, or neck cancers. The FDA has not approved it for those cancers, which predominately affect men.

The federal government is seeking to increase uptake among boys in many ways. Merck claims that the vaccine is 100 percent effective in preventing the most common genital warts. Gardasil 9's website states: "Every hour, there are an estimated 40 new cases of genital warts."[69]

While not as frothy as the initial marketing campaign to teenage girls, Merck's marketing to boys is still impressive. Nobel laureate Dr. Harald zur Hausen exhorts that vaccinating boys is "of the utmost importance" to protect them.[70] The NIH has funded social media campaigns, including posters, television announcements, and Internet sites to increase uptake.

The US is ahead of the international curve in making gender-neutral recommendations. A few other countries, including Australia, Austria, and Liechtenstein, joined the US in 2014, recommending HPV vaccines for boys.[71] Even though most European Union countries have continued to recommend it to girls only, that may be changing. In the past, European cost-effectiveness research did not support vaccinating boys.[72] In 2017, however, Italy announced it would make HPV vaccines available to boys. A similar campaign is underway in the UK and Ireland, with these countries expecting to introduce the male program in 2018.[73]

The cost-benefit question for boys is especially doubtful. One study seeking to show cost-effectiveness for boys suggests that the throat cancer cases averted when men are 30-50 will cover the costs of vaccination today. This study is highly speculative, however.[74] Once again, there have been no clinical trials on the vaccine for throat cancer, which mainly affects men over 50. Smoking tobacco, drinking alcohol, and a diet low in fruits and vegetables seem to be the key risk factors.[75]

The hype about preventing anal cancer also seems misleading, with a total of about 480 anal cancer deaths per year in the US among men.[76] In fact, in a Merck-funded study of 4,055 males, the authors acknowledged that HPV vaccine "efficacy against precancerous lesions was not observed."[77] In other words, the vaccine did not do a better job than the trial control in preventing anal lesions, let alone anal cancer. As Jeanne Lenzer, a medical investigative journalist, pointedly asked, "[I]s it worth the risk of exposing millions of youth to the as yet uncertain harms of the vaccine?"[78] Dr. Angela Raffle told the *New York Times*, "If we give it to boys, then all pretense of scientific worth and cost analysis goes out the window."[79]

SUMMER 2016 GARDASIL 9 AD CAMPAIGN

In summer 2016, Merck launched a new television ad campaign aimed at both male and female preteens and their parents. The ad opens with an actor playing a young woman who has cervical cancer. She earnestly asks her parents if they knew that they could have prevented her cancer if they had vaccinated her when she was 11 or 12. Then the ad cuts to a young man who says he has an HPV-related cancer. Had his parents known about the vaccine, they could have protected him when he was 11 or 12. The actors ask: "Did you know? Mom, Dad?" The ad ends with the message to parents: "What will you say? Don't wait. Talk to your child's doctor today. Learn more at HPV.com."[80]

Playing on parents' guilt and children's fears, the ad reinforces the meme that "good parents vaccinate" with Gardasil 9. Yet the ad gives virtually no information about the virus, cancer, vaccine, doses required, possible adverse effects, or how continued cancer screening remains essential. The ad, directing itself squarely to children and parents, would be illegal almost everywhere else, but it remains on the air in the US.

HPV vaccines already generate over $2.5 billion annually, with the prospect of new markets to come: low- and middle-resource countries, boys and men, older teens, adults, and potential booster shots. With speculation about giving the vaccines even to babies, no demographic seems off the table. Without question, HPV vaccines have been money-making blockbusters.

14.

THE UNITED STATES:
SELLING AND
COMPELLING

"This [the HPV vaccine] is it. This is the Holy Grail." [1]
Dr. Eliav Barr, senior director of Clinical Research
Merck Research Laboratories, Boston Globe, 2007

The Holy Grail for vaccine manufacturers is to have governmentments mandate their products. People generally obey; the vast majority of parents comply with childhood vaccination mandates. According to the CDC, upward of 90 percent of US children receive state-mandated vaccines; a mere 1.7 percent of parents assert the right to exempt their children from specific vaccines on medical, religious, or other grounds.[2] Thus, in the US, once all fifty states mandate a particular vaccine, about four million children have to buy that product annually. Four million vaccine customers every year, without liability, is an extraordinary incentive. To be able to dispense with the marketing Merck had to do initially—to be able to simply have states compel students to take its product or lose the opportunity to attend school—that was the goal.

As we've noted, the Gardasil three-dose series had an initial price tag of $360, not including doctor visits. The Gardasil 9 series, not including doctor visits, is at least $410.[3] If every state mandates Gardasil 9, that would be $1.64 billion per year for each birth year cohort in the US market (4 million x $410). Think about that–$1.64 billion in revenue annually with no marketing and no liability. The states compel, the doctors administer, and the school districts enforce. Getting states to mandate the HPV vaccine creates huge, guaranteed markets with minimal expense and virtually no liabilities, stretching out *ad infinitum*.

Mandates don't materialize out of thin air, however. The best way to create mandates is through lobbying, first by lobbying credible third parties, and then by having those groups lobby state legislators and opinion leaders. The more indirect it appears, the better. The pitch should be about health, not profits. Although Merck's efforts to mandate Gardasil have had their ups and downs since 2006, the quest for the Holy Grail still beckons.

THE KEYS TO THE MANDATE KINGDOM: ACIP AND VACCINES FOR CHILDREN

The CDC's Advisory Committee on Immunization Practices is a group of medical and public health experts who recommend vaccines to the public. ACIP includes fifteen voting members, fourteen of whom are from a medically related profession. One member represents the public. In addition to the voting members, eight people represent other federal agencies, and 30 are from so-called liaison organizations, although they do not have voting rights.[4]

Essential to Gardasil's financial success would be the ACIP recommendation and approval for the Vaccines for Children program. In February 2004, more than two years before Merck completed clinical trials and FDA approved Gardasil, preparation began within ACIP toward an HPV vaccine recommendation. These preparations began seven months before Merck took Vioxx off the market. At that time, an HPV vaccine working group formed, with representatives from relevant government health agencies, as well as the American Academy of Pediatrics, the American Academy of Family Physicians, and other professional membership groups. The working group met monthly from 2004 to 2006.[5]

FEBRUARY 2006 ACIP MEETING ON HPV VACCINES

At the February ACIP meeting, the lion's share of time went to Gardasil, even though the FDA, the first gatekeeper, had yet to approve either Gardasil or Cervarix. Presenters came from the National Cancer Institute, Merck, and the CDC, among other institutions. They explained that studies for the vaccines had "surrogate endpoints" of cervical lesions, rather than cervical cancer. They noted that vaccinated women had fewer abnormal Pap tests, based on up to five years' study. Merck's clinical trials involved 27,000 women and children on four continents.[6]

CDC's Dr. Anne Schuchat asked perhaps the most probing question, wondering about HPV-type replacement when types 16 and 18 are no longer common because of the vaccine.[7] Given that today we know of over two hundred HPV types, this was an extremely important question. The presenter answered that there was no evidence of replacement over the four-year trial period. Cervical cancer develops, however, over approximately twenty to thirty years. So, what was the relevance of the four years of data? No one asked.

At the end of the meeting, the Committee heard public comments supporting Gardasil. The President of Women in Government (WIG) noted that its members had already introduced "cervical cancer prevention legislation" in 44 states, in line with Merck's strategy of "disease branding." She wanted to be sure that the vaccine would be available to all women, regardless of socioeconomic background.[8]

There was no discussion of possible conflicts of interest given the National Institutes of Health's patents related to the vaccine, the vaccine's short demonstrated efficacy period of just four and a half years, the use of surrogate endpoints, the use of fauxcebos, and sketchy cost-effectiveness compared with routine Pap tests. All these issues required discussion for a thorough evaluation, but that didn't happen.

JUNE 2006 ACIP MEETING

ACIP unanimously voted to recommend Gardasil for routine administration to 11- and 12-year-old girls in June 2006 and resolved that the government should purchase and distribute it for free to qualifying children.[9] The presenters all spoke glowingly.

While the Committee recommended that girls aged 11 to 12 get three doses of Gardasil, it gave permission for doctors to start the series on girls as young as 9.[10] ACIP recommended vaccination for girls and women up to age 26 but failed to recommend screening them prior to vaccinating to see if they had already been exposed to any HPV types, in which case the vaccine would be ineffective. ACIP also made slightly different recommendations for girls and women with previous abnormal Pap tests, positive HPV tests, or genital warts, as well as specific recommendations for nursing mothers. But it urged these precautions and different recommendations for only a tiny fraction of women.[11] With this first ACIP recommendation, Gardasil was truly on its way.

LATER ACIP MEETINGS ON THE HPV VACCINES

ACIP has made many more HPV vaccine recommendations since 2006, but not a single safety warning. In October 2009, it recommended GSK's Cervarix to girls and young women and made a permissive recommendation for Gardasil for males aged 9 through 26.[12] Merck's primary pitch to boys was that the vaccine could prevent genital warts and anal and penile cancer, as well as protect future sexual partners from HPV transmission. In October 2011, ACIP expanded its recommendation for 11- and 12-year-old boys and males up to 21, with the condition that the vaccine could be given through age 26.[13] In February 2015, ACIP recommended Gardasil 9 for routine vaccination of all 11- and 12-year-old girls and boys.[14]

Since the initial 2006 recommendation, ACIP members have voiced virtually no concerns about safety, but they have worried greatly about lower-than-expected uptake.[15] By 2012, over 50 percent of parents reported that they were not likely to have their children vaccinated. Parents' reasons varied, including lack of knowledge, no need, no recommendation by parents' healthcare provider, cost, and safety concerns.[16] Among parents of girls with no intent to vaccinate, safety concerns grew from 5.4 percent in 2008 to 19.3 percent in 2011.[17] Still, parents' safety concerns did not provoke ACIP discussion.

By October 2013, ACIP noted that "improving vaccination coverage among US adolescent girls has stalled," although coverage among boys was still increasing.[18] Girls were not getting vaccinated despite the vaccine's insurance coverage under the Affordable Care Act and most private insurers.[19]

ACIP remains concerned about low uptake. The government has funded a speakers' bureau, eleven marketing organizations, and new pages on the CDC website to encourage physicians and parents to administer the HPV vaccine.[20] Dr. Schuchat reported that the CDC was reaching out to cervical cancer survivors to help it better market the vaccine.

Another HPV vaccine uptake strategy at ACIP was called the "3-star visit" approach, where a medical office gives teenagers three vaccines at once: meningococcal, TDaP, and HPV. If the teen walks out the door having received all three vaccines, the nurse gets three stars: "What you measure, you accomplish."[21]

STATE MANDATES: THE HOLY GRAIL

Once again, the ticket to big money in the US is state mandates. HPV vaccine advocates, however, sharply disagreed initially on whether Merck should pursue mandates. Dr. Jon Abramson, the ACIP Chair who recommended HPV to 11-to-12-year-old girls, publicly opposed mandates, reasoning that states had better ways to spend their healthcare money.[22]

Merck was in a hurry, however, and made contributions to political campaigns and legislative organizations. Just three months after ACIP recommended Gardasil, Michigan lawmakers introduced a law to mandate it.[23] By February 2007, 24 states plus the District of Columbia had introduced mandate legislation, while 41 states had drafted legislation to provide school-based education about cervical cancer and the vaccine against it.[24]

In its quest for mandates, Merck hit a roadblock in Texas. Governor Rick Perry issued an executive order in February 2007 to mandate that all sixth-grade girls get Gardasil with only limited exemptions. The Governor circumvented the legislature, which would ordinarily be the body to decide. When it became public that Merck had contributed $6,000 to Perry's gubernatorial reelection campaign and that Merck employed Perry's former chief of staff, Mike Toomey, the order was dead. Toomey had committed to raise $50 million for Perry's presidential campaign, with a hefty chunk likely to come from Merck and its executives.[25]

The legislature voted 181 to 3 to overturn Perry's executive order.[26] After this legislative drubbing, Merck announced that it would stop pressing for mandates, at least for the time being. Dr. Richard Haupt, a Merck executive, told the *New York Times* that school mandates "are being viewed as a distraction."[27] Another doctor from ACIP told the press that while the vaccine was useful, more information was necessary before mandates would be desirable.[28]

After the 2007 turning point in Texas, Gardasil began to generate somewhat more controversy. Commentators started to ask questions about its safety, cost, and actual benefit. Some noted that Merck had not made out a clinical or cost-effectiveness case. Although Merck had sought to mandate the vaccines for 11- and 12-year-old girls, out of the more than 20,000 clinical trial participants, fewer than 1,000 girls 12 or younger received Gardasil in the trials.[29] Dr. Diane Harper stated that "giving it to 11-year-olds is a great big public health experiment. . . . After all, the drug only has five years of clinical trials behind it and has never been actually shown to prevent cervical cancer, only precancerous lesions."[30]

On cost, too, commentators were dubious. One 2007 editorial in *Nature Biotechnology* noted that Merck would have to show that a $30 billion initial investment (4 million children in an annual cohort x $360 for three doses of Gardasil x 20 years for likely diagnoses of cervical cancer) would be worthwhile before a single life would be saved.[31] The editorial concluded that Gardasil cannot be the whole solution—there needs to be greater awareness of disease risk, safe sex, condom use, and cervical cancer screening. Another 2007 editorial, in *American Journal of Bioethics*, opined, "[J]ust as pizza bearing cheerleader drug reps are a poor substitute for medical education, pharmaceutical company lobbying is a poor substitute for well-reasoned public health policymaking."[32]

Despite Merck's tactical retreat, state HPV vaccine mandates are still the Holy Grail. And Merck has had several successes, too. Virginia's legislature passed a mandate in 2007 that girls entering sixth grade must receive the HPV vaccine.[33] Not surprisingly, Merck has significant economic interests there. In December 2006, Merck announced that it sought to invest $57 million to expand its Elkton, Virginia, plant to manufacture Gardasil. Two months later, the Governor announced mandate legislation. Four months after that, Merck pledged $193 million more. A spokeswoman for the Governor noted that children's parents have broad opt-out rights and said that the mandate decision was "completely separate" from Merck's investment decisions.[34]

Since 2007, Washington, DC, has required sixth-grade girls to get an HPV vaccine, with an opt-out clause. This bill passed the DC City Council, and Congress then approved it.[35] Because DC's schools are 79 percent African American, scholar Malika Redmond has argued that this early Gardasil mandate "triggered historical concerns of the exploitation of African American bodies."[36] With few other mandates, she raised concern that African American children in the District of Columbia might be being used as almost clinical trial subjects to see early safety and effectiveness signals. With the history of other experimentation on African Americans in mind, and especially the Tuskegee experiments related to sexually transmitted diseases, she flagged the DC mandate as one that especially raised questions of equal treatment.

The latest state to join Virginia and the District of Columbia is Rhode Island. As of September 1, 2015, it requires all seventh graders, both girls and boys, to receive one dose of Gardasil.[37] Interestingly, although there is a meningitis booster vaccine requirement for the twelfth grade, there is no requirement for a second dose of the HPV vaccine.[38] With vaccine effectiveness seemingly predicated on two doses and yet no requirement for a second dose, the mandate is irrational, at best. Rhode Island imposed this new mandate by administrative means, without debate or legislative action.[39] Merck does significant business with Rhode Island; it sold Rhode Island $5.6 million of vaccines in 2015 and maintains close ties with lobbyists. The new mandate increases Merck's Rhode Island sales, requiring each new seventh-grade cohort to buy the vaccine, either directly or at taxpayer expense. The new requirement has sparked growing opposition and controversy.[40] Like DC and Virginia, Rhode Island permits parents to opt out on religious and medical grounds.[41] Legislative attempts to remove the religious exemption died in committee.[42]

Although the vast majority of states have not yet passed HPV vaccine mandates, Merck and its allies are working to change that.

THE HARD SELL

Even without mandates, HPV uptake among adolescents is substantial. As of 2016, the CDC reported that 65 percent of teenage girls and 56 percent of teenage boys had received at least one dose of an HPV vaccine.[43] By contrast, uptake for the TDaP booster, a mandated teen vaccine, is over 88 percent.[44] From the CDC's perspective, the gap between HPV and TDaP uptake in this age group shows that "[w]e are missing crucial opportunities to protect the next generation from cancers caused by HPV."[45]

The CDC recommends many ways to increase uptake, including PR campaigns, emails and robocalls, as well as physician and parent trainings.[46] These initiatives display a remarkable level of private-public partnership, with federal tax dollars literally selling Merck products.

Most physician organizations have rallied behind the vaccine. The list of prominent medical organizations endorsing HPV vaccination is long but includes the American Academy of Family Physicians, the American Academy of Pediatrics, the American College of Obstetricians and Gynecologists, the American Medical Association, the American Pharmacists Association, the Infectious Diseases Society of America, and Planned Parenthood.[47] Legislative groups, such as Women in Government, also play critical roles in third-party marketing.

In January 2016, 69 US cancer centers joined the team to sell HPV vaccines.[48] The 69 centers include most major US university medical centers, including Harvard, Yale, Stanford, NYU, Johns Hopkins, and UCLA, as well as other hospital medical centers, such as the Mayo Clinic. According to Mount Sinai Hospital's press release, the joint statement emerged out of a summit to "identify barriers to increasing [HPV] immunization rates in pediatric settings across the country."[49] The joint statement echoes earlier marketing points: the vaccine is for cancer prevention, not sexually transmitted infections. The total number of HPV infections, about 14 million annually in the US, is the reference point, despite the fact that over 90 clear on their own.[50] The cancer centers' pitch is that the vaccine is not just for cervical cancer, but for all HPV-related cancers.[51]

What's new is the portrayal of relatively low vaccine uptake compared to other vaccines as a "serious public health threat." These federally funded centers state that they were "compelled to jointly issue this call to action" in view of the "tragically underused" vaccine. They assert that current low vaccination rates are "alarming." The Centers urge parents and guardians to complete the series before children's 13th birthdays and to complete it as soon as possible for those between 13 and 26 for women and 13 and 21 for men. They call on all healthcare providers "to be advocates for cancer prevention" and ask providers to "join forces," as HPV "is our best defense." They conclude: "The HPV vaccine PREVENTS CANCER."[52] (Capitalization in original.)

This joint statement takes HPV vaccine marketing rhetoric of a "serious public health threat" to a new level, using military images and vocabulary from the "war against cancer" and paving the way to mandates. The engagement of these centers further fuses the "war on cancer" with HPV vaccine marketing.

VACCINATING THE VULNERABLE

In addition to the quest for universal mandates, vaccine promotion focuses on particularly vulnerable populations—preteens and teens, immigrants seeking citizenship, those in the military, those who go to Medicaid-funded clinics, and even those in juvenile detention.

Several states, while not adopting HPV vaccine mandates, have passed laws to allow preteen children to "consent" to treatments and vaccination against sexually transmitted infections, including HPV, without parental knowledge or consent. In January 2012, California passed AB 499, giving children age 12 and up the right to consent to confidential medical services to prevent sexually transmitted infections. Parents may not access children's medical records for these confidential visits, and the children may receive vaccines for free.[53]

There may be compelling public policy rationales to allow sexually active minors access to contraception and treatment for sexually transmitted infections without parental consent. The case for granting children access to a vaccine to prevent cancer twenty to thirty years in the future is dubious, however. Because the vaccine does not have a well-established history of safety or effectiveness, and its reported side effects are severe, it is troubling to consider preteens making these medical decisions alone. Many consider these laws an infringement on parental rights and reasonably question whether preteenagers can exercise informed consent on such questions.[54]

The National Vaccine Information Center, a national vaccine watchdog, called California Governor Jerry Brown's decision to sign this into law "a violation of parental rights and federal vaccine safety law." Director Barbara Loe Fisher lamented that "California parents, who will not be informed before their minor children are given vaccines, will be the ones left to deal with the consequences legally and financially if their child becomes vaccine injured."[55]

Federal law requires that a parent or guardian receive a vaccine information sheet before consenting to a vaccine.[56] The CDC website has clear instructions to medical staff on this.[57] Some states are circumventing this federal law by allowing minors to get the vaccine without parental knowledge or consent.

California is not alone in permitting minors aged 12 and up to consent to medical care without parental knowledge or consent. North Carolina has an even broader law: "Any minor may

give effective consent . . . for medical health services for the prevention . . . of venereal disease and other [reportable] diseases."[58]
Vaccine rights lawyer Alan Phillips calls the California and North
Carolina laws "stealth vaccine laws," as they allow children to "consent" to vaccination without ever using the polarizing words "vaccine" or "immunization."[59]

One New York State county offered children free headphones
and speakers if they consented to HPV shots on their own. The
New York Department of Health issued a regulation in 2016 to allow minors to consent to sexual health treatment, including HPV
vaccines, without parental knowledge.[60] Thus the goodies were attractive, lawful incentives, clearly aimed at the children themselves.
Many public-private partnerships, including Planned Parenthood,
supported the regulation.[61] Ironically, those under age 18 cannot go
to an R-rated movie or buy cigarettes without parental consent, but
they can consent to a potentially life-altering vaccine.[62]

MANDATES FOR YOUNG IMMIGRANT WOMEN

After the 2006 ACIP recommendation, one automatic mandate
went into effect: the mandate for immigrants applying for visas to
enter the US or to adjust their immigration status. Under a 1996
law, the US immigration service required immigrants to receive all
ACIP-recommended vaccines for their age group. Thus, as of July
2008, this meant that all immigrant girls aged 11 to 26 were required to receive at least the first dose of Gardasil, the only ACIP-
approved HPV vaccine available at the time.[63]

The 1996 law accomplished what many states are now trying to
achieve: automatic requirement of all ACIP-recommended vaccines
by age. These young women were not eligible for free vaccines, however, so the vaccine requirement involved out-of-pocket payment for
each dose, costing at least $120, not to mention doctors' fees.[64]

The National Coalition for Immigrant Women's Rights described
the mandate as "essentially a surcharge applied only to young immigrant women that will effectively block them from immigrating
to the US or becoming US citizens."[65] It further argued that the

"requirement violates a woman's basic right to self-determination, creates additional barriers for immigrant families seeking adjustment of status, and unfairly forces immigrant women to subject their bodies to a new treatment with known side effects."[66]

The policy ended in December 2009, when the CDC adopted a federal rule removing the HPV vaccine mandate for immigrants.[67] The CDC adopted new criteria for immigrants: (1) the vaccine must be age-appropriate, (2) it must protect against a disease that has the potential to cause an outbreak, and (3) the disease must have been eliminated or be in the process of elimination in the US.[68] Because HPV was not the target of outbreak control or elimination, the CDC could not require immigrant women to get it.[69]

The HPV vaccine mandate for young immigrant women was an unusual case where the federal government abandoned a mandate on principled grounds. Were US states to adopt these same criteria, no state legislature would be able to mandate the HPV vaccine.

UPTAKE IN THE MILITARY

Like in any business, big clients are attractive—they can buy a lot of product, and their purchases often sway others. Thus, having the military on one's side to recommend medical products is a decided advantage, both for direct sales and persuasive power. Shortly after ACIP recommended Gardasil to girls and young women, the military followed suit to recommend the vaccine to its women and girls. In March 2007, the Department of Defense health insurance plan, Tricare, started covering Gardasil for young women.[70] By 2012, following ACIP recommendations, it offered the vaccine to all military service personnel, male and female.[71] Despite military insurance coverage, the uptake among female military personnel is low. An article reviewing women's HPV vaccine uptake from 2006 to 2011 found that only 22.5 percent of all eligible women took at least one dose while in the military but offered no explanation for low uptake.[72] As those in the military often are mandated to receive many vaccines to serve in different parts of the world, perhaps they are more cautious than civilians when it comes to recommended vaccines.

HPV Vaccination in Juvenile Detention Facilities

In April 2010, *Science Daily* ran a story that 39 US states already offered HPV vaccines to detained or arrested adolescent girls.[73] In most states, a facility superintendent may consent to vaccination "with the adolescent's agreement." The *Science Daily* article succinctly described the findings of a research study on HPV vaccines in the juvenile justice system: "The health of this high risk population could be significantly improved with health care programs based in the juvenile justice setting."[74] Can incarcerated girls voluntarily "agree" to HPV vaccination?[75] How can juvenile facilities possibly know the girls' family health histories? Increased uptake should not be at the expense of the right to informed consent.[76]

To date, most states do not mandate the HPV vaccine, nor is it mandatory in the military, for immigrants, or for girls in detention. But the sales strategy is clear: have third parties endorse the vaccine, have institutions and physicians urge uptake, and ultimately secure universal mandates through state laws. These sales techniques work.

15.

INJURY REPORTS FLOOD IN

By 2010, Norma Erickson, a freelance reporter, had been writing about health for Examiner.com, an Internet newspaper out of Washington, DC, for some time. She wrote about diet, exercise, and other paths to wellness. In her research, she began to come across inexplicable stories about perfectly healthy teenage girls receiving the Gardasil vaccine and then suffering bizarre and terrible symptoms: pain, heart palpitations, dizziness, vomiting, personality changes, seizures, and even death. Norma was puzzled and started contacting the parents to ask for more information. She asked Examiner.com if she could be their Vaccines Examiner, and they said yes. She started the online series "Meet the Gardasil Girls."

Norma supported vaccines. She'd raised three children on her own, vaccinating each precisely as doctors recommended. But she was independent-minded and had a drive to get to the bottom of things. Something with this particular vaccine just seemed terribly wrong. Moms were reporting that their perfectly healthy teenage girls were becoming seriously injured after vaccination, and no one seemed to know why.

In several stories for Examiner.com, Norma chronicled Merck's aggressive ad campaign to convince moms and their daughters that Gardasil was the best way to prevent cervical cancer. She carefully reviewed the Gardasil package insert, which seemed to raise more questions than it answered.

Norma was certainly aware that cervical cancer is a truly devastating disease. She had known women who had suffered from cervical cancer and knew that it could be lethal. In her research, she learned that women in lower income countries were at a much higher risk of developing cervical cancer. While she had no issue with a safe, effective vaccine, Norma also knew that Pap tests were incredibly effective at detecting early-stage abnormal growths. Her primary concern was for the girls she'd read about, whose stories of HPV vaccine injury were appearing online. So in 2010, Norma published her first Gardasil Girl story.

ALEXIS: CHANGING DREAMS TO NIGHTMARES

In spring of 2007, Alexis was a happy, shy, well-adjusted 13-year-old living in New Mexico with her mom, Tracy, her dad, and younger sister Kimber. She was on the honor roll at school and had a sweet disposition. She had been diagnosed with type 1 diabetes a year before, but Alexis took that in stride, teaching her peers about her insulin pump and diabetes.

Alexis wanted to go to Germany for the summer to visit her maternal grandparents. Tracy was worried about letting Alexis go on her own because of her recent diabetes diagnosis, but Alexis's pediatrician thought it was fine because Alexis was handling it in such a mature way.

In March 2007, before Alexis went to Germany for the summer, the pediatrician insisted that she get Gardasil, explaining that because she had diabetes, it was "very, very important to get her vaccinated for EVERYTHING that came up because of her weakened immune system."[1] No one noticed any problems or reactions from the shot she got in her thigh.

Alexis got her second shot in June 2007, right before leaving for Germany. Again, there were no immediate reactions, so she went to Germany as planned. Her grandparents thought she acted a bit out of character, but nothing serious. When Alexis came home to New Mexico, however, Tracy, like any mom, noticed the little things: Alexis didn't seem to get jet lag as she had the last time she'd gone to Germany. Although she had always been very sensitive, she didn't cry when she learned that the family dog of twelve years had died while she was away.

In the fall of 2007, Alexis's behavior became stranger. She started getting into trouble at school and couldn't concentrate. She went into rages and screamed at the family. She would say she wanted to go to an orphanage or to be adopted by another family, which greatly upset Tracy. Doctors didn't think much of this and told Tracy that Alexis was testing boundaries like a typical teen. But Tracy knew this wasn't typical; she knew in her gut that something was terribly wrong.

Alexis soon started having massive panic attacks, where her heart would race so fast that Tracy could see her chest thumping. Alexis started saying, "Things look funny or strange," and that people's faces made her sick to her stomach.

Tracy started to realize that Alexis couldn't sleep. She stayed up in her room all night writing nonsense on little notes. Then Alexis became obsessed with eating. In retrospect, Tracy realized that Alexis's seizures must have begun around this time.

Tracy took her daughter to see the endocrinologist they had been seeing for her diabetes, and he sent her to a psychologist. The psychologist's only explanation for Alexis's odd behavior was that she must have been sexually molested in Germany. Tracy grilled Alexis and her parents and was convinced that the psychologist's theory was wrong. Then Tracy and Alexis were sent to another psychologist and psychiatrist, and the new psychiatrist prescribed antipsychotic medications. Nothing worked, and Alexis only got worse. By January 2008, Alexis was starting to throw up all the food she ate, but at the same time she was ravenously hungry, so she would vomit and then want to eat again.

Still not knowing what was causing her symptoms, they went back to the pediatrician for Alexis's third dose of Gardasil in January 2008. Tracy asked the pediatrician if Gardasil could have anything to do with her daughter's bizarre behaviors. The pediatrician reassured her. "No, but if she didn't finish the series, then it could cause more problems."[2] The doctor never explained what those problems might be. Tracy trusted her doctor, so Alexis got the third dose.

This time, Alexis's reaction to the shot was swift and clear. She immediately lost five pounds, could not keep any food down, and could not sleep. Alexis's pediatrician sent her to the hospital. She was admitted for four days so the doctors could do an extensive battery of tests. Everything came back normal, and again, doctors told Tracy that Alexis had no medical problems and that everything must be psychological.

As a result, doctors sent Alexis to a behavioral hospital where the new doctors and other staff put her on more antipsychotic medications, none of which helped her sleep or stopped the vomiting.[3] Believing that her unwillingness to eat was psychosomatic, the doctors at the hospital refused to feed Alexis if she vomited. Nurses observed her eating her own vomit because she received no other food. After five days, the hospital released Alexis, saying all was well, although Alexis still could barely hold down food or sleep.

Doctors next sent Alexis to a children's psychiatric hospital where, finally, a psychiatrist realized that she was having seizures. From an electroencephalograph he learned that Alexis was having seizures in the frontal lobe of her brain, in the part that controls personality. She had likely been having seizures for many months.

Alexis then spent the next six months at this hospital while undergoing many different medical tests: EEGs, CT scans, MRIs, spinal taps, muscle biopsy, blood tests, and more. All the results were normal, although she was feeling anything but normal! Finally, the doctors came to the conclusion that Alexis had recently been exposed to a virus, even though she didn't show typical symptoms of a viral infection. The virus seemed to have led to brain inflammation and then to seizures, causing serious brain damage. By the end of 2008, just a year and a half after the first dose of Gardasil, Alexis—who had been a good student—was now testing at a 4th-grade level, although she should have been in high school. She had been unable to attend school since the fall of 2007. She was only fifteen years old.

At this point, Alexis had seizures almost constantly, day and night. She was in relentless pain, and no medications helped. New symptoms appeared as the months went by—numbness in her arms and legs, headaches, loss of bladder control (she had to start wearing diapers), vision problems, brain fog, chronic fatigue, rapid heart rate, high blood pressure, and memory loss.

In 2009, Alexis went to yet another hospital because of a racing heart and very high blood pressure. Perplexed, the doctors said they had never seen anything like this before but offered no help. By 2010, when Tracy met Norma, she was trying to obtain some government-funded services for Alexis for her brain injuries. Tracy found out that Alexis would have to wait for years in New Mexico before she would receive any benefits. Alexis joined a waiting list of over 47,000 people with traumatic brain injuries from various causes, all hoping to get services.

Alexis's condition put enormous strain on the family. Tracy devoted herself full-time to keeping Alexis alive. Her once-vibrant daughter became "a toddler, a little old lady, and a teenager combined."[4] Alexis's younger sister Kimber wrote: "Being nine or ten years old and watching your older sister slowly dissolve and someone completely different taking her place is simply wrong. It is pretty much the exact same thing as watching a hit man kill her before your eyes. It is—just knowing the fact that you will never see your sister again. The only difference is, through my experience, it was slower, I didn't understand what was happening, and I didn't know I was never going to see the real her, or should I say the old her, ever again."[5]

Like so many of the moms Norma interviewed, Tracy was adamant that other parents needed to know. Tracy ended one of her Internet posts on Alexis: "Gardasil changed everything! Our perfectly normal lives have been forever transformed into a living nightmare. Please, learn from our story. Do not let your child become 'One More Girl' like Alexis because of Gardasil."[6]

Through her extensive reporting, Norma was aware that Alexis's story was not isolated; some stories were even more chilling. Norma also interviewed Emily Tarsell, whose daughter Christina died shortly after receiving her third dose.

CHRISTINA: GONE AFTER GARDASIL

Emily Tarsell, Christina's mom, is a licensed clinical counselor in Maryland who is incredibly proud of her daughter, Chris. Emily liked to say that Chris had insight, compassion, and self-determination beyond her years. But Chris never got the chance to fulfill her potential.

Chris was an honors student throughout high school and college. She had just completed her junior year majoring in Studio Art with a minor in philosophy at the prestigious liberal arts Bard College in the Hudson River Valley in New York. She liked to cook and hang out with friends and was looking forward to returning to a summer job there at Bard's Hessel Museum of Art. Chris was a passionate, talented artist. She served as art editor for two literary magazines and had won awards in several juried exhibitions. She was also an avid and accomplished athlete. She excelled in baseball on the boys' team in middle school, on varsity softball during high school, and played on an award-winning tennis team in college.

Chris also devoted herself to community service through her church, Girl Scouts where she earned a Gold Award, the National Honor Society, and Amnesty International. Any organization Chris participated in was proud to count her as a member. That all ended 18 days after Chris received her third dose of Gardasil.

In August 2007, when Chris was twenty years old and not yet sexually active, Emily took her to see a gynecologist for the first time and to see a primary care doctor for adults. Chris was perfectly healthy. At the first appointment with the gynecologist, the doctor recommended the HPV vaccine, saying it was safe and effective and would prevent cervical cancer. The doctor did not mention any adverse side effects or provide any written information about risks and benefits. As a mom, Emily's initial gut response was to decline this novel vaccine, but decades earlier she had lost a sister to uterine cancer. Even though that is very different from cervical cancer, Emily was inclined to consider the vaccine. Chris had gotten all recommended childhood vaccines, and Emily had always accepted that they were safe and effective, as advertised.

Chris was indifferent about the vaccine and looked to her mom for advice. Based on the gynecologist's recommendation and the understanding that Chris should be vaccinated before any sexual exposure to HPV, Emily and Chris agreed that she would start the 3-dose series.

After Chris's first shot at the end of August 2007, she went back to college. Emily didn't see Chris again until she came home for Thanksgiving break.

Chris saw her primary care doctor and gynecologist on the same day during the break. The gynecologist gave her the second Gardasil shot. During the routine physical with the primary care doctor, the doctor detected an arrhythmia in Chris's heartbeat. This was totally new; in the 20 years of Chris's life, she had never had any reports of an arrhythmia or any kind of chronic illness. They were very surprised, but the doctor reassured them that it might be a false positive. The doctor suggested that they come back again at the end of December, when Chris would be home for the winter break.

As instructed, Chris went with her mom to the primary care doctor when she returned in December. The doctor again picked up the arrhythmia. After consulting with colleagues, Chris's doctor advised her to get an echocardiogram. In addition, Chris had developed persistent sinus congestion, so Emily and Chris saw an ear, nose, and throat specialist. The doctor saw no structural issues but suggested that she might be having an allergic reaction to something. Emily and Chris planned to do some follow-up testing for possible allergies.

When Chris went back to school after the holidays, she got an echocardiogram. The results of the heart test were normal; there were no structural problems. They thought everything was fine, since the doctor did not prescribe any medication or request further follow-up. Emily later learned that the echocardiogram was not the right test for Chris's problem. To test for a timing problem like an arrhythmia, Chris should have worn a Holter monitor for a period of time, which could have picked up her heart condition. Chris resumed her spring semester activities. She had some complaints about joint problems in her arm but thought, "Well, maybe

I won't play tennis next year." But as far as Emily knew, everything was okay.

Chris came home at the end of the semester in late May 2008. Her mom was out of town, so Chris's dad, Richard, took her for the third Gardasil shot on June 3. A few days later, when Chris picked Emily up at the airport, Chris said, "Mom, I'm feeling really tired." Chris continued to complain of tiredness for days. She said she felt faint and dizzy when she stood up, and she had a rash on her neck. It all seemed peculiar, but they never imagined these symptoms were related to the vaccine.

Emily thought that these unusual complaints would probably be temporary and might be due to fatigue following the semester, or perhaps a result of low blood pressure. She suggested that Chris stay home a couple more weeks to rest before going back to start her summer job. But Chris was scheduled for an orientation at her new job, and she didn't want to miss it or disappoint her employer. She was also eager to get back to school to join her roommates, who had just moved to off-campus housing. And she was looking forward to having a car at school for the first time, since she had just been given her mom's old car. Pushing herself, Chris drove back.

Emily was worried about her daughter, though; she asked Chris to call her after the six-hour drive back. Chris arrived safely, but Emily said, "I'll come and see you in a couple weeks as soon as my summer break begins. I want to help you set up your new place, and I want to follow up on your symptoms." Emily was a therapist in a school for special needs children at the time, so she was able to take a few weeks off in June to be with Chris. If the symptoms persisted, Emily could help Chris figure out what was going on.

Before Emily got that chance to see her daughter, though, there was a knock at Emily's front door. It was late in the evening; it was the police. Emily's first thought was, "Yikes, what did I do wrong?" But she quickly sensed that it must be about Chris. Emily nervously asked the officer, "Is this about Chris; is something wrong with Chris? Oh my God, was my daughter in an accident?" There was an anxious silence, and then the officer answered, "No, Chris was not in an accident." Then after another tense silence, the officer said,

"Ms. Tarsell, Chris was found dead in her bed, at school. We're terribly sorry." They could offer no explanations.

In denial at first, Emily kept repeating, "No, you have the wrong address; this can't be possible." She had just seen Chris; she couldn't believe it. She seemed to have a few new health complaints, but they didn't seem life-threatening. Emily paced around the house, yelling repeatedly, "No, no, no, this can't be." Emily had been alone when she got the news; she called Chris's dad. He too couldn't believe it. "Stop kidding. This is a bad joke." Eventually, as their new reality set in, though, they both had to accept the tragedy. Their entire world fell apart.

Emily and Richard went to Bard to bring Chris's remains home. Emily spoke with the pathologist and urged her to please find out what had happened. She shared with the pathologist the previously reported arrhythmias and asked that they pay special attention to the heart. Was there something about Chris's heart that could have caused her death? The pathologist spent extra time investigating Chris's heart and consulted with other colleagues. But the pathology team couldn't find any structural issues. They ruled out narcotics and violence and found nothing that would explain Chris's sudden death.

At that point, Emily really had no idea what had happened. It was not until sometime later that Richard mentioned that he had heard on television that there were reports of deaths related to Gardasil. That's the first time that it dawned on Emily, "Could it be? Could Gardasil have caused Chris's death?"

Emily was driven to find out what had happened to her only child. She called the primary care doctor to report Chris's death, and the doctor prompted Emily to file a report to the federal Vaccine Adverse Event Reporting System (VAERS). Emily did so and asked the gynecologist to file one, as well. The pathologist had already done so.

Emily imagined that the FDA and CDC would want to interview her to understand more about what had happened, but they did not; they asked only for the name of Chris's doctor. The CDC did obtain Chris's medical records and slide specimens from her autopsy. They did one test to see if she had had streptococcus virus. She had not. They also noted that there were no inflammatory infiltrates in the myocardium. That was the full extent of their investigation, so the cause of death was still undetermined. The CDC's lack of diligence astonished Emily.

At the time, the CDC website said that it investigated death reports to VAERS. Emily was skeptical. They had hardly looked into Chris's death at all. Furthermore, through a Freedom of Information Act request, Emily obtained copies of all VAERS reports for her daughter and discovered that Merck had submitted an unsubstantiated report that Chris had died from a viral infection. Merck had also recorded this misinformation about Chris's death on its Worldwide Adverse Experience System, a repository for safety information on Merck products. The Merck report was untrue.

Emily pursued Merck to ask where they had gotten their information. Merck claimed the report came from the gynecologist. Emily pursued this further and obtained written documentation that neither the gynecologist nor anyone in her office had ever reported to Merck that Chris's death was due to viral infection. Emily corresponded with Merck at length to withdraw the erroneous statement.

After several months, Merck submitted another VAERS report saying that "the mother says the death was not due to viral infection." Merck never admitted its statement was in error and unsubstantiated. To Emily's knowledge, Merck has never changed its entry on its own reporting system. Once a report is made to VAERS, it cannot be deleted, only supplemented. The original remains, but new material can be added. Therefore, Merck's initial false entry is still there and seemingly always will be.

Emily felt abandoned by the government officials who were supposed to investigate vaccine safety. The thought that her daughter's death would be dismissed as "unexplained" was unbearable. Just as these feelings swept over her, Emily learned that Judicial Watch was tracking post-Gardasil adverse events; they were interested in talking with her about Chris's case. Sinclair Broadcasting Group (David Sckrabulis and Toni Randle) interviewed Emily. She also learned of the National Vaccine Information Center (NVIC) and felt much-needed support from its cofounder, Barbara Loe Fisher. Other interviews followed, with NBC News (Lauren Dunn); the *New York Post* (Susan Edelman); an evening news special on WBAL-TV (Jane Miller); videos by Duty to Inform; documentaries by Gary Null, Joe Ferdman, and Channel 1 France; several radio interviews with Peter Tucker on Spectrum Today; and interviews for *Good Housekeeping* and *Newsweek* magazines. The latter two interviews and the French documentary were later denied publication and airing by their respective editors and producer. But Emily was grateful to those seeking the truth about Gardasil and who had the courage to share Chris's story.

Emily then joined NVIC as a volunteer director for Gardasil network development. In that capacity, Emily took phone calls and gathered information from mothers reporting serious adverse events following Gardasil vaccination. With one exception, she was astounded to find that the CDC and other authorities did not adequately investigate reported deaths. There was no standardized questionnaire or checklist of symptoms to compare pre- and postinoculation symptoms. Such a checklist would be particularly helpful with Gardasil. Because women received three consecutive shots over several months at that time, she could be her own baseline to see whether or not symptoms appeared or worsened after each inoculation. Emily suggested that NVIC create such a checklist and that they use the data for a study to explore a possible dose-response relationship after Gardasil. NVIC embraced the idea and created such a checklist. After hosting a major conference about HPV vaccines with expert speakers and working on the documentary *The Greater Good*, NVIC decided to turn its resources toward preserving vaccination choice rather than reporting on injuries from specific vaccines.

Wanting to continue to investigate Gardasil, Emily left NVIC and created her own website at www.gardasil-and-unexplained-deaths. com. She also later networked with Norma Erickson and Freda Birrell at SaneVax.org. A statistician and friend, Jim Garrett, had previously volunteered to analyze the data from the NVIC questionnaires. The analysis found a dose-response relationship for reports of chronic fatigue, headache, dizziness, joint/muscle pain or weakness, chest pain, skin disorders, heart disorders, problems concentrating, menstrual problems, and seizures. Emily posted the pilot survey on her website and wrote a letter to the CDC, imploring it to conduct a large-scale study. It was the first of several letters of concern Emily sent to the CDC. The rote responses were always that the CDC and FDA closely monitor safety and that "there is no evidence that the vaccine has been associated with any specific health outcome."

The symptoms from the survey results were consistent with those Chris had experienced. Emily now knew in her heart that Gardasil had caused Chris's death. Much remained to be explained, however, and Emily realized that the onus was on her to investigate her daughter's death. This was true for the other families of injured girls with whom she had spoken, as well. They began to network and share information, exchange autopsy reports, compare lot numbers, identify research, consult experts, find attorneys, and offer one another emotional support. Emily had thought that all vials of the vaccine had the same purity and content but learned that this is not true. The FDA allows a fairly wide range of acceptable contamination, so there was variability in the purity of different vaccine lots. Also, lot numbers change in different countries. Families compared lot numbers and found some in common. They reported these to the CDC but got no response.

There was a special bond among the six other mothers Emily knew that had, at about the same time, lost their daughters: Megan Hild, Jessica Ericzon, Santana Valdez, Amber Kaufman, Jenny Tetlock, and Annabelle Morin. Having learned they could not sue Merck directly, a group of families, including Emily's, initially filed cases in the VICP with the same law firm. But after a period of time, the firm decided not to represent Gardasil cases, leaving some families scrambling to find an attorney before the statute of limitations expired. Emily was fortunate to find attorney Mark Sadaka. Although Emily could have gone with more established firms, she went with her gut feeling. Sadaka Associates filed her petition in April 2010.

Emily felt great partnership with her attorney and the world-class immunologist Dr. Yehuda Shoenfeld and electrophysiologist and cardiologist Dr. Michael Eldar, who were able to testify in great detail about how Chris died. For over seven years, through ups and downs, they pushed forward with Chris's case. More about Chris's precedent-setting case is in Chapter 16.

In August 2009, the FDA and CDC published a postlicensure safety surveillance report on Gardasil.[7] This again spawned an upsurge of media interest. Videographers, reporters, and radio stations across the country interviewed Emily and others. Emily was skeptical of the CDC's claim of few serious adverse reports and 32 deaths. Following Chris's death, which had been the 23rd death reported, Emily read thousands of VAERS reports on www.wonder.cdc.gov/vaers; it certainly seemed that the incidence of serious injury reports from HPV vaccines was much higher than what CDC was asserting. Emily also found a discrepancy in the way that serious injuries were coded. She set about to test her hunch with a pilot study. She enlisted the expertise of fourteen volunteers, including doctors, university researchers, a statistician, and an attorney. The study took several years, in part because the participants did their work when time permitted, but it has been submitted for publication in 2018. Emily feels that the thousands of hours devoted to the project will have been time well spent if the study proves helpful to others.

There was another upsurge of media interest in Gardasil during the 2011 Republican Presidential debate between Rick Perry and Michele Bachmann. Bachmann criticized Perry for having signed an executive order for mandatory Gardasil vaccinations in Texas. Under pressure from constituents, Perry had to withdraw the mandate. During the debate, Bachmann reported the story of a mother whose daughter deteriorated cognitively after Gardasil, suggesting the vaccine had seriously injured the girl. Bachmann and the mother were ridiculed in the media for associating the vaccine with injury. Emily could identify with the feeling of being dismissed, attacked, belittled, and ignored, as happened when Emily testified against approval of Gardasil for boys at a National Vaccine Advisory Committee meeting or when she testified in DC against mandatory Gardasil vaccinations for school girls. The most vicious attacks, however, followed an episode of Katie Couric's TV show on Gardasil.

SaneVax invited Emily to participate as one of the guests to talk about Chris and her loss. The fallout in the media for suggesting that Gardasil can cause injury and death was brutal.

Troubled by the CDC's seeming indifference to reports of serious adverse events from Gardasil, Emily turned many times to her federal legislators, Senator Barbara Mikulski, Senator Ben Cardin, and Congressman Elijah Cummings, asking for a Congressional hearing. Sometimes other victims, activist groups, or scientists accompanied her. Legislators often promised follow-up, but nothing ever came of it. Emily's state legislators were more responsive. Along with state activist groups, Emily testified in several hearings, one of which succeeded in putting a consumer on the state vaccine advisory committee. She and others succeeded many times in preventing HPV vaccine mandates in Maryland. But Emily believes it will take a tsunami of public pressure to force Congress and state legislatures to adequately investigate HPV vaccines.

Emily is grateful to those who educate the public, advocate for truth and justice, and support people like her who have suffered an HPV vaccine-related tragedy. She has a website at www.gardasil -and-unexplained-deaths.com.

Norma wrote many other "Gardasil Girls" stories, about girls who survived, like Alexis, and girls who died, like Chris, and how their families struggled to find truth, justice, and healing. While there were striking similarities among the accounts, each one was as distinct as it was heart-wrenching. Each was the story of a normal girl who suffered catastrophic injury or death apparently from an HPV vaccine. Although causation wasn't clear, the girls seemed to get significantly worse with every dose. Neither the moms nor the doctors understood what was going on, but the HPV vaccine was the common denominator.

Norma felt compelled to learn more about how and why this was happening. She was in close touch with several activists who had been able to arrange a meeting with the FDA in March 2010 about the safety and efficacy of the two HPV vaccines then on the market, Gardasil and Cervarix.

THE MARCH 12, 2010, FDA WEBINAR ON GLOBAL PARENTAL CONCERNS ABOUT THE HPV VACCINES

After many parents and activists had been in touch with the FDA, it formally invited a group of parents and activists to make a presentation. The officials said that they wanted a "listening session" to better understand concerns. The FDA scheduled a webinar on March 12, 2010, to hear out six activists: Karen Maynor, mother of the late Megan Hild of New Mexico; Rosemary Mathis, whose daughter Lauren of North Carolina was injured; Freda Birrell, a political activist and lobbyist from Scotland; Leslie Carol Botha, a broadcast journalist from Colorado; Cynthia Janak, a research analyst from Illinois; and Janny Stokvis, a research analyst from the Netherlands.[8]

The group issued a press release about the meeting and then made a well-documented PowerPoint presentation to FDA representatives with hundreds of pages of research, data, and information on parental concerns.[9] They hoped to alert the FDA and the public to the terrible problems that had occurred in the four years since the HPV vaccines had been in wide use: there were credible reports of death, paralysis, seizures, blindness, infertility, amenorrhea, miscarriages, and more. They were dismayed that not only were authorities not questioning the vaccine's safety, but that in October 2009, the FDA approved its use in boys and young men ages 9 to 26.

The group's press release noted that VAERS already had reports of 64 deaths and over 17,500 reports of adverse events. The presenters noted similar reports of deaths and injuries from around the world. They had started a new website that said simply, "We have got to do something about this. These girls need our help!"[10]

The group represented a growing global community of parents, journalists, and researchers trying to help families desperate to understand what had happened.[11]

The 2010 presentation emphasized that the adverse effects were similar: seizures, heart problems, paralysis, menstrual changes, vision loss, joint aches, headaches, brain inflammation, and chronic fatigue. While acknowledging that cervical cancer is a serious health issue, particularly in low-resource countries, the presenters pointed to major gaps in the science for HPV vaccines.[12]

The activists' slides also analyzed VAERS information. They showed that, since Gardasil came on the market, the HPV vaccines were accounting for a disproportionate number of life-threatening injuries and emergency room visits compared to all other vaccines administered to girls and young women.[13] The presenters even provided insights into why certain types of girls—those who were athletic, overweight, or menstruating at the time of vaccination—seemed most likely to be injured.[14] The activists hypothesized that the connection to testosterone and other endocrine factors might be at play, especially during menstruation or if the child was overweight. Not only did they present information on the possible effect of the vaccine on the endocrine system, they went further, associating a possible link between the vaccine and reduced blood flow to the heart. The activists believed that young people around the world were at risk.[15] They sounded alarms to the FDA.

News of this meeting inspired Norma. The presenters had done an excellent job, and the FDA had heard them out. The activists hoped that the FDA would jump on this new information. The webinar cited many scientific studies. The women were confident that the FDA would investigate. Norma couldn't wait to hear the FDA's response and to write about it. Yet she waited and waited. While the FDA had appeared to listen, as the end of 2010 approached, more than nine months later, the FDA had not replied at all.

HPV VACCINE INJURY?

"The side effects of the vaccine are similar to those of other vaccines, and so the benefit vs. risk ratio is very high on the benefit side."[16]
Drs. Lowy and Schiller, LEONARD LOPATE RADIO SHOW

With over 270 million doses of HPV vaccines distributed in over 129 countries, and with the backing of medical organizations and governments around the world, few parents would worry that HPV vaccines are unsafe.[17] The world's leading health institutions give HPV vaccines glowing reports and reject HPV vaccine injury claims as "unfounded" and "psychogenic." They argue that the HPV clinical trials and monitoring of them after licensure have proven the vaccines safe and effective.

But hundreds of scientists and doctors around the world, unaffiliated with the pharmaceutical industry, believe that HPV vaccine injuries are real and devastating. They believe that governments should urgently reevaluate their recommendations for use. We review information below from multiple sources to assess HPV vaccine safety.

CDC

The CDC's website states "HPV Vaccine is Safe–(Gardasil)."[18] This webpage links to information for parents that states: "Prelicensure clinical trials and data collected after the vaccine was made available show that it is very safe."[19] The bulletin describes mild side effects, including pain at the injection site, fever, dizziness, nausea, and occasional fainting. It states: "CDC has carefully studied the risks of HPV vaccination. HPV vaccination is recommended because the benefits, such as prevention of cancer, far outweigh the risks of possible side effects."[20]

The CDC information bulletin then reviews several studies to prove Gardasil safety. The studies assert no association between Gardasil and anaphylaxis, Guillain-Barré Syndrome, stroke, blood clots, appendicitis, seizures, autoimmune conditions, or multiple sclerosis. The bulletin contains no reference to reported deaths.[21] It also carries the logos of the Department of Health and Human Services, the American Academy of Family Physicians, and the American Academy of Pediatrics, the main players in US children's healthcare. After reading this, most people would feel confident that the risks are minimal.

WHO

The World Health Organization, the most important global health organization, suggests the same safety profile. On December 17, 2015, the Global Advisory Committee on Vaccine Safety (Safety Committee) issued its most recent statement on HPV vaccine safety.[22] It reports that it has "not found any safety issue that would alter its recommendation for the use of the vaccine."[23] The Safety Committee referenced a large study in France of 2 million girls, suggesting no association between HPV vaccination and autoimmune conditions, except possibly an association with Guillain-Barré Syndrome, a disease that causes paralysis. That study suggested a small risk of 1 per 100,000 girls.[24]

The Safety Committee singled out Japan because Japan had suspended its proactive national health ministry recommendation for the HPV vaccine. (See Chapter 24.) It said that in Japan, "young women are being left vulnerable to HPV-related cancers that otherwise could be prevented. Policy decisions based on weak evidence, leading to lack of use of safe and effective vaccines, can result in real harm."[25] While the Safety Committee suggests that adverse event reporting is important, "[t]he greatest health benefit globally is anticipated in countries without routine cervical cancer screening, where the vaccine is yet to be introduced."[26]

The WHO issued a position paper on HPV vaccines in May 2017 to reinforce the Safety Committee's assessment.[27] It claims that "[d]ata from all sources continue to be reassuring regarding the safety profile of all 3 vaccines [i.e., Gardasil, Gardasil 9, and Cervarix]."[28] "In pre-licensure trials, no serious adverse events attributable to the vaccine were recorded for either the quadrivalent or bivalent vaccine."[29] On the issue of complex regional pain syndrome (CRPS) and postural orthostatic tachycardia syndrome (POTS), adverse events that are frequently reported, the WHO states that there is no evidence that they are a "direct effect of the HPV vaccines."[30] It concludes that "[a]ll 3 licensed HPV vaccines—bivalent, quadrivalent and nonavalent—have excellent safety, efficacy and effectiveness profiles."[31]

MEDICAL ASSOCIATIONS

In the United States, the overwhelming majority of medical associations recommend the HPV vaccine to preteens.[32] The American Academy of Pediatrics and the American Association of Family Physicians join with the CDC to recommend universal use. In 2017, the American College of Obstetricians and Gynecologists issued an official opinion, advising members to talk to women about getting the vaccine for themselves and their children. The opinion also recommends giving the HPV vaccine to lactating mothers and does not recommend screening for pregnancy, even though the package insert does not recommend the vaccine for pregnant women.[33]

The FDA pointed to this opinion letter to bolster its view that it is safe to give the HPV vaccine to women who might be positive for vaccine-targeted HPV types. In a letter to the authors, the FDA spokesman wrote:

> [not testing for HPV infection before vaccination is] consistent with the March 2017 recommendations and conclusions of the American College of Obstetricians and Gynecologists, which notes: Testing for HPV DNA is not recommended before vaccination. Vaccination is recommended even if the patient is tested for HPV DNA and the results are positive.[34]

As we discussed earlier, the clinical trials suggest that the vaccine will not be effective in those who test positive, and it may have "negative efficacy," i.e., enhance the risk of cervical lesions. Nonetheless, the international medical consensus stands behind the safety and efficacy of HPV vaccines.

SCIENTISTS' AND DOCTORS' VIEWS

Many scientists, too, recommend HPV vaccines as safe cancer prevention. In 2016, ten years after Gardasil's approval, Merck put out a press release based on a new meta-analysis, showing Gardasil's real-world effectiveness. The data from nine countries, which had introduced Gardasil vaccination, showed lower rates of genital warts and cervical abnormalities than if those same children had not received the vaccine. The press release acknowledged that there was no decrease in cervical cancer cases reported, as the children had not yet reached the age when cervical cancer typically occurs. The president of Merck Vaccines, Dr. Jacques Cholat, noted that "the full public health potential of HPV vaccination of males and females is not yet realized even after a decade of use."[35] The underlying article, written by an international team of scientists, had appeared two days earlier in *Clinical Infectious Diseases*.[36] The authors screened 903 articles in medical databases and selected 58 studies for analysis.[37] Although results varied by country, age of vaccination, and number of doses, they found decreases in genital warts, cervical abnormalities, and cervical lesions. The authors dismissed safety concerns, stating that "[u]nfounded notions about vaccine-related adverse experiences" have derailed HPV vaccination programs in some countries.[38] They recommend universal adoption of HPV vaccine programs to improve global public health.[39] Acknowledging that "no intervention is without some risk," they urge public health officials and caregivers to "counterbalance the *perceived* vaccine-safety concerns" against the weight of HPV-related cancers.[40] (Emphasis added.)

This study had fourteen coauthors, of whom nine were employed full-time by Merck or Sanofi Pasteur, Merck's former joint venture partner in Europe. The article points out that all the other authors have been Merck investigators, and many have even closer affiliations. The lead author, Dr. Garland, received funding to do HPV vaccine studies for Merck and GSK, fees for board membership on the Merck Global Advisory Board, and honoraria for being in its speakers bureau.[41] Three additional people who assisted with the literature review were also on Merck or Sanofi payrolls. Because of those authors' overt conflicts of interest, one cannot accept their conclusions uncritically.

Dr. Diane Harper also recently published a ten-year retrospective on HPV vaccines.[42] Unlike the authors above, Dr. Harper and her colleague listed no financial conflicts of interest, but they too saw population-based effectiveness of HPV vaccines. The takeaway from their retrospective, though, was that "vaccination does not replace screening. Prevention of cervical cancer must still rely on participation in ongoing screening programs."[43] Unfortunately, this study did not address safety at all.

FOCUS ON SAFETY

Scientists who focus on safety have a different perspective from those focusing on effectiveness. Perhaps the best overview of safety concerns about the HPV vaccines is a chapter in the groundbreaking 2015 textbook *Vaccines and Autoimmunity*, the result of decades of work in vaccinology, immunology, and autoimmunity. In its introduction, the editors, including Dr. Yehuda Shoenfeld, state that they are "quite confident that vaccinations represent one of the most remarkable revolutions in medicine."[44] Yet the book details the growing body of science on vaccine adverse reactions and injuries.

The textbook focuses first on the role of vaccine adjuvants in stimulating autoimmunity. It also looks at genetic factors, which may predispose some individuals to vaccine-induced autoimmune disorders. With contributions from over seventy scientists, the book analyzes the connections between vaccines, autoimmune conditions, narcolepsy, Type 1 diabetes, and other serious health problems. Scientists Lucija Tomljenovic and Christopher Shaw contributed a chapter on adverse reactions to HPV vaccines.[45] They acknowledge that cervical cancer is a serious disease that affects millions of women. But they understand HPV vaccine adverse events to be real and requiring serious analysis, as well. They examine reports to VAERS and case reports in the medical literature, documenting serious adverse events. The percentage of adverse events reported to VAERS from 2007 to 2013 for the HPV vaccine represented between 42 percent to 80 percent of adverse events for all vaccines administered to the same age group, i.e., females aged 9 to 29.[46] They observed the same unusually high frequency of adverse events related to HPV vaccines in similar reporting systems in Australia and worldwide.

One study analyzed VAERS adverse reports for Gardasil compared to the Menactra vaccine against meningitis, which is given to the same age group. Gardasil had 8.5 times more emergency room visits, 12.5 times more hospitalizations, 10 times more life-threatening events, and 26.5 times more disabilities than Menactra.[47] Tomljenovic and Shaw argue that this pattern of injury is "somewhat difficult to dismiss."[48]

Tomljenovic and Shaw note ways in which the scientists "gamed" the studies to avoid uncovering autoimmune reactions. The techniques employed to mask problems included: (1) making the population sample less susceptible to adverse reaction (participants had to have only one dose of Gardasil, and there was no notation of how many doses each participant had); (2) failing to include any immunologists or neurologists on the safety review committee to study adverse events; and (3) reporting only systemic autoimmune diseases, like multiple sclerosis, acute demyelinating encephalomyelitis, and Guillain-Barré Syndrome, but excluding typical short-term autoimmune symptoms, such as joint pain, fatigue, numbness, weakness, and cognitive disturbances, which can often lead to more serious autoimmune conditions.[49]

Tomljenovic and Shaw assert that HPV vaccines likely cause autoimmune disorders because of their strong immune-stimulating ingredients.[50] They conclude that HPV vaccines have a "troubling safety profile" and that the recommendations for HPV vaccines should "urgently and accurately [be] reassessed."[51] In their view, because healthy teenage girls face an almost zero percent risk of death from cervical cancer, it is completely unjustifiable that the vaccine carries any substantial risks, let alone a risk of death. Because cervical screening is still needed regardless of vaccination, and because the risk of death appears real, they conclude that the "risks from the vaccine . . . seem to significantly outweigh the as yet unproven long-term benefits."[52]

HPV VACCINE PACKAGE INSERTS

HPV vaccine package inserts, which doctors receive with the vaccine vials, also suggest real risks. In the United States, pharmaceutical companies are required to list reported adverse events, even if these reports have not been proven.[53] The package inserts, which doctors do not give out but which are available on the Internet, in fact provide a great deal of important information.[54]

The Gardasil insert states, "GARDASIL has not been evaluated for the potential to cause carcinogenicity or genotoxicity."[55] Similarly, the Cervarix package insert states, "CERVARIX has not been evaluated for its carcinogenic or mutagenic potential."[56] These are important disclosures: the vaccines sold as anticancer products might themselves cause cancer or genetic changes that could lead to cancer. The failure to investigate if vaccines may cause cancer is especially worrisome, as Gardasil's clinical trial data show that Gardasil may elevate a woman's risk of serious cervical lesions if she is already infected with HPV 16 or 18 when vaccinated.

The package inserts contain adverse events that people have reported, even if no causal link is clear. While reported events are by no means proof of causation, they are important information, especially as teenagers and young adults are among the healthiest people in any society. In Gardasil's long list of adverse events, buried between the relatively minor symptoms of "chills" and "fatigue," is death (emphasis added):

> Blood and lymphatic system disorders: Autoimmune hemolytic anemia, idiopathic thrombocytopenic purpura, lymphadenopathy. Respiratory, thoracic and mediastinal disorders: Pulmonary embolus. Gastrointestinal disorders: Nausea, pancreatitis, vomiting. General disorders and administration site conditions: Asthenia, chills, **death**, fatigue, malaise. Immune system disorders: Autoimmune diseases, hypersensitivity reactions including anaphylactic/anaphylactoid reactions, bronchospasm, and urticaria. Musculoskeletal and connective tissue disorders: Arthralgia, myalgia. Nervous system disorders: Acute disseminated encephalomyelitis, dizziness, Guillain-Barré syndrome, headache, motor neuron disease, paralysis, seizures, syncope (including syncope associated with tonicclonic movements and other

seizure-like activity) sometimes resulting in falling with injury, transverse myelitis. Infections and infestations: cellulitis.
Vascular disorders: Deep venous thrombosis.[57]

Cervarix's package insert contains a shorter list but includes disorders of the blood and lymphatic system, immune system, and nervous system. Notably, it does not list death, although deaths after
Cervarix have occurred.[58]

HPV Vaccine VAERS Reports 2006–2017

In 1986, Congress created VAERS under the 1986 National
Childhood Vaccine Injury Act, as a database for keeping track of
vaccine injuries. While it is far from perfect, it is the best repository of US vaccine injury information available. Below is information in VAERS (Wonder Database) as of May 2018 for injuries and
deaths following the HPV vaccine.[59] As of that date, there have been
57,620 reports including 420 deaths.[60]

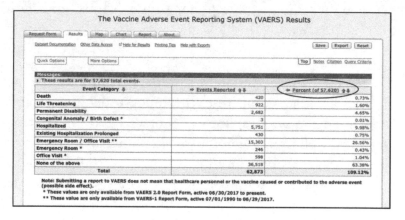

Source: CDC Wonder Database VAERS[61]

Individual Injuries

Accounts of HPV vaccine injury, like those below, have been
circulating since the HPV vaccine clinical trials. Norma and her

colleague Freda Birrell have been helping families since 2010, putting them in touch with other families and publishing injury accounts on the website for SaneVax, the advocacy organization they created. Every family's account is different, but collectively these stories convey the trauma families are living through.

EMMA AND JULIA: ONE FAMILY'S EXPERIENCE[62]

Emma, 21, has classic good looks: she's tall and athletic and has long, wavy blonde hair and blue eyes. Seeing her, one would never guess that she suffers from extremely disabling health conditions. Before going away to college in August 2014, Emma got a first Gardasil shot when she was 18. She got the HPV vaccine together with a hepatitis A vaccine based on her pediatrician's recommendation. Emma had been a competitive swimmer for twelve years and had been recruited to college. Ill health was not a concern, although she had been living with Type 1 diabetes since age five.

Emma had a wart on her knee, and the pediatrician suggested that the HPV vaccine would "help with the wart," as well as prevent cervical cancer. The pediatrician didn't warn Emma or her mother, Deborah, of any possible side effects, except that Emma might faint. This seemed odd to Emma, as she'd had many shots in the past and had never passed out nor thought the pain of a needle extreme. But immediately after getting the HPV vaccine, Emma lost consciousness and almost fell to the ground. Her blood pressure dropped precipitously, and she wasn't able to get up for twenty minutes. The doctor said this was normal, so she and her mom didn't think much of it.

Once Emma got to college, though, she couldn't sleep at night and had panic attacks, pounding heart episodes, and intense fatigue. Even going up the stairs was a struggle. Worst of all, Emma was retching 20–30 times per day. Oddly, even though she could barely hold down food, she had already gained fifteen pounds.

Emma came home for the summer after her freshman year, determined to lose weight. Over the summer, she worked as a lifeguard, jogged every day, and kept a strict diet of no sugar or gluten. Just as she was starting to feel better and getting ready to go back to school, Emma and her younger sister, Julia, went back to the pediatrician to get HPV shots. Not recognizing any link between Emma's condition and the vaccine, a year after her first shot, Emma got her second HPV shot and Julia got her first one in August 2015. They both received flu vaccines, as well.

The injections themselves were uneventful. But within 24 hours, Julia was convulsing on the floor, gasping for air, and was saying good-bye to her family as if she were dying. An ambulance rushed Julia to the emergency room. There, doctors tried to tell them that Julia's seizures were psychosomatic.

Deborah found the doctors' explanations ridiculous. As an oncology nurse and mother of four, Deborah was smart, confident, medically savvy, and not easily intimidated. There was no way Julia's seizures were in her head. Soon Julia was also suffering from throat infections, extremely painful menstrual periods, severe constipation, rapid heartbeats, and fainting incidents. In one incident, Julia was paralyzed from the waist down for 24 hours. These symptoms were hardly psychosomatic.

After several days with Julia in the hospital, Deborah started her own research. She wondered if perhaps Julia had caught something while on a trip to Nicaragua. All the tests for infectious diseases came back normal. Deborah then came upon literature about symptoms like Julia's right after Gardasil. Although in retrospect it seemed strange, it took Deborah a while to put together what was happening.

Deborah had worked at a major New York City hospital, so she started reaching out to doctors there to request literature on HPV vaccines. She started getting science: articles in journals like *Immunological Research, Lupus,* and *Vaccine.* By 2015, there was considerable scientific literature about adverse reactions. Despite this, doctors openly mocked Deborah for suggesting that Julia might be suffering an adverse vaccine reaction. Yet for the next eight months, Julia had at least one or two seizures a week.

At this point, Deborah still did not imagine that Julia's and Emma's severe health problems were related. But as soon as Emma got back to college, she called to say that her skin felt like it was burning, and she started retching 40–50 times a day, even more than freshman year. She was getting even more severe headaches, fatigue, anxiety, and pain. At first, Deborah simply imagined that Emma was really upset about her sister Julia's condition. Eventually, though, Deborah began to piece things together.

She realized that Emma's more severe symptoms began shortly after the second dose of Gardasil. She realized that there was a dose-response relationship in Emma's symptoms and that Julia's nearly fatal reaction happened within 24 hours of injection. The connections were becoming clear. Since recognizing that the girls suffered injury from the HPV vaccine, Deborah has done exhaustive research on the vaccine and recovery. She has been in touch with medical researchers around the world.

The vaccine affected Julia's heart. To evaluate her condition, she wore a heart monitor for 14 days. At times, her heart rate was over 200, even when she was sleeping. This was a serious risk, as a normal heart rate is between 60 and 100.[63] In the hospital, Deborah would watch the heart monitor as Julia's heart raced from 30 to 200 in seconds. Every time Julia would stand, she would get dizzy. Julia has been diagnosed with postural orthostatic tachycardia syndrome, or POTS, a disorder associated with HPV vaccines. Scientists in Japan have also reported on girls who suffer seizures like Julia's.

Deborah uncovered reports that premature ovarian failure is a side effect of HPV vaccination. She worried because Emma was having very painful menstrual periods, long stretches with no periods, and then nonstop bleeding. They went to gynecologists to do cervical screening, but bleeding was so heavy that they couldn't do a Pap test. Then the gynecologist did an ultrasound and found two large polyps, requiring immediate surgery. Emma's ovaries were not functioning properly.

Before Gardasil, Deborah had two healthy honor students—a recruited athlete and an opera singer. Although Emma had had diabetes from age five, she'd started her own foundation and traveled every year to Nicaragua to help kids with diabetes. The girls had no history of psychological disorders. These young women had their whole lives ahead of them, but serious health problems now cloud their futures. And part of the sadness is that their injuries are silent. The daughters are still beautiful and don't appear sick. But one moment they could be walking down the street and the next moment could be on the floor with a seizure or in the hospital because of bleeding or a throat infection.

Through her research, Deborah realizes that her daughters might have had genetic predispositions that made their HPV vaccine injuries more likely. Sadly, neither the manufacturer nor the pediatrician informed Deborah and her daughters that the vaccine might trigger them. In an interview, Deborah spoke at length. She said, "There is science out there linking these vaccines with genes and autoimmune responses. Why aren't they testing before they give something that may trigger a strong autoimmune response? We have new autoimmune disorders in these kids. They already have revved up immune systems, and then we give them an antigen with an adjuvant. And worst of all, no doctor will admit that this is what's happening. Doctors will say, 'Oh, well, that has never been proven.'

"It's a sin that these kids get hurt by something that the government recommends. The government doesn't say, 'Let's look at that, why did that happen to her? Let's prevent this from happening to anybody else.' Instead, they say, 'No, it didn't happen from that. No, no.'

"And then they look at the statistics, and say it's one in a million or one in a hundred thousand people. That's not enough to say the government isn't going to stop doing it anymore. But how do we know it's only one in a hundred thousand people, or one in fifty thousand, or one in a million, when no doctor will acknowledge that a vaccine has injured anyone?

"If your kid was injured, then as a parent you start to meet other parents of kids that were injured. I've been made fun of by doctors who say, 'Oh, what did you find, a blog on the Internet that made you think that your kid was affected?' I say, 'No, actually I found peer-reviewed, scientific literature discussing symptoms that are identical to my daughters.' And I've seen videos of people from across the world with the same exact seizures and arrhythmias that

Julia had 24 hours after Gardasil. I don't even know these people, or know anything about them, but we have videos of our kids, yet we are all being told that our kids have psychogenic issues.

"There's something wrong with the whole system—the system in which the government and doctors are pressuring you to take a vaccine when it's well established that there is a potential risk of harm. That's why Congress created the National Vaccine Injury Compensation Program. But no doctor will ever admit that there's been a vaccine injury, and doctors don't really know how to help once there is one. And then once you prove to doctors that you have facts, they won't look at them. They tell you that you're crazy, your child is crazy, it's a conversion disorder and a thousand other things. But don't let anyone snow you."

Deborah is an inspiration to other parents fighting for their children's health after HPV vaccine injury. She continues her research and also moderates social media groups, so that families can connect and help one another.

JOEL GOMEZ

Joel Gomez was a healthy 14-year-old boy who died in his sleep on August 20, 2013, the day after receiving his second dose of Gardasil.[64] Joel was training for his high school football team, playing four to five hours per day for the two months before he died. He had visited his pediatrician regularly since birth with no evidence of any preexisting health issues, including cardiac abnormalities, psychological problems, or substance abuse. He received the first dose of the vaccine on June 19, 2013, with no adverse reactions. On August 19, 2013, he received the second injection at the doctor's office. On August 20, 2013, his family found him dead in his bed.

The Los Angeles medical examiner's office performed an autopsy on August 23, 2013. They opined that Joel had died of myocarditis, or heart attack, of unknown cause. Joel Gomez's family filed a compensation claim for his death in the National Vaccine Injury Compensation Program. Their counsel retained Dr. Sin Hang Lee, a pathologist, as an expert. Dr. Lee's expert report, written following his examination of the evidence and the scientific literature, found that that Gardasil caused Joel's death. Dr. Lee had already published several articles on HPV vaccine injuries, as we discuss later in Chapter 19.

After examining three slides from the coroner, Dr. Lee explained why he disagreed with the coroner's theory of a heart attack of unknown cause. He concluded that "[t]he only plausible mechanism causing the sudden unexpected death of this teenager is the physiopathologic events induced by injection of the second dose of Gardasil."[65] Because Joel had not taken any other drugs or suffered any other injuries, "the only known factor that might cause his death on August 19, 2013, is the second Gardasil injection given to him shortly before he went home and went to sleep."[66]

Special Masters, the acting judges in the compensation program, often criticize petitioners' experts and give their reports little weight. But that was not the case here. Special Master Millman called Dr. Lee's report "extremely thorough and well written."[67] While HHS did not fully concede that Gardasil caused Joel's death, it settled the case, awarding the Gomez family $200,000 in damages,[68] while the maximum amount when someone has died is $250,000. One can draw the inference that HHS believed Joel's family deserved compensation, even though the Joint Stipulation states that it "shall not be construed as an admission . . . that Joel's death, or any other injury, was caused by his HPV vaccinations."[69]

Joel's death was tragic. There were no signs that Joel might die from his second dose. He was healthy, athletic, and showed no obvious adverse reaction after the first dose. Based on his report, Dr. Lee explained that "[t]eenagers vaccinated with Gardasil should stay away from competitive sports such as football for at least two months, and should have an electrocardiogram to rule out silent myocardial infarction if there is any incidence of syncope, chest discomfort, tachycardia, or hypotension within two months after Gardasil vaccination."[70] In other words, vaccination with Gardasil is a serious medical intervention that requires close monitoring and restriction of athletic activities.

MADDIE MOORMAN: A LIFE ENDED AT 21

"Sometimes I can't believe she's gone. If not for Gardasil, none of this would have happened."[71] *Tracie Moorman, Maddie's Mother*

Maddie was a typical fifteen-year-old high schooler. She was a great student and she loved more than anything to play the guitar and hang out with friends. Aside from problems with irregular menstrual cycles, she was very healthy. Her pediatrician recommended Gardasil on numerous visits, but Tracie was hesitant. When she brought Maddie to her gynecologist for a second opinion on Maddie's menstrual cycle problems, it came up again. The gynecologist told Tracie that it was a vaccine to prevent cervical cancer and Maddie was due to get it. Tracie finally consented to Maddie getting the vaccine, a decision she deeply regrets.

After the first dose, Maddie had symptoms immediately, although Tracie wasn't sure they were related to the vaccine because the gynecologist had also prescribed a drug at the same time. Maddie continued to feel poorly, but, for the most part, she was able to go to school and seemed OK.

In April 2012, after Maddie received the second dose, she was bedridden for five days, almost unable to talk. She said, "Something is happening to my brain." She complained that she couldn't think or read, even though she was a topflight student with a photographic memory. She had excruciating migraine headaches every day. She missed more than a half year of school and had to get a home tutor. Exhaustion took over, even though she slept as much as fourteen hours a night but never felt rested.

As the time for the third dose approached, Tracie and her husband began to research the vaccine and if it could be the reason Maddie was so ill. After preparing a timeline of the two HPV vaccinations and when Maddie's symptoms began, the connection became clear. Tracie and her husband explained their conclusions to the pediatrician, who dismissed Maddie's reactions as coincidental. The gynecologist's office also warned Tracie against forgoing the third dose, admonishing that the insurance company then might not reimburse the first and second doses. Nonetheless, they refused the third dose.

By September 2012, Maddie and her mother had seen a succession of physicians to try to recover her health. They saw a neurologist, psychiatrist, gynecologist, allergist, pediatrician, ENT doctor, and even an ophthalmologist. They received prescriptions for all kinds of drugs. None of them seemed to help.

Finally, they found a chiropractic internist who did offer some hope. Maddie started taking nutritional supplements and went on a very strict hypoallergenic, organic diet. They also pursued a number of detoxification protocols. Although Maddie was homebound for most of her junior year in high school, she was able to complete her senior year at school and graduated. Tracie was beginning to feel hopeful that her daughter was getting better.

Tracie was extremely grateful, even though her daughter continued to suffer from anxiety and had to limit stress. Filing a claim in the vaccine injury compensation program was important to Tracie, because to not do so was almost collusion. So they did file a claim, even though they knew the process took many years. In the meantime, Tracie and Maddie helped other families suffering from HPV vaccine injury who looked to them for guidance from Maddie's recovery.

Maddie entered the University of Kansas in 2014 on a scholarship that she maintained for three years. She had many interests, including psychology, gender studies, music, and Spanish. She ultimately settled on Spanish as her major and opted to spend the second semester of her junior year in Salamanca, Spain. She traveled to Spain in January 2017 and had a wonderful time there, even saying that she did not want to return home. But she did come back in early May 2017. Sadly, shortly after returning home, Maddie died on June 24, 2017. She had taken her own life, which was an enormous shock to her friends and family.

After her death, Tracie looked at Maddie's recent college notebooks. Although most of the pages were in Spanish, they were interspersed with journal entries in English about how Maddie's brain "buzzed." She wrote about her brain injury and suicidal thoughts.

She wrote that she was never able to stop the constant buzzing sound in her head since the vaccine. Tracie was learning all this for the first time.

To her mom, Maddie was an incredible girl, wise beyond her years. Tracie can't stop herself from asking, "what if, what if, what if . . ." Tracie remains in disbelief that what happened to Maddie can happen in this country. She consoles herself daily with her personal ode to Maddie: "Fiercely loved. Forever free. Maddie Marie."

COLTON BERRETT: GONE TOO SOON

"We mourned with my son . . . we mourned every teenage event that didn't happen."[72] *Kathleen Berrett, Colton's mother*

Any parent would be proud to have Colton Berrett as a son. He was always smiling. An exuberant, friendly, and popular teen, he was quick with a joke. The Church of Jesus Christ of Latter-day Saints was a big part of Colton's life. His family was everything to Colton: his mom, Kathleen; a dad, Rob; his younger brother, Gavin; and his younger sister, Kaitlyn. She and Colton had a special bond. When she was born, he was seven and would help Kathleen take care of her. Always the helper in the family, Colton wanted to make everyone happy.

Strong, athletic, and an avid outdoorsman, Colton camped, skied, swam, road mountain bikes, hiked, and played basketball and other sports. When he was six, he learned to ride a motocross bike and got his first full-size bike for Christmas. Motocross was a family sport; Colton inherited his passion for it from his parents. Sports and the outdoors were an integral part of growing up in the Berrett household, whether participating or watching favorite teams play.

At thirteen, Colton was healthy; he was growing and becoming a typical teenager. On February 1, 2014, just before his fourteenth birthday, Colton received his third dose of Gardasil. The injection site hurt a lot, and Colton felt like he had a fever in his arm, but he seemed all right after a while. Two weeks later, it was a different story. On Saturday, February 15th, Rob took Colton for his first ride on his new motocross bike. Colton was excited, but his neck had begun to hurt the day before. On the 15th, it felt worse; Colton was very tired. They had the best day they could; Colton was a natural on the bike. Looking back at a photo from that day, Kathleen can see that Colton was not himself. "He looked droopy. Not like the hyper and happy kid he was."

When Colton got home that day, he immediately crashed on his bed, dirty clothes and all, too tired to even shower. He felt nauseated, exhausted, and weak. He had a fever; it seemed like he was coming down with the flu. By Sunday, he didn't want to get out of bed. His head ached, and his neck hurt even more. The right side of his body was weakening. Dizziness set in, and he could barely lift his head. Kathleen worried about meningitis, but the symptoms didn't quite fit. She gave him bread, ibuprofen, and tried to keep him hydrated.

Monday Feb. 17, 2014, was Presidents' Day, a school holiday, and Colton was supposed to go skiing with his best friend. Instead, as his condition deteriorated, Rob had to hold Colton's head for him to walk to the car to go to an urgent care center. The urgent care staff immediately called an ambulance to transport Colton to Primary Children's Hospital in Salt Lake City. The weakness was now paralysis, slowly progressing from his neck all the way down to his toes. With fear on his face, Colton told Rob, "Dad, I don't want to be paralyzed!" Rob was scared too but tried to stay strong for Colton. As the medical team at Primary Children's ran tests, the doctor asked if Colton had been sick in the past few weeks, asking particularly about any viruses or infections. When Kathleen mentioned that Colton had received Gardasil on February 1, the doctor appeared concerned and said he would make a report to VAERS. The doctor explained VAERS to Kathleen and told her that because of the timing of Colton's symptoms with his vaccination, he had to make a report. She was taken aback. Colton's primary care doctor had told the Berretts that Gardasil was safe.

The medical team at Primary Children's diagnosed Colton with transverse myelitis, from c-1 (the top of the spine) to the cauda equina (near the lower end of the spinal cord). This inflammation of the spinal cord interrupted the signals that the spinal cord nerves send through the body and caused his paralysis. Even though he had to be intubated and was on a ventilator, he could answer yes/no questions with his left hand—until the spreading paralysis took away that way of communicating. Always resourceful, Colton then used his eyebrows to answer questions. After four more days, he was completely paralyzed. Eleven days after he was admitted, doctors performed a tracheotomy. Colton remained on a ventilator for the rest of his life.

He was in the hospital for a total of 88 days; his daily routine was grueling. Because of his paralysis, Colton went to occupational, speech, and physical therapies. The hardest, though, was respiratory-assisted "cough" therapy. Due to his paralyzed diaphragm, Colton couldn't clear mucous on his own. A respiratory therapist had to treat him every few hours to keep his airways clear to prevent pneumonia. It was painful; Colton hated it. His parents were trained to do the cough assist, as well. When Colton went home, they and his nurses continued this treatment several times a day.

Colton's doctors and parents were honest with him about the diagnosis and prognosis: about a third of transverse myelitis patients have a full or close to complete recovery; a third regain some function; but the final third don't progress much, if at all. Kathleen and Rob remained positive. Kathleen kept hoping that at the end of his hospital stay, a recovered Colton would come home. No one wanted to think that such a young, vibrant boy might not recover.

With perseverance, Colton beat many of the odds. After only a couple of months in the hospital, he was taking a few steps. After several more months at home, with intensive outpatient therapy, he regained use of his legs and the lower half of his left arm and hand. He even learned to write adeptly with his left hand. He wore a brace to support his head, neck, and upper torso, with a sling attached for his right arm to rest in. His family offered tremendous support, helping with his care and taking him to therapy. His friends, especially his best friend Josh, were there for him, too.

Colton missed the active life he had before Gardasil and was frustrated to need round-the-clock care from his parents and nurses, without the privacy and independence teens crave. This was not the life Colton had envisioned, but he was determined to keep a positive attitude and recover as much as possible. His parents did everything they could to keep him engaged in some of the activities he loved. He got a recumbent trike with adapted controls. The trike allowed him to be in a safe, reclined position and with a basket behind the seat for his ventilator. On nice days, he could go a few miles. The family continued taking many camping trips but now needed to run a generator at night to power Colton's equipment. They even got a Polaris RZR UTV (utility task vehicle) that Colton could operate off-road on sand dunes, in the mountains, and in the desert in Utah and Idaho. He participated in adaptive skiing using a sit-ski, sailed an adaptive boat on a lake, and rode horses. But it wasn't the same. He missed not being able to fully use his body and be in control. Colton hated the constant stares in public, as well as having someone with him all the time to carry his ventilator.

Colton received Gardasil because he and his parents were told it would prevent his future wife from getting cervical cancer. Now Colton believed that his dream of having a wife and family would never happen. Despite the fact that he was a popular, handsome young man, he didn't think girls would want to date him. Realizing he couldn't go on a Church mission like his friends was another harsh blow. Even when he became a high school senior, in the 2017–18 school year, going to college seemed like an unattainable dream.

Colton maintained a happy demeanor for the world, but his parents now realize he was struggling with the uncertainty of his future. When surgery to implant a device to help him breathe without his vent didn't work, he was devastated. He had been so hopeful about leaving behind the heavy, cumbersome ventilator that he relied on 24/7. He was so determined, despite his physical dependency, not to be a burden. Often he apologized to his parents that they had to care for him. They reassured him that they loved him and were there for him no matter what and that he was never a burden.

On January 5, 2018, almost four years after Colton received the Gardasil vaccine, once again tragedy turned the Berretts' lives upside down. That night was a rare time when Colton was alone. Rob and Gavin went to ride motocross, Kathleen and Kaitlyn went to a movie, and his nurse was given the night off. Colton wanted to watch a movie at home; nothing seemed out of the ordinary. Colton could now be alone for short periods of time, and his parents wanted him to have some independence and privacy like other 17-year-olds.

When the Berretts returned home a few hours later, Colton wasn't in his chair. At first, they thought he might have been teasing them, hiding quietly in a closet waiting to be found. As they continued to rush to find Colton, something felt wrong. Feeling helpless and dependent, he took his own life. He had been the helper to others his whole life before his paralysis. Kathleen and Rob believe Gardasil first took Colton's physical health and then ultimately his life. He was just two months away from his 18th birthday and about to graduate high school, a huge accomplishment he worked so hard for with all his challenges.

His family's faith and the outpouring from those who knew Colton personally or had read his story on social media have been a great solace to them. They continue to share his story, and his legacy continues to inspire. Echoing the words of a popular song his best friend played at his funeral, Colton truly walked through Hell with a smile!

Most people want to base their views about HPV vaccines on the science, but the science today is inconclusive. There are studies that allegedly both prove and disprove safety and effectiveness. Unquestionably, the preeminent medical bodies of the day—the WHO, CDC, FDA, EMA—consider the vaccine safe.

But who has the most at stake? Who has the greater conflicts of interest? What do children and families have to gain from asserting

HPV vaccine injury? Wealth? Fame? Prestige? Hardly. Indeed, families who have suffered injuries or death usually suffer further trauma from the institutions and doctors that consider their pain "psychogenic." Society often shames and silences them as "antivaccine."

By contrast, industry, government, and medicine have a great deal to gain in defending HPV vaccine safety. They have wealth, fame, credibility, and prestige on the line. And more. Some in industry, government, science, and medicine may have more than "gamed" the system; they may have lied to regulators, falsified data, intentionally misrepresented facts, and failed to disclose material information to human subjects, investors, and consumers. If this is so, they may be looking at civil and even criminal liability.

16.

SEEKING JUSTICE

THE PROMISE OF VACCINES

Although controversial, vaccines have played a prominent role in Western public health for almost three hundred years, since Edward Jenner started vaccinating against smallpox in England in the eighteenth century. Most vaccines are injections given to healthy people to protect against infectious diseases. The injections typically contain a weakened form of the disease-causing agent, usually a virus or bacterium, as well as other biological and inorganic materials.

In the 1950s and 1960s, universal vaccination against many childhood infectious diseases—including measles, mumps, and rubella—became routine. By the 1970s, vaccines had become standard pediatric medicine. The situation started to change somewhat in the 1980s. Most children in the US by then were receiving vaccines against seven different diseases—polio, diphtheria, tetanus, pertussis, measles, mumps, rubella—and some children were suffering severe injury and death as a result. Families began suing doctors and manufacturers for catastrophic vaccine injuries based on legal theories of failure to warn, unreasonably unsafe products, and negligence. Most plaintiffs were unsuccessful, because proving causation of injury is extremely difficult. When plaintiffs did succeed, however, defendants had to pay substantial damage awards—sometimes in the millions of dollars.[1]

Representatives of industry and healthcare became concerned about liability and insurance costs. Corporations threatened to stop producing vaccines unless the government agreed to help. Congress stepped in to try to resolve the problems between vaccine producers, healthcare providers, the federal government, and injured families.

In 1986, Congress passed the National Childhood Vaccine Injury Act, intending to achieve three goals: (1) ensure a stable vaccine supply; (2) compensate those injured; and (3) improve vaccine safety. The 1986 Act made it impossible to sue vaccine manufacturers or healthcare providers for vaccine injury without first filing in a federal compensation program. About two-thirds of all claims in the compensation program lose, and only 0.5 percent then file claims in ordinary courts.[2] Although intended to be simple and quick, the compensation program is complex, slow, and extremely adversarial.

Congress intended for the 1986 Act to make vaccines safer. Many, including vaccine inventor Jonas Salk, thought that giving liability protection to industry would diminish its incentives to make vaccines safer.[3] If an injured victim can't sue a corporation for harm from its product, why make it safer? Litigation risk has always been a spur to product innovation and safety. Removing this element was a radical change. This extraordinary liability protection for vaccines, considered biologics, is completely different from that of drugs. Litigation has led to major changes and recalls of many drugs, including several by Merck and GSK, the HPV vaccine manufacturers.

Only a small fraction, less than 1 percent of the total federal vaccine budget, goes toward vaccine safety research.[4] While manufacturers have to go through lengthy processes for vaccine government approval and recommendation, there is little required safety surveillance after the initial licensure. And manufacturers themselves oversee most, if not all, of that safety monitoring.

Once Congress passed the 1986 Act, manufacturers had real financial incentives to add vaccines to the federally recommended childhood vaccine schedule. While seven vaccines were federally recommended in 1986, the CDC now recommends 69 doses of 16 vaccines to children up to age 18, vastly increasing the number of vaccines and doses they receive.[5] Whereas vaccines were a low-margin medical product in 1986, profit margins are now in double digits. The market value of childhood vaccines in the US is approximately $17.4 billion in 2018.[6] Vaccines moved from being liability-laden, backwater products in 1986 to now being almost liability-free, lucrative biologics at center stage, with over 260 vaccines in development.[7] No vaccine better exemplifies this transformation than the HPV vaccine.

COMPENSATING HPV INJURIES

Most Americans do not know about the court that exclusively hears cases on vaccine injury. If you suffer a vaccine injury or death in the US from a vaccine that ACIP recommends, then you cannot directly sue a pharmaceutical company or doctor. Under the 1986 law, you must first sue in the Compensation Program. Ninety-nine percent of petitioners do not elect to pursue claims in civil court after having litigated there. Because petitioners believe that further litigation will likely be expensive and futile, they end their legal journey. So for 99.5 percent of those injured by vaccines, the Compensation Program is the only way to seek legal justice.

The first step in the process is to file a claim in the Compensation Program against the Department of Health and Human Services within three years of the first symptoms from the injury, not three years from when you connected the symptoms to the vaccine. The statute of limitations trips up most would-be petitioners who learn about the Compensation Program only after three years have elapsed.

Department of Justice lawyers represent HHS, which is the defendant in all cases. The manufacturers and doctors don't have to show up at all. Congress passed the 1986 Act to shield industry and doctors from liability, but also to ensure compensation in the event of injury.[8] The program was supposed to be no-fault so that families could receive compensation "quickly, easily, and with certainty and generosity."[9] But Congress left the door open so that individuals might be able to sue later in civil court.[10]

Congress created a "Table of Injuries" as part of the Compensation Program, listing injuries that would presumptively lead to compensation. If an individual suffered a "Table Injury," then the person would be able to make that case simply, and HHS would be obliged to pay compensation unless HHS could prove a more likely cause of injury. The Secretary of HHS, charged with keeping the Table updated, has added a handful of presumptive injuries since 1995.[11]

Today, over 98 percent of all cases in the Compensation Program are "off-Table," meaning that petitioners have to prove that the vaccine caused the injury by a standard of "more likely than not."[12] Petitioners must provide medical and scientific evidence to meet this standard. And proving causation for any medical injury is very difficult. It is even harder in the compensation program, where petitioners are not entitled to discovery from the manufacturer.

Human biology is complex. How vaccines affect the body is poorly understood. This is especially so for the HPV vaccine. Scientists themselves acknowledge that its mechanism to induce immunity is not clear. The WHO's most recent position paper states that "[t]he mechanism of protection conferred by HPV vaccines is *assumed,* on the basis of data from *animal models* to be mediated by . . . antibodies against the major viral coat protein, L1."[13] (Emphasis added.) In other words, WHO scientists do not understand how the vaccine works; they rely on assumptions. So to ask vaccine victims to "prove causation" when so little is clear is a tall order indeed.

According to one legal scholar, either the HHS Secretary should have amended the Table to add new injuries associated with the vaccine or should have removed Gardasil from the Table, thus permitting victims to sue the manufacturers directly in civil court. Under either of these scenarios, victims might have gotten a fair shot at compensation. As neither route has been available, however, HPV vaccine victims have been at a particular disadvantage because of this byzantine legal regime.[14]

To gain compensation in an off-Table claim, a petitioner must establish three criteria: (1) close timing between the vaccine and injury; (2) a credible medical theory about how the injury or death occurred; and (3) a logical sequence of events related to that theory.[15] Although this may sound like an easy threshold to meet, it's not. About two-thirds of all petitioners lose. Objective observers find the program to be slow, cumbersome, and highly adversarial.

A 2014 Government Accounting Office report, which followed two other government-commissioned studies of the program, confirms these impressions.[16] Perhaps the primary benefit of the Program to petitioners in off-Table cases is that they do not have to pay their own attorneys' fees. The Special Masters award attorneys' fees after the case out of federal funds.

The Court of Federal Claims appoints Special Masters to hear cases of vaccine injury in the Compensation Program and to make factual findings about whether the vaccine likely caused the injury. Almost all Special Masters are former government attorneys who previously worked in the military, the Department of Justice, or another federal agency.[17] The Special Masters serve four-year terms; even the Court of Federal Claims judges serve only fifteen-year terms.[18] Because of their relatively insecure positions and prior work histories, many petitioners question their impartiality.

As of early 2018, there have been 280 cases filed in the Compensation Program for HPV vaccine injury, and 156 cases have been dismissed.[19] When petitioners receive compensation, it is usually pursuant to a "joint stipulation," where HHS does not agree that the injury is the result of the vaccine but is willing to settle. Most people infer some level of responsibility when HHS agrees to pay substantial compensation, but the settlement agreement nonetheless specifies that the award implies no liability. To date, the Compensation Program has only entered a verdict in one case that an HPV vaccine caused death, and that's in the case of Chris Tarsell that we discussed above in Chapter 15.

Judicial Watch, a nonprofit organization, researched HPV vaccine injury awards in the Compensation Program. In 2013, they found that the Program had already paid out $5.9 million in awards and annuities to 49 HPV vaccine victims.[20] Judicial Watch's president said, "Public health officials should stop pushing Gardasil on children."[21]

A handful of compensation decisions for HPV vaccine victims from the US Vaccine Injury Compensation Program are below. Some of the compensation amounts are "proffers," which HHS offered, or "joint stipulations," when the parties settled without complete adjudication. The judgment in Chris Tarsell's case was a verdict by a VICP Special Master. Her case regarding death from HPV vaccination lasted eight years, but the Special Master ultimately ruled that Gardasil more likely than not caused Christina's arrhythmia leading to her death.

The vast majority of HPV vaccine injury claims receive no compensation for failure to prove causation. Those compensation amounts included below are among the largest ones to date, suggesting that the VICP has acknowledged significant evidence of HPV vaccine harm. These awards also give some sense of the wide range of injuries that have occurred.

Decisions from the US National Vaccine Injury Compensation Program for Injuries and Deaths from HPV Vaccination

Petitioner	Year	Medical Condition	Type of Compensation	Compensation
D. Angell	2016	Seborrheic dermatitis	joint stipulation	$225,000
Rosalinda Cruz	2013	Limbic encephalitis	joint stipulation	$200,000
Shermian Daniel, MD	2016	Multiple sclerosis (MS), Aggravated acute demyelinating encephalomyelitis (ADEM)	joint stipulation	$350,000
Cory Danielson	2016	Pancreatitis	joint stipulation	$95,000
Bailey Day	2017	Neuromyelitis optica	proffer	$1.53 million

Angela Disanto	2015	Encephalitis	joint stipulation	$135,000
Jane Doe 89	2010	MS	joint stipulation	$500,000
Jessica Ericzon	2015	**Death**	joint stipulation	$200,000
Joel Gomez	2016	**Death**	joint stipulation	$200,000
V. Huerta	2014	Complex Regional Pain Syndrome	proffer	$162,000
Susan Ibarra	2011	**Death**	joint stipulation	$240,000
Brittney LeClair	2011	ADEM, Transverse Myelitis	joint stipulation	$150,000
Kevin Lopez	2012	ADEM, Guillain-Barré syndrome (GBS)	joint stipulation	$1.23 mil.
A. McCulloch	2016	Limbic encephalitis	proffer	$1.47 mil.
Megan Morgan	2016	Ulcerative colitis	proffer	$800,000
A. Olund	2014	GBS	joint stipulation	$185,000
Amanda Ratner	2013	Macrophagic myofasciitis	joint stipulation	$350,000
Sherry Salmins	2015	GBS	proffer	$1.4 mil.
Karen Stark	2013	Syncope, head trauma	joint stipulation	$175,000
Christina Tarsell	2017	**Death**	adjudicated concession of the maximum death award	$250,000

The chart above paints one picture; individual accounts provide another.

EMILY TARSELL'S SEARCH FOR JUSTICE

After Emily Tarsell reported her daughter Chris's death to VAERS, she retained attorney Mark Sadaka to file Chris's case in the VICP. He in turn hired two world-class experts, Dr. Yehuda Shoenfeld and Dr. Michael Eldar. Their expertise spanned immunology, cardiology, and electrophysiology. It took more than four years from the time Emily filed the petition in April 2010 until the hearing occurred November 13–14, 2014. There was no jury or judge in robes. The only people present at the hearing were the attorneys for Emily and HHS, their respective experts, the Special Master in plain clothes, and Emily.

Experts on both sides agreed that Christina died from an arrhythmia. In a day and a half of testimony, Emily's experts explained the mechanism by which Gardasil could have caused the fatal arrhythmia by molecular mimicry at the cellular level. Because of this mimicry, the HPV 16 L1 protein that Chris's immune system produced after vaccination targeted not only the HPV virus, but also her own proteins that shared structural similarities. In Chris's case, the L1 protein shared structural similarities with the L-type calcium channel receptor in her cells. Thus autoantibodies bound to the L-Type calcium channel receptors caused them to dysfunction and fail to regulate the influx of calcium into her heart cells. Increased concentrations of calcium in Chris's heart cells caused premature ventricular contractions, triggering a fatal arrhythmia. Emily's lawyers filed peer-reviewed scientific articles to support their experts' testimony and exhaustive documentation about Chris's medical history. HHS's experts challenged Emily's experts but failed to offer any alternative explanation for Chris's death.

SPECIAL MASTER MORAN'S FEBRUARY 2016 RULING[22]

After waiting a year and four months after the hearing, Emily received word in February 2016 that Special Master Christian J. Moran denied compensation. First, he challenged that Chris's arrhythmia started after the first HPV shot. He opined that the arrhythmia might have started earlier, although there was no evidence for such an inference. To the contrary, medical records showed that Chris had no observed heart problems over the six years before her HPV shots. Emily had six exhibits from doctor visits where Chris's heart rate was normal. In addition, electrocardiograms taken three months after Chris's first injection and one month after her second injection showed a wave pattern characteristic of premature ventricular contractions for the first time. Such premature beats are capable of triggering fatal arrhythmias. Despite no evidence of a preexisting heart condition and documentation of initial symptoms after Gardasil vaccinations, Special Master Moran inferred that Chris's condition might have been preexisting, so he considered that there was insufficient proof that the vaccine caused the arrhythmia.

Next, Special Master Moran gave no credence to Emily's experts' theory that Chris developed an autoimmune disorder from the HPV shots, causing Chris's own antibodies to attack the calcium channel of her heart and leading to its dysfunction and fatal arrhythmia. He challenged the authority of the four peer-reviewed scientific articles Emily's experts introduced by Dr. Darja Kanduc, explaining the theorized mechanism of injury. He also put great store by the CDC autopsy report of Chris's heart tissue, which stated that there were no "conspicuous inflammatory cell infiltrates," even though experts on both sides acknowledged that this indicator was not particularly meaningful. The Special Master acknowledged that Chris's case could suggest a possible dose-response or challenge-rechallenge sequence with declining health after each dose, culminating in death after the third dose. But he rejected the challenge-rechallenge theory, arguing that Emily's lawyers had not proved it sufficiently.

The Department of Justice attorneys relied on epidemiological studies to rebut Emily's evidence. In essence, they argued that because millions of Gardasil shots had been given, and they did not find an increased rate of sudden death following HPV vaccination, Chris's death from one of those doses was implausible. HHS offered no alternative explanation, but the law does not require them to do so unless a petitioner asserts a presumptive injury or has proved, by a preponderance of the evidence, that the vaccine caused the petitioner's injury. Because no serious HPV vaccine injuries are on-Table and because the Special Master did not accept that Emily had met her burden, the government did not have to prove causation. The case tested only Emily's claim.

Special Master Moran stated that he was not requiring scientific certainty, but merely a more-likely-than-not standard. He concluded, "[w]e do not know the reason why apparently healthy young people die, and, in the context of Ms. Tarsell's claim in the Vaccine Program, the Secretary [of HHS] does not bear the burden of supplying a reason for Christina's senseless death."[23]

Emily and her lawyers believed that Special Master Moran had not applied the required legal standard fairly. They appealed his decision to the Court of Federal Claims, which hears appeals from the Compensation Program, arguing that the Special Master had ignored key evidence, distorted petitioner's theory of causation, misread Chris's records, made unsupported factual inferences, and thus had decided the case in an arbitrary and capricious manner that violated the law.

THE DECISION VACATING THE SPECIAL MASTER'S DECISION[24]

Over a year later, Emily received a decision from the Court of Federal Claims. Judge Mary Ellen Coster Williams vacated Special Master Moran's decision and sent the case back to him for reconsideration in keeping with the higher court's ruling. Judge Williams found that Special Master Moran had not applied the correct legal standards.[25] She identified many shortcomings in his decision, in particular explaining that he had applied the key legal test incorrectly.

Special Master Moran improperly ruled that the onset of Chris's arrhythmia was unknown. On the contrary, although the exact moment of its start was uncertain, Judge Williams provided a chart of thirty pulse rate records, showing that from 1996 through 2006, before Chris's HPV shots, her pulse had never indicated an arrhythmia.[26] Furthermore, there were two consecutive electrocardiograms recorded three months after the first shot and one month after the second one that indicated irregular heartbeats. This made it more likely than not that the arrhythmia developed after the HPV vaccines, since it was first detected after these shots. Judge Williams also held that petitioner's experts had provided a plausible medical theory linking the vaccine to Chris's death that even the government's experts acknowledged was possible.

Finally, Judge Williams argued that the Special Master had failed to review the totality of the evidence, including Chris's history of potential autoimmune disease, the opinions of her treating physicians, and evidence of a challenge-rechallenge phenomenon, where each dose provokes a more severe reaction. Thus, she vacated the Special Master's ruling and sent the case back.

RULING ON REMAND FINDING ENTITLEMENT[27]

On September 1, 2017, Special Master Moran issued his second judgment, following Judge Williams's order, finding that Emily was entitled to compensation for Chris's death.[28] He reconsidered previous evidence about Chris's autoimmunity, the plausibility of the medical theory, and evidence of challenge-rechallenge. This subsequent decision, besides reviewing the evidence in a more searching way, seemed more empathic, calling this a "tragic case about a woman, Christina Tarsell, who died much too young." Because HHS did not appeal this decision, it is now final. It is the first case to unequivocally establish that Gardasil vaccination caused a young woman's death, and thus it will serve as an important precedent in future death cases in the Compensation Program. Finally, on February 26, 2018, Special Master Moran awarded Emily Tarsell $250,000 for Christina's death and $60,000 for her past pain and suffering.[29]

For Emily, the process has been a test of faith. She has had to persevere mightily to find truth, validation, and accountability. The way the pieces came together to prove Chris's case was nothing short of miraculous. Her extraordinary team prevailed: the HPV vaccine more likely than not caused Chris's arrhythmias, which in turn led to her sudden, unexpected death. There is no alternative explanation that makes any sense; indeed, the government never even proposed one. But still, it took eight long, hard years to resolve Chris's case. And this in a forum that Congress intended to be simple, quick, generous, and nonadversarial!

Emily had to fight HHS every step of the way. She discovered that the agency is riddled with conflicts of interest, impeding truth, safety, and accountability. She no longer believes that government health agencies adequately investigate vaccines before or after licensure. And she believes that the public is inadequately informed about vaccine risks, inadequately protected against them, and inadequately compensated in the event of injury. She has learned all this the hard way.

Most families of vaccine-injured children never get as far as Emily did because of the many stumbling blocks. Chris's case was much stronger than many because Chris received the HPV vaccines separate from any other vaccines; she was not on any other medications; her death was eighteen days after her last HPV shot; and Emily had medical evidence both before and after vaccination showing that postvaccination symptoms did not exist before vaccination. Emily knows that other children may have died from the vaccine, but they are less likely to receive compensation and acknowledgement because of the short three-year statute of limitations and because of other complications, including the inability to find the right experts and science.

For Emily, the purpose of this legal nightmare was not the money. Congress capped the award for death at $250,000 in 1986 and has never raised it. For Emily, it was about accountability for Chris's death and shedding light on the deadly side effects of this vaccine. People are not getting the information about the true risks and benefits. People are unaware that the vaccine has caused death and many serious injuries. They are also unaware that it has never prevented a single case of cervical cancer. To Emily, this is simply wrong. So she works every day to raise awareness and to ensure that her daughter's tragic death might save another young person's life.

THE NONCOMPENSATION OF JASMYNE GRAMZA

Jasmyne Gramza was twelve when she received her first HPV vaccine in her hometown of Phoenix, Arizona.[30] She received all three doses and seemed fine after each one. Two months after the last dose, though, Jasmyne started to bruise easily. In February 2014, Jasmyne's mother Tarah Gramza, a labor and delivery room nurse, took Jasmyne to see the pediatrician. The doctor took Jasmyne's blood, and Tarah didn't expect to hear back for some time.

The doctor called her urgently the next morning, telling Tarah to take Jasmyne to the emergency room right away. He had detected that Jasmyne's platelet level was 23,000, when it should have been about 200,000. Doctors diagnosed Jasmyne with idiopathic thrombocytopenic purpura (ITP) and antiphospholipid syndrome, both blood disorders preventing her blood from clotting properly. For months, Jasmyne was extremely ill. She could not attend school, had frequent nose bleeds that would not stop, irregular and heavy menstrual periods, small red dots all over her body, and suffered severe fatigue. Her platelet level went down to as low as 4,000 before she went into remission in July 2014 after significant treatment.

Fortunately, Jasmyne has recovered, but she remains at high risk for chronic ITP. Symptoms include low platelet count and bleeding, which can lead to fatal complications.[31] Jasmyne's antiphospholipid profile will likely make it difficult or impossible for her to become pregnant.

The first doctors who treated Jasmyne thought her case was rare and made no connection to her vaccination. Tarah, however, started doing her own medical research and learned that there was significant literature linking ITP and antiphospholipid syndrome with vaccines.[32] She then located an experienced lawyer in the Compensation Program to handle the case. He was familiar with vaccine injury and put Tarah in touch with leading scientists for Jasmyne's condition. The lawyer, in fact, knew far more than Jasmyne's treating physicians about potential vaccine injuries.

Tarah filed her daughter's claim on March 10, 2015; the hearing for the case took place in June 2017. Tarah was fortunate that Dr.

Shoenfeld, a leading expert on autoimmune conditions, published a case report on Jasmyne's development of ITP with antiphospholipid antibodies and agreed to write an expert report and to testify.[33] He opined that the HPV vaccine led to her ITP.[34]

The two HHS experts claimed that Jasmyne had lupus, not idiopathic thrombocytopenia purpura, and that lupus was unrelated to the vaccine, even though Jasmyne's treating physician ruled out lupus at her first diagnosis and throughout her treatment, as did Dr. Shoenfeld. Despite peer-reviewed science and world-class experts, HHS lawyers refused to settle. The Gramzas had already spent countless hours and over $200,000 dealing with Jasmyne's medical trauma.

In a letter to a Congressional Oversight Committee, Tarah urged it to reform the Compensation Program. "[W]e have found the Vaccine Court to be a program designed not to help families provide relief, but a program designed to give refuge to the vaccine manufacturers." She wrote that while it was put in place to help families, it instead primarily serves to shield vaccine makers.[35]

More than seven months after the hearing, the Special Master denied compensation, finding that the timing of Jasmyne's symptoms did not fit the recognizable profile for vaccine-induced ITP. Although the Special Master acknowledged that vaccines, and HPV vaccines in particular, could induce ITP, he found that "Petitioner has not demonstrated that the July 2013 onset of her ITP occurred in a medically-acceptable timeframe six months after receipt of the third HPV dose in January 2013."[36] As the decision hinges on factual findings, Tarah had little legal basis for appeal. It would be difficult for the Gramza family to argue that the Special Master's decision was arbitrary and capricious, the standard they must meet to have the decision overturned on appeal.

Although in theory the Gramza family could try their case in civil court, they would have to find and compensate their own lawyers and experts, and they would face the same hurdles in proving causation. So this decision, to Tarah Gramza, highlights how far this program had strayed from Congress's initial vision of a simple, quick, nonadversarial, generous program for injury victims. Tarah knows well that medical conditions don't follow legalistic timing rules and that individuals vary greatly in their biological makeups.

There is no absolute certainty today that Jasmyne's ITP occurred because of her HPV vaccines. Perhaps in the future, biomarkers will constitute more definitive proof. But in common-sense terms, Jasmyne's symptoms started after the vaccination and worsened within a reasonable time period after the last dose. To the family, the HPV vaccine is by far the most plausible explanation why Jasmyne got this rare blood disorder. Because few legal precedents provide a "medically-acceptable timeframe," Jasmyne's case lost. Of course, the family is grateful that Jasmyne largely recovered; they know that not all families are so fortunate. But this experience left Tarah unconvinced of justice for vaccine injury victims.

WHAT ABOUT OTHER COURTS?

Until 2011, it was possible to sue the manufacturer of a vaccine for a "design defect" if the plaintiff had first filed in the Compensation Program. Few cases were filed under this theory, and only certain state and federal courts permitted such claims after the 1986 Act. But in 2008, the Supreme Court of Georgia unanimously ruled that an individual could bring such a claim in a civil court.[37] The federal Third Circuit Court of Appeals ruled that a person could not bring such a claim.[38] The US Supreme Court decided to hear the two cases to reconcile the issue. It joined the cases, even though they were about different vaccines with different alleged design defects.

Bruesewitz v. Wyeth (2011)

In a 6–2 decision, the Supreme Court ruled that individuals may not bring vaccine design defect claims to civil courts.[39] The Court ruled that only the FDA has the authority to decide if a vaccine design is defective, although the FDA has never done this. The dissent strongly disagreed with the majority's interpretation.

This 2011 Supreme Court decision has direct impact on those injured by the HPV vaccine. If it were possible to sue Merck for vaccine design defect, plaintiffs' lawyers would have done so already. But the Supreme Court's 2011 decision forecloses them. Many assert that the HPV vaccine is defectively designed, harming an unacceptably high proportion of those who receive it.

This legal situation is different in countries of the European Union, however. A 2017 decision of the European Court of Justice, *N.W. v. Sanofi Pasteur*, reaffirmed the rights of petitioners to bring claims against manufacturers for defective products, including vaccines.[40] The European Court's decision, contrasting *Bruesewitz v. Wyeth*, may play a role in future HPV vaccine litigation in the European Union.

Robi v. Merck

One US plaintiff, Jennifer Robi, has sued Merck in a California state court for fraud and deceit, negligent misrepresentation, and inadequate warnings and information about the HPV vaccine. She has also sued the medical office and doctors where she received HPV shots for malpractice and battery. Filed in 2016, *Robi v. Merck* has the potential to uncover important information about Gardasil through legal discovery.[41]

Jennifer Robi first filed a petition in the Compensation Program in 2013, as she was required to do, alleging that her acquired demyelinating neuropathy and the aggravation of her existing fibromyalgia occurred because of three HPV shots she received in 2010 and 2011. Special Master Moran, who presided over her case, just as he did over Chris Tarsell's, dismissed it for insufficient proof. He ruled that her medical records did not support her claim.[42]

Her complaint in a California court states that her complex medical conditions include Postural Orthostatic Tachycardia Syndrome and a small fiber neuropathy. She asserts that Merck's disclosures to the FDA "wrongfully and deceitfully failed, during the preapproval processing period and thereafter, to disclose . . . material facts and information relating to the effectiveness and safety of Gardasil."[43] Further, she argues that Merck wrongfully and deceitfully manipulated fear of cancer by repeatedly stating and implying that to prevent cervical cancer, it was imperative for girls to get the vaccine.

She argues that Merck sold these products knowing that if consumers had been fully informed of the risks and benefits, most would have chosen not to vaccinate.[44]

Furthermore, Robi claims that the medical providers who gave her the Gardasil shots were negligent both in administering them and in failing to diagnose the nature of her underlying immunological condition afterward, making the causal relationship between Gardasil and her serious medical conditions "unascertainable" before February 2016.[45] She and her parents were negligently deprived of their right to informed consent. Had she and her parents received the necessary material facts and information, they would have rejected Gardasil. Because the shots were without her parents' and her informed consent, they constituted medical batteries.[46] If in fact the court finds that Merck engaged in fraud toward the FDA, the liability protections of the 1986 Act fade away. Robi's case will be one to watch.

Families all over the world are seeking justice after HPV vaccine injuries. People have filed lawsuits in France, Spain, Australia, Japan, Colombia, Israel, India, the US, and doubtless other countries, as well. Later chapters follow the HPV saga in several countries where the pursuit of justice continues.

17.

Controlling the Message

"Above all, the experience of tobacco shows how powerful profits can be as a motivator, even at the cost of millions of lives and unspeakable suffering."[1] *Kelly Brownell and Kenneth Warner*

Superficially, Big Tobacco and Big Pharma would seem to have little in common. Big Tobacco markets dangerous "lifestyle" products, whereas the pharmaceutical industry markets drugs and treatments that can be lifesaving. Looking deeper, though, there are important similarities.

Big Pharma's vaccine marketing parallels Big Tobacco's marketing in several ways: (1) significant public relations framing; (2) influence over government regulators; (3) silencing or discrediting any science that suggests harm; and (4) marketing products, particularly to youth.[2] Big Pharma has had the added advantage of not just marketing, but compelling, its products to children. Big Tobacco's framing focused on smokers' personal enjoyment, choice, and personal responsibility. Big Pharma's framing for HPV vaccines has several similarities:

- Focus on responsibility—"Community Immunity" (collective vs. personal);

- Play on fears (infectious disease vs. government usurpation of freedom);

- Vilify and silence critics as "quack scientists" or "junk journalists" or "antivaccine;" and

- Dismiss legitimate concerns about safety and industry practices.[3]

As former FDA director David Kessler explained about Big Tobacco:

> Every tobacco company executive in the public eye was told to learn the script backwards and forwards, no deviation was allowed. The basic premise was simple—smoking had not been proved to cause cancer. Not proven, not proven, not proven—this would be stated insistently and repeatedly. Inject a thin wedge of doubt, create controversy, never deviate from the prepared line. It was a simple plan and it worked.[4]

In the HPV vaccine marketplace, industry goes to great lengths to discredit and silence those who assert that the vaccine is causing harm. Big Pharma has successfully silenced scientists, news broadcasters, and print journalists, crying "not proven, not proven, not proven," just like Big Tobacco before it. Big Pharma's version, though, seems to go even further when it comes to vaccines—certain questions simply cannot be asked.

Over the years, Big Pharma has silenced or discredited HPV vaccine critics on many specific occasions. By sowing doubts about injuries as "anecdotes" and "psychogenic" stories of hysterical girls, Big Pharma has cynically followed Big Tobacco's footsteps.

PRINT JOURNALISM: *TORONTO STAR*'S RETRACTED 2015 EXPOSÉ

On February 5, 2015, the *Toronto Star*, a major newspaper in Canada, ran a front-page story on the HPV vaccine by two seasoned investigative journalists, Jesse McLean and David Bruser. It focused on well-documented accounts of injury and death. The article's subtitle read: "Although hundreds of thousands of girls in Canada have safely taken Gardasil, at least 60 Canadians experienced debilitating illnesses after inoculation."[5] The in-depth story, featuring interviews with parents and young women as well as somber photos, noted at the outset that "[t]here is no conclusive evidence showing the vaccine caused a death or illness."[6] The article reached girls in the story through Health Canada, the country's public health agency, which had received more than 50 reports of serious HPV vaccine injury since 2007. The girls and their families reported conditions including fibromyalgia, heart attack, migraines, weakness, and death. They also said that doctors often dismissed their symptoms or characterized them as psychological.[7]

The article prompted a swift backlash. On February 11, 2015, an editorial signed by 69 physicians under the title "Science shows HPV vaccine has no dark side" ran in the newspaper.[8] The doctors alleged that the "litany of horror stories and its innuendo give the incorrect impression that the vaccine caused the harm."[9] The editorial argued that correlation is not causation and that "[t]o attribute rare devastating occurrences to a vaccine requires evidence of causation, of which the international scientific community and the *Star* article have none."[10]

The next day, February 12, 2015, *Toronto Star*'s investigative editor defended the story in a statement.[11] He noted that it was based on "serious reports on a government health database" that physicians and others had reported. He argued that the newspaper had given "a balanced account of concerns" and that the story was "no different than other stories" that the *Star* had done. Despite accounts of injury, the article went to "great lengths to explain the benefits of Gardasil."[12]

Then on February 20, 2015, the publisher offered a wan defense of the piece but wrote that "we have concluded that in this case our story treatment led to confusion between anecdotes and evidence," and as a result, the publisher retracted the original article from the *Star*'s website.[13] The publisher acknowledged that there had been no misinformation and no mistakes, yet he retracted it allegedly because it had caused "confusion" in the minds of readers.

The *Washington Post* piled on in a February 25, 2015 op-ed, noting that the *Star*'s HPV article had "epitomized the failure to strike . . . [the right] balance."[14] It cited critics who characterized the piece as "everything wrong with vaccine reporting in one dangerous package."[15]

What induced the *Star*'s publisher to retract a factually accurate piece that its editorial staff stood behind is impossible to know. We can surmise, though, that the pressures must have been real, whether from advertisers, government agencies, the medical community, influential individuals, or all of the above.

THE EXCORIATION OF KATIE COURIC

Since 2009, there has been scant investigative journalism about the HPV vaccine in the US. Until then, mainstream newspapers had expressed some reservations about the HPV vaccine, its cost-benefit ratio, and injury profile. But since then, there has been little coverage of reported injuries or controversy abroad. This changed when Katie Couric announced in 2013 that she would air a program about the HPV vaccine, including conversations with those who alleged injury and death.

SaneVax was instrumental in arranging for HPV vaccine victims to participate in the show alongside HPV vaccine advocates. Couric is a well-known American talk show host and current Yahoo news anchor. Her own lifestyle and news show, *Katie*, ran on ABC from 2012 to 2014.[16] Reportedly, Katie Couric was one of the best-paid media anchors in the US in 2012; she was called "America's Darling."[17] The show that she aired December 4, 2013, included two mothers and accounts of two girls: one girl who died shortly after receiving the vaccine and the other who said she couldn't get out of bed for three years. Couric went to great lengths to give positive information about the vaccine, as well; she noted that she had vaccinated her own daughters.

Putting the HPV vaccine controversy on a nationally syndicated TV show was unprecedented. The ABC website received 12,000 comments.[18] Print journalists attacked Couric immediately. *Time* magazine's Alexandra Sifferlin wrote, "[t]here is no 'HPV Vaccine Controversy'. . . .The bottom line is that there is no scientific evidence that the HPV vaccine causes adverse effects beyond normal vaccine side effects, such as dizziness, nausea, and pain and redness at the injection site."[19] Michael Hiltzik of the *Los Angeles Times* wrote that the show portrayed false balance and was wrong to suggest that the vaccine was controversial. "Merely to ask the questions [about the vaccine's safety] is to validate them [doubts]," he wrote.[20]

Like the *Toronto Star* publisher, Couric then offered a mea culpa for having hosted the show. On December 10, 2013, she wrote in the *Huffington Post*:

> Following the show, and in fact before it even aired, there was criticism that the program was too anti-vaccine and anti-science, and in retrospect, some of that criticism was valid. We simply spent too much time on the serious adverse events that have been reported in very rare cases following the vaccine. More emphasis should have been given to the safety and efficacy of the HPV vaccines.[21]

In reality, Couric didn't really cover the HPV vaccine story at all. She didn't look broadly at the claims of injury and death; she didn't examine Japan's decision to withdraw its recommendation for the vaccine; she didn't look at the legislative and judicial proceedings against HPV manufacturers in India or elsewhere. All she did was ask questions.[22] But she asked questions that Big Pharma censors in mainstream media. On December 19, 2013, Couric and ABC agreed to terminate her show in summer 2014 for undisclosed reasons.[23]

SUPPRESSING HPV VACCINE SAFETY SCIENCE

Even more dangerous than censorship of public discourse is suppression of science. The retraction of a scientific study about the HPV vaccine in mice by Romen Inbar et al., published in January 2016 in the journal *Vaccine*, brought the issue into sharp focus. Led by internationally renowned autoimmunity expert Yehuda Shoenfeld, nine scientists collaborated to look at the effects of Gardasil and its aluminum-based adjuvant in mice.[24] They divided the mice into four groups: (1) mice injected with Gardasil; (2) mice injected with an aluminum-containing adjuvant (because Merck claims AAHS is proprietary, the researchers were unable to obtain AAHS and substituted a different aluminum-containing adjuvant); (3) mice injected with Gardasil plus an additional vaccine; and (4) mice injected with a true saline placebo. The findings suggested that both Gardasil and the adjuvant injections caused long-term behavioral and cognitive abnormalities. The article concluded that "Gardasil, both through its aluminum adjuvant and its HPV antigen types, triggers neuro-inflammation and autoimmune reactions leading to behavioral changes, including cognitive and psychological impairments."[25] The article raised serious questions about Gardasil safety and the use of false placebos in vaccine trials in general. The article called for new guidelines for placebos in all vaccine clinical trials.[26]

The authors submitted their manuscript to *Vaccine* in September 2015. They made revisions based on the journal's peer reviewer comments and resubmitted it on December 15, 2015. The journal accepted the revised article on December 31, 2015, and published it online January 9, 2016. Within days, the journal removed the article from its website and within weeks posted a notice that it had retracted it. *Vaccine*'s statement, on PubMed,[27] the central medical online library, stated:

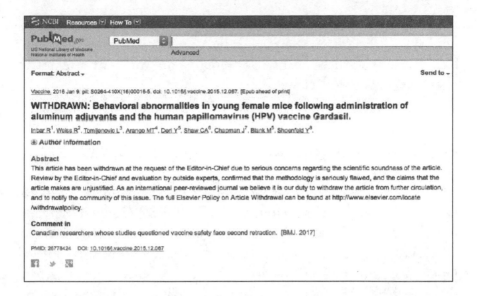

Source: PubMed, see note 27.

Retraction of a scientific article creates a stigma that the article contains serious errors, fraudulent data, or both. The article in this case had passed the journal's standard peer review process, and the authors had no reason to imagine that the journal would change its mind. The journal's statement about why it retracted the article failed to clarify why the article's methodology was "seriously flawed" or why the journal had not appreciated these allegedly serious shortcomings during its lengthy peer review process.

Dr. Shoenfeld told the Canadian newspaper *The National Post* that the authors were considering legal action. He wrote in an email exchange, "To simply retract a paper, which reports a result that one does not like, makes a mockery of the whole review process."[28] Several sources pointed out that *Vaccine* Editor-in-Chief Dr. Gregory Poland has serious conflicts of interest resulting from his obligations to Merck, Gardasil's manufacturer, as chairman of a safety evaluation committee for vaccine trials and as a consultant for new vaccine development.[29] He has also consulted on vaccine development for several other pharmaceutical companies, including CSL Biotherapies, Avianax, Sanofi Pasteur, Dynavax, Novartis Vaccines and Therapeutics, PAXVAX, and Emergent Biosolutions.[30]

Fortunately, another scientific journal, *Immunologic Research*, re-published it.[31] Still, the retraction by *Vaccine's* editor-in-chief, who has obvious conflicts of interest, remains an apparent attempt to censor inconvenient science.

INTERGOVERNMENTAL AND GOVERNMENTAL COVER-UPS?

Perhaps the most serious allegation of suppression on HPV vaccine science comes from Dr. Sin Hang Lee. On January 14, 2016, Dr. Lee sent an open letter to the WHO Director General Margaret Chan about its Global Advisory Committee on Vaccine Safety (GACVS). Dr. Lee claimed the Committee had deliberately misled Japanese health authorities on HPV vaccine safety. He suggested that the WHO officials' acts required Dr. Chan to "act quickly and decisively regarding this critical public health issue."[32]

Based on detailed correspondence between GACVS Chairperson Dr. Robert Pless with other scientists before a February 26, 2014, meeting in Japan, Dr. Lee alleged that GACVS intentionally misled Japanese regulators to think that the HPV vaccine does not elevate "any cytokine associated with reactogenicity."[33] In fact, GACVS affirmatively knew from one of its own experts that HPV vaccination does increase cytokines, including tumor necrosis factor (TNF), particularly at the injection site, compared to other vaccines. Dr. Lee showed, through careful review of emails, that they "chose to suppress this information at the [Japanese] public hearing."[34]

Dr. Lee went on to explain the mechanism by which the HPV vaccine provokes cytokine release, including TNF cytokines. Dr. Lee stated that "there is a known molecular mechanism to explain why serious adverse reactions occur more often in people injected with HPV vaccines than with other vaccines, and why certain predisposed vaccinees may suffer a sudden unexpected death as the result of Gardasil vaccination."[35] Dr. Lee still has received no response to his open letter, and the WHO has initiated no public investigation or inquiry into his allegations.

COMPLAINING TO THE EUROPEAN MEDICINES AGENCY

In July 2015, Denmark requested the European Medicines Agency to investigate HPV vaccine adverse effects based on reported cases of postural orthostatic tachycardia syndrome (POTS) following vaccination. In Chapter 25, we get a sense of the background to this complaint and the doctors whose data initiated the investigation. In response to Denmark's request, the EMA launched a study, leading to a report to assess the safety of the vaccine in the European Union, and particularly the high number of reports from Denmark, where many young women were suffering from unusual symptoms. The EMA report dismissed safety concerns and reports of suspected HPV-related complex regional pain syndrome (CRPS) and POTS. The report surveyed existing scientific data from vaccine manufacturers and information from Danish clinics, which treat HPV vaccine injury patients, concluding that the data "do not suggest a causal link" between CRPS, POTS, and the vaccines.[36]

The EMA report went on to say that the authors consulted with a Scientific Advisory Group, which purportedly opined that "the reports to date do not constitute a signal which would warrant further investigation."[37] In other words, not only did the EMA not find injuries, but it recommended against any further investigation into causal relationships. The report concluded that the risk-benefit balance for Cervarix, Gardasil, Gardasil 9, and Silgard, the European trade name for Gardasil, "remain[ed] favourable."

Researchers at the Nordic Cochrane Centre, a nonprofit medical research group in Denmark, filed a complaint with the EMA in May 2016 for "maladministration" because of its 2015 report.[38] The complaint alleged that the EMA, giving the impression of consensus, had misrepresented the facts. The complaint relied on a 256-page confidential report that had been leaked to them.[39] That internal report reflected sharp disagreements among EMA scientists and suggested that their review had been substandard and biased to favor manufacturers.

The Cochrane Centre described the EMA dismissal of research from Denmark as "unfair, misleading, partly erroneous and pejorative" and came close to "an accusation of scientific misconduct."[40]

In many places, the Cochrane complaint stated that the EMA's methods were "totally unacceptable," including the revelation that the EMA experts were not only anonymous, but also bound to a supposed duty of life-long confidentiality.[41]

It wrote: "We find it unacceptable that the EMA in its official report did not make it clear that it allowed the drug companies to be their own judges when evaluating whether the vaccine is safe, particularly since there is a huge amount of money at stake: The global expenditure so far on HPV vaccines can be roughly estimated at 25 billion Euros."[42] In addition to overall criticism, it continued: "[w]e believe this constitutes scientific misconduct, but the EMA accepted it nonetheless, without reservations."[43]

In the internal report, some EMA experts compared the HPV vaccine clinical trials to those for Vioxx, the drug Merck had taken off the market in 2004 under pressure. Merck scientists knew of the adverse Vioxx reactions in clinical trials, but "the medication was brought into circulation. For HPV now, the same seems to occur. We are . . . reporting a particularly large number of cases [of injury] for a vaccination, for which a zero tolerance regarding the side effects should prevail."[44] The EMA's official report brought none of this to light. The Nordic Cochrane Centre also pointed to Merck's use of false placebos and alleged a potential cover-up.[45] It described the EMA's report as "outright scientific misconduct."[46]

Mincing no words, it concluded:

> The bottom line for the EMA seems to have been that the vaccine should be protected from criticism at all costs because it is believed to save lives by protecting against development of cervical cancer. . . . The EMA accepted uncritically substandard research performed by the [vaccine manufacturers] and produced a superficial, substandard official report that was clearly flawed and unrepresentative, considering the serious concerns raised in internal discussion, which were sealed by life-long confidentiality agreements.[47]

In July 2016, the EMA responded, refuting Cochrane's claims.[48] It did not address the Centre's major criticisms, though. Dissatisfied, the Centre filed a complaint in October 2016 with the European Ombudsman so that a third party could evaluate the issue.[49] The Ombudsman responded in June 2017, seven months after the complaint was filed, dismissing the Centre's accusation of maladministration and stressing that its office was not a "scientific body" and could not judge the merits.[50] The Ombudsman dismissed claims of conflicts of interest and accepted that the EMA's retention of internal documents was reasonable.

The Nordic Cochrane Centre then again critiqued the EMA, arguing that all its procedures and information should be public, and that citizens should decide for themselves whether to take any particular vaccine, drug, or other medical intervention.[51] To date, though, the EMA has not released any internal documents related to its 2015 assessment of HPV vaccine safety. The EMA continues to stand behind its 2015 decision that the HPV vaccines have been thoroughly assessed by their agency and are safe.

MUST THE WORLD ACCEPT THAT HPV VACCINES ARE SAFE?

In 2015, Heidi Larson, an anthropologist and lecturer at the London School of Hygiene & Tropical Medicine, published a paper in *Nature* titled "The World Must Accept That The HPV Vaccines Are Safe."[52] Dr. Larson asserts that children's adverse reactions are all psychosomatic. She asks the world to ignore the reports of unexplained illnesses after HPV vaccination and instead trust that the conditions are unrelated to the vaccine.

In making this case, Dr. Larson ignores the body of science relating to aluminum toxicity, DNA contamination, and effects of other vaccine ingredients that we discuss at length throughout this book. She ignores the adverse event reporting systems such as VAERS and Vigibase, and even the clinical trial data. She sows doubt in children's accounts of harm attributable to a product, just as the cigarette industry did for more than a century.

The way Big Pharma manages scientific and public discourse around HPV vaccines draws on Big Tobacco's playbook. HPV vaccine discourse is even more troubling, though, because it involves physicians, international and national health organizations, and children and their families. We must ask the same question about Big Pharma that others asked about Big Tobacco: "Who are these persons who knowingly and secretly decide to put the buying public at risk solely for the purpose of making profits and who believe that illness and death of consumers is an apparent cost of their own prosperity?"

18.

AUSTRALIA: FIRST TO INJECT

Australia is at the center of the HPV vaccine universe, although most people in the US are completely unaware of it. Australia conducted clinical trials for both HPV vaccines and was one of the first countries to recommend it for girls in 2007. It recommended the vaccine for boys in 2013. Cervical cancer is rare in Australia, with mortality rates even lower than in the Unites States, at 1.8 deaths per 100,000 women.[1] Even before introducing the vaccine, Australia had the second-lowest cervical cancer rate in the world. But there are around 900 new cases annually, and tragically, around 250 women die of it each year.[2]

In indigenous communities where screening rates are low, cervical cancer rates are much higher.[3] Only about 50 percent of indigenous women get regular Pap tests. As a result, they are four times more likely to die from the disease.[4]

The HPV vaccine is an Australian invention, at least based on the 1990s patent wars. Professor Ian Frazer and Dr. Ian Zhou led the research team from University of Queensland that first produced an HPV VLP in a lab. Zhou died in 1999 before the world would see his invention. Professor Frazer continued their work, though, with the help of critical investment from Commonwealth Serum Laboratories (CSL), an Australian biotech company. Frazer and Zhou's family own a general patent on VLP technology and also earn royalties on all HPV vaccines sold in the developed world.[5] CSL has the exclusive rights to sell Gardasil in Australia and New Zealand, sharing profits with Merck.[6]

Due to the international acclaim associated with the vaccine's launch, Frazer became an Australian celebrity and the unofficial Australian spokesman for HPV vaccines. He is considered a "National Treasure" and received the "Australian of the Year" award in 2006, among other honors. One magazine even dubbed him "God's gift to women," for his contribution to women's health.[7]

As the FDA got closer to approving the vaccine in 2006 in the US, stakeholders in the Australian vaccine program assumed that regulators would approve adding the HPV vaccine to the national schedule without hesitation. In a surprising turn of events, however, Australia's drug approval board, the Pharmaceutical Benefits Advisory Committee, rejected the Gardasil application in November 2006.[8] The Advisory Committee based its decision on cost and efficacy. The then-Minister for Health, Tony Abbott, justified the decision by saying that the Committee had unanswered questions. According to an article in *The Australian*, he even floated the "bizarre idea that a misplaced confidence in the effectiveness of the vaccine might actually result in an increase in cancer rates."[9] He also said on a national radio show that he would not vaccinate his own daughters.[10]

The media reacted quickly to condemn Minister Abbott. Within 24 hours, Prime Minister Howard stepped up to allay public fears over what the Health Minister had said. The prime minister reassured the public that this "wonderful drug" that the public had been waiting for would be available without delay.[11] In an unprecedented move, Prime Minister Howard stepped in to assure the Advisory Committee that the vaccine manufacturer would lower the cost if the Committee approved it. This assurance posed an ethical challenge to the Committee's independence. Nonetheless, the Committee quickly reversed its previous decision and approved Gardasil. Prime Minister Howard then asked for the vaccine school program to begin in April 2007, six months ahead of schedule. CSL, which distributes the vaccine, agreed to accelerate the rollout. Australia would be the first country in the world to make it available as part of a national school immunization program, despite its low rate of cervical cancer.

This decision was not without controversy. The prime minister's unusual intervention in the Committee approval process led to an oversight review the next year. The Committee's Health Policy Monitor Marion Haas noted that a perceived willingness to interfere in the recommendation process might incentivize manufacturers and lobbyists to attempt to influence future Committee decisions.[12] This would result in a loss of public confidence in the Committee and would undermine its independence. In the case of Gardasil, however, Ms. Haas did not recommend any corrective action or policy changes, as the public largely supported the Committee's decision.

The Committee immediately endorsed the HPV vaccine, stepping over the controversy. Australia's swift action showed the world its confidence in what they believed to be a lifesaving tool to prevent cervical cancer, developed by an Australian team. National pride helped lift the vaccine to market after fifteen years of hard work, and Ian Frazer himself injected the first girl in Australia, outside of the clinical trials. The stage was now set for other countries to follow suit. Many Western countries adopted national HPV vaccine programs within a few years.[13]

Australian schools introduced the vaccine in April 2007. With uptake rates currently over 70 percent, the program is seen as a success.[14] Since 2013, boys have been getting the vaccine too, with a consistent uptake of around 70 percent, as well. In 2013, the *New York Times* ran the headline "HPV Vaccines Showing Successes in Australia," detailing reductions in warts and some high-grade cervical abnormalities after only four years. The article heralded Australia as a shining example of HPV vaccine uptake in contrast to lower uptake in the US.[15]

Soon after the vaccine's arrival at schools, however, reports of adverse reactions began to surface. By May 2007, over AU$1 billion had been wiped from CSL's share price in a jittery market reaction to the media reporting alleged adverse events.[16] In one Melbourne school, 25 girls reportedly became sick, and five girls were hospitalized. By this time, the former Health Minister, Tony Abbott, who had famously criticized the vaccine's introduction, was now prime minister. In a remarkable turnaround, he was now urging parents to continue to vaccinate their children, reassuring the public that the vaccine was safe.[17] Physicians treating the children echoed the prime minister, saying that the children's health problems were not related to the vaccine. A CSL spokesperson announced that the girls had suffered a collective anxiety attack, not physical reactions.[18] Ian Frazer too was quick to dismiss the girls' reactions as psychosomatic and urged the public to appreciate the "cancer-preventing vaccine."[19] The share price recovered.

CSL has played an important role in introducing HPV vaccines in Australia. It is one of the country's top twenty companies, now worth almost AU $50 billion (around US $40 billion). It earned AU$183 million (around US $140 million) from royalties and licensing fees in 2016–17, largely from Gardasil sales worldwide.[20] The company earns 7 percent in royalties from Merck and 2 percent in royalties from GSK for licensing their HPV vaccine technology to the pharmaceutical giants.[21] In a strange twist of fate, some girls who report autoimmune disorders following the HPV vaccine are recommended by their doctors to receive CSL's IVIG (intravenous immunoglobulin) to treat their symptoms. IVIG products are a "key growth driver" at CSL.[22] Who's to say if this is a coincidence?

REPORTS OF RARE CONDITIONS EMERGE

Australia is committed to reporting and studying the side effects to HPV vaccines through the Department of Health's Therapeutic Goods Association (TGA) using its Database of Adverse Event Notifications, or DAEN, system.[23] From April 2007, when the vaccine was first introduced in schools, to March 2018, there were around 4,300 reported adverse events, including one death.[24]

Just as in other countries with documented reports of serious adverse events after vaccination, the TGA denies any causal association.[25] But like in the US, UK, and Ireland, the TGA receives critical funding from industry in licensing fees. This funding may create conflicts of interest, despite the promise of regulatory oversight.[26]

In 2015, the TGA published Australia's most recent in-depth report on adverse events following the vaccine for the year 2013.[27] The adverse event rate in girls was 122 per 100,000 and 101 per 100,000 in boys 12-to-13-years old.[28] Interestingly, for boys aged 14 to 15, the rate decreased to 44 per 100,000 doses, with no reason given as to why.[29] Is there a reason why younger boys have more than twice the reactions that older boys have? The reaction rate for girls is *seventeen times* the incidence rate for cervical cancer throughout the life span, but this is not examined. All adverse events were considered mild, and the report only looked for acute reactions in 2013 and did not consider long-term ones. The report also looked only at anaphylaxis, fainting, allergic reactions, and conditions that required hospitalization. The TGA did not review other conditions or clusters of symptoms in the 748 reports filed that year.[30]

When the TGA published this information on its website, it prefaced the data by mentioning three other conditions of interest in 12- and 13-year-olds: demyelinating disorders, complex regional pain syndrome (CRPS), and premature ovarian failure (POF).[31] The TGA stated that it looked at "a few" cases of demyelination disorders, such as multiple sclerosis, reported after Gardasil. However, it found "no evidence that the incidence of demyelination disorders after Gardasil vaccination is higher than would occur by chance."[32] There were three cases of CRPS following the vaccine, but CRPS was considered to be "a very rare adverse event associated with the injection rather than the vaccine itself." Since CRPS is an autoimmune condition, its causal association with injection rather than the vaccine is incomplete at best. Finally, the TGA looked at three POF reports and stated that the "condition is known to occur naturally in this age group" and that there was no evidence to suggest that Gardasil is the cause.[33]

There may be no conclusive evidence that Gardasil is the cause, but the TGA statement that POF occurs naturally in this age group has no basis in fact. POF, meaning in essence permanent infertility in many cases, is a devastating diagnosis. To say that it is "known to occur naturally" at 13, which is the age group the TGA looked at, is simply a distortion of the truth. Dr. Deirdre Little, with over thirty years of clinical experience in New South Wales, published an article on POF cases she observed in her practice, which we discuss in Chapter 10. She wrote that the "age-specific incidence of idiopathic POF in early to mid-adolescence is so rare as to be unknown."[34] Despite Dr. Little's best efforts to bring the TGA's attention to these cases, the Australian government and scientific community have largely ignored her research.

AUSTRALIA'S HPV VACCINE CRITICS

Professor Ian Frazer denies that there are any long-term problems following HPV vaccination. Stephen Tunley, the Australian father of an injured daughter, disagrees. Stephen's daughter received the vaccine in 2009; she became seriously ill after her second shot. He is dedicated to finding out how the vaccine may have caused the cascade of events leading to his daughter's severe and chronic illness.

Steve's research quickly took him to SaneVax, where he became acquainted with Norma Erickson and Freda Birrell. Steve agreed to join the SaneVax board in 2011 and has been an outspoken campaigner for HPV vaccine safety ever since. He has been featured in several media articles and has published comments in *Lancet* criticizing HPV studies.[35]

Media heavyweights like the online research group *The Conversation*, to which Ian Frazer is a contributor, quickly attack any voices of dissent.[36] Because of its support from thousands of universities and research institutes, *The Conversation*'s articles have been widely cited since 2010.[37] Government agencies and industry also lend support to the vaccine, making dissent almost inaudible.

One critic who managed to get her voice heard was University of Wollongong PhD candidate Judy Wilyman. In 2015, she published a controversial doctoral thesis on Australia's vaccination policies.[38] Wilyman dissected the arguments for universal HPV vaccination and the assumptions underpinning the decision to adopt a national program. She highlighted the disparity between incidence and mortality in high versus low-resource countries, exposing the fallacy that HPV infection poses equal risk to all women. She criticized the

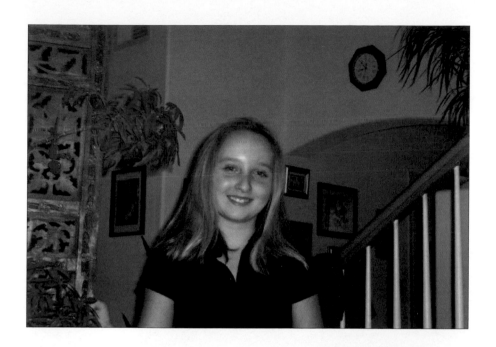

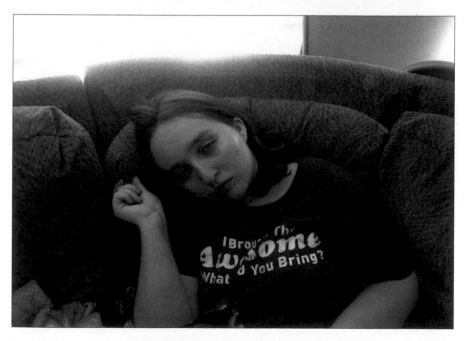

In Chapter 15, we learn about Alexis Wolf, who suffered permanent, serious neurological injury after HPV vaccination. These are before and after photos.

In 2010, Chris Tarsell died shortly after her third Gardasil shot. In Chapter 15, we learn how Emily Tarsell, Chris's mother, took the case through the Vaccine Injury Compensation Program, which determined that Gardasil vaccination likely caused Chris's death.

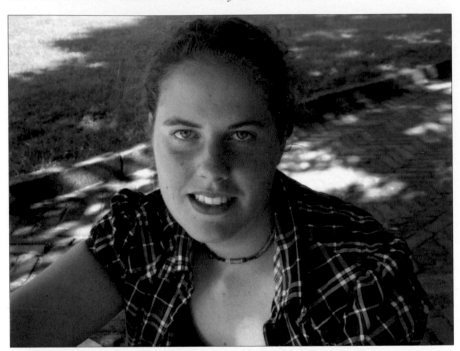

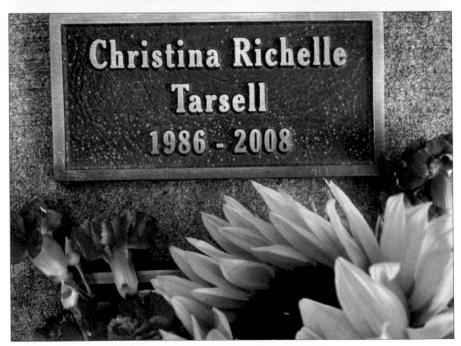

Christina Richelle
Tarsell
1986 - 2008

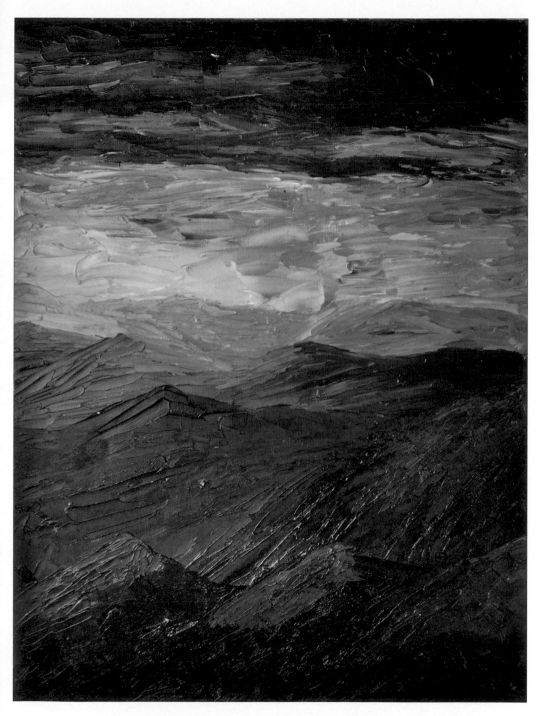

As we discuss in Chapter 15, Chris Tarsell was a talented young artist. Above is one of her paintings.

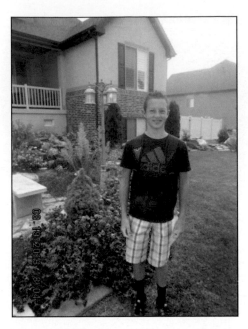

Colton Berrett had a reaction within two weeks of his third Gardasil shot in 2013. He became paralyzed and dependent on a ventilator 24/7. Colton took his own life in 2018, shortly before his 18th birthday. His story is in Chapter 15.

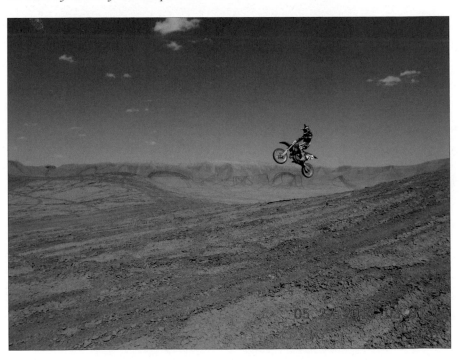

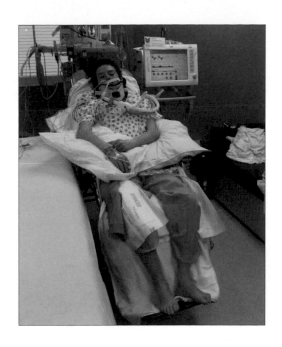

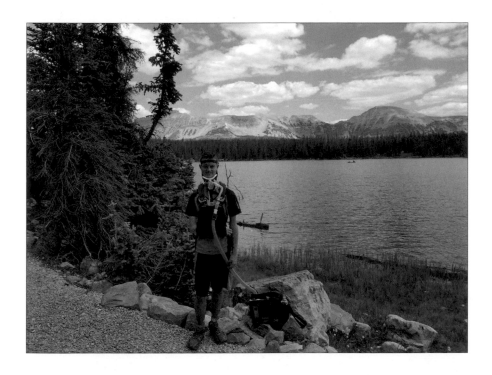

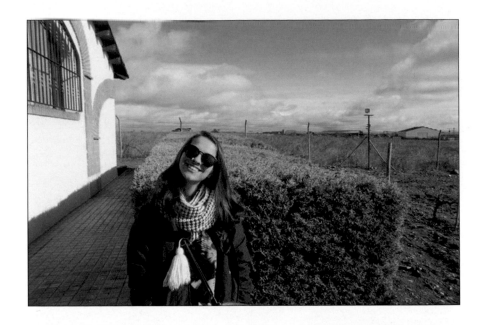

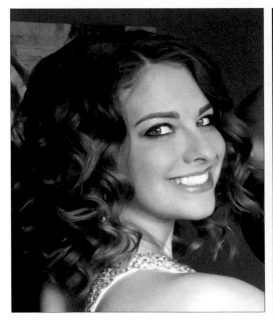

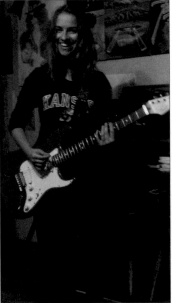

We learn in Chapter 15 of the painful shock Maddie's family suffered when she took her own life, unable to endure the silent pain of her lasting adverse effects from HPV vaccination.

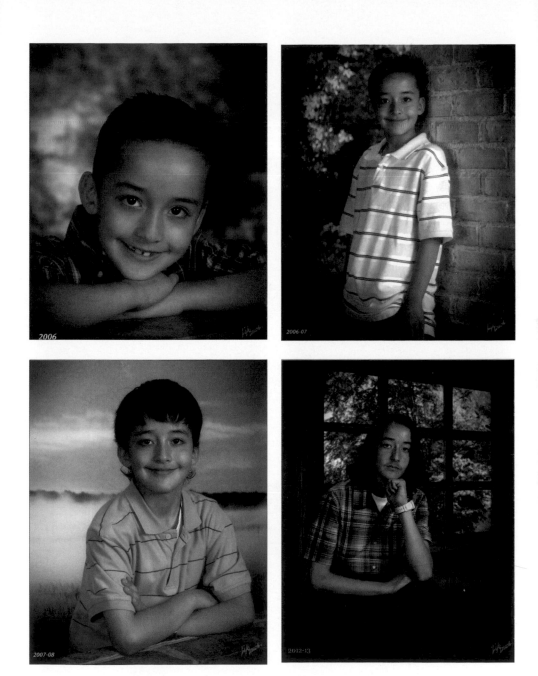

Joel Gomez died within hours of receiving his second Gardasil dose. In Chapter 15, we delve into the case Joel's parents brought to the Vaccine Injury Compensation Program for his death.

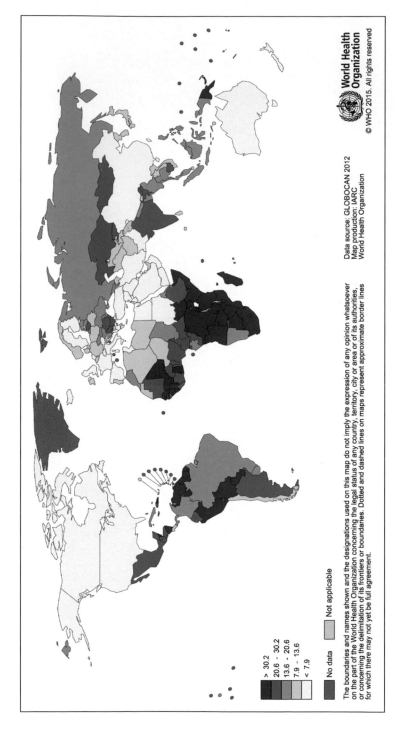

The legend reads:

> 30.2
20.6 - 30.2
13.6 - 20.6
7.9 - 13.6
< 7.9

No data   Not applicable

Data source: GLOBOCAN 2012
Map production: IARC
World Health Organization

World Health
Organization

The incidence of cervical cancer predominantly affects low resource countries. We explore the many factors influencing cervical cancer incidence in Chapter 4.
(Source: http://globocan.iarc.fr/old/FactSheets/cancers/cervix-new.asp)

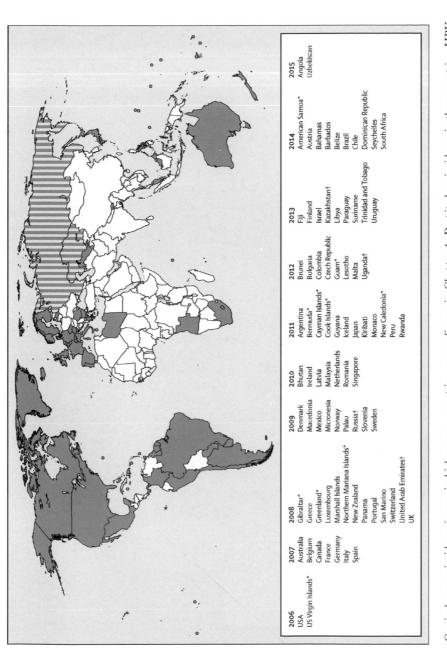

2006	2007	2008	2009	2010	2011	2012	2013	2014	2015
USA	Australia	Gibraltar*	Denmark	Bhutan	Argentina	Brunei	Fiji	American Samoa*	Angola
US Virgin Islands*	Belgium	Greece	Macedonia	Ireland	Bermuda*	Bulgaria	Finland	Austria	Uzbekistan
	Canada	Greenland*	Mexico	Latvia	Cayman Islands*	Colombia	Israel	Bahamas	
	France	Luxembourg	Micronesia	Malaysia	Cook Islands*	Czech Republic	Kazakhstan†	Barbados	
	Germany	Marshall Islands	Norway	Netherlands	Guyana	Guam*	Libya	Belize	
	Italy	Northern Mariana Islands*	Palau	Romania	Iceland	Lesotho	Paraguay	Brazil	
	Spain	New Zealand	Russia†	Singapore	Japan	Malta	Suriname	Chile	
		Panama	Slovenia		Kiribati	Uganda†	Trinidad and Tobago	Dominican Republic	
		Portugal	Sweden		Monaco		Uruguay	Seychelles	
		San Marino			New Caledonia*			South Africa	
		Switzerland			Peru				
		United Arab Emirates†			Rwanda				
		UK							

Cervical cancer incidence is rare in high resource countries, as we discuss in Chapter 4. Despite low incidence in these countries, HPV vaccine producers market there aggressively, as indicated by the green shading above. (Source: The Lancet, "Global estimates of human papillomavirus vaccination coverage by region and income level: a pooled analysis," https://www.thelancet.com/journals/langlo/article/ PIIS2214-109X(16)30099-7/fulltext; license agreement: https://creativecommons.org/licenses/by/4.0/.)

As we learn in Chapters 13 and 14, the CDC strongly promotes the HPV vaccine. The US government earns substantial royalties from sales, as we analyze in Chapter 3.

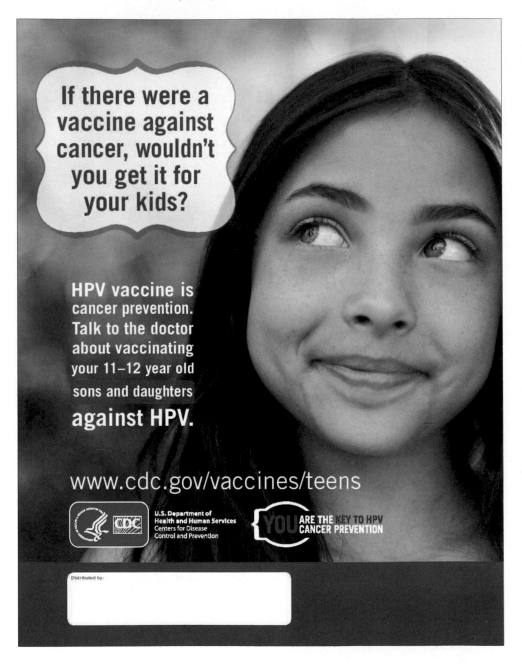

HPV Vaccination

can **prevent** an estimated

28,500 new **cancers** per year.

That's more than the average attendance at one of the largest pop concert tours of last year.

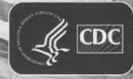

U.S. Department of Health and Human Services
Centers for Disease Control and Prevention

CS267081

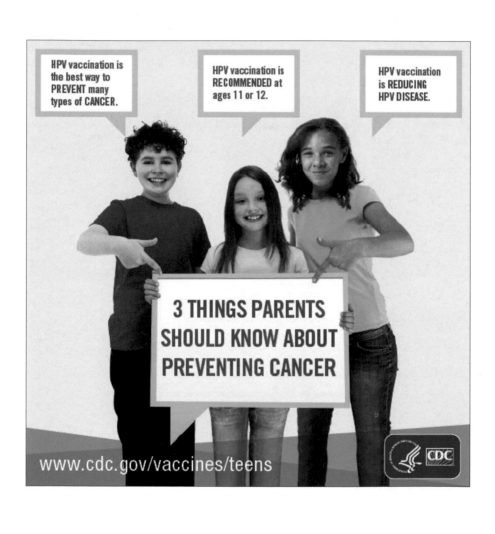

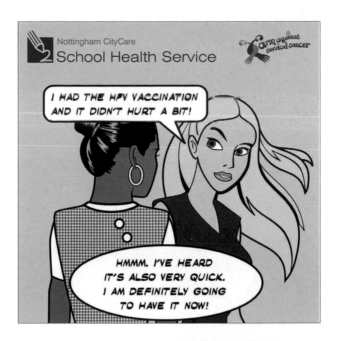

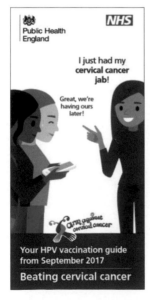

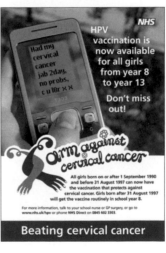

The UK has one of the highest uptake rates of HPV vaccines in the world. In Chapter 27, we examine how UK direct marketing to school children may explain why.

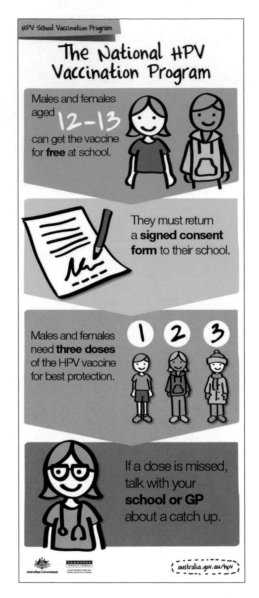

Boasting one of the HPV vaccine co-inventors, Australia was one of the first countries to approve the vaccine. We discuss the vaccine's invention in Chapter 3 and Australia's role in it. Australian children receive HPV vaccines in school, as we discuss in Chapter 18.

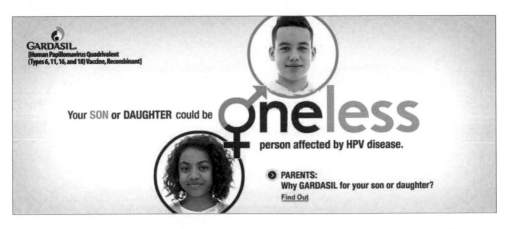

This is a Merck ad for Gardasil, using the signature tag line "Be One Less," which we discuss in Chapter 13.

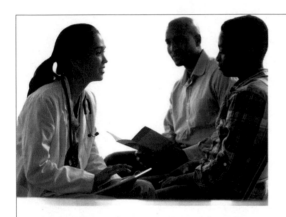

Merck markets HPV vaccines to parents and children alike. This 2018 flyer from an insurance company urges parents to vaccinate their preteenage children. We discuss marketing in Chapters 13 and 14.

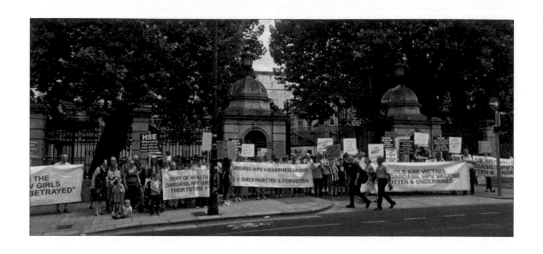

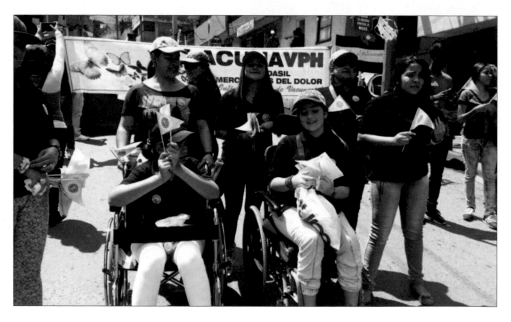

Parents in Ireland (top) and Colombia (bottom), literally continents apart, took to the streets to protest government neglect in the face of severe HPV vaccine injuries. In Chapters 26 and 28, we discuss what happened in these two different countries. Girls suffered the same adverse reactions, yet their injuries were labeled "psychosomatic," and the girls and their families were branded "antivaccine." We discuss the marginalization of injury in Chapter 15.

Australian government's involvement in marketing the HPV vaccine as cancer prevention when the clinical trials could not show this.

The University accepted her thesis and granted her a doctoral degree, but a media backlash ensued. A public petition with over 2,200 signatures demanded that the Australian Department of Health intervene and issue "unequivocal condemnation of this travesty," amid accusations of "gross academic misconduct at the University of Wollongong."[39] The petition accused the University of supporting "dangerous myth-making." An article in *The Australian* criticized her "antivaccine" stance and, by association, the University.[40] Her doctoral supervisor, Professor Brian Martin, vigorously supported Dr. Wilyman's research and intellectual freedom.[41] Professor Martin published many retorts to accusations from *The Australian* and other blogs on his private website, defending her thesis and the University's doctoral procedures.[42]

GARDASIL 9 IN 2018

In late 2017, at a dramatic press conference on Australia's Bondi Beach, Prime Minister Malcolm Turnbull announced that Gardasil 9 would replace Gardasil in schools beginning the following September.[43] He proclaimed, with Ian Frazer by his side, that it was possible to completely eliminate HPV through vaccination. Mr. Turnbull seized the moment to promote the vaccine against the backdrop of the world-famous surfing beach, repeatedly referring to the vaccine as "lifesaving," just like the lifeguards behind him.[44] Adopting Gardasil 9 also coincides with a new two-dose schedule to bring Australia into line with other countries that had reduced the number of doses from three to two in 2015–16.

Australia has succeeded in maintaining relatively high HPV vaccination rates, at least in part because of an effective public relations apparatus. The vaccine is a source of pride for the Australian government, and it is using this invention to promote the country as a center for excellence in scientific research and development. With Professor Frazer leading the campaign toward universal Gardasil 9 uptake in 2018, the voices of the injured will likely remain all but unheard.

PART III

A DEEPER LOOK AT HPV VACCINE SCIENCE

19.

CHALLENGING THE SCIENTIFIC CONSENSUS: THE MAVERICKS

In 2010, Norma Erickson, whom we met in Chapter 15, joined with others to create SaneVax to promote only Safe, Affordable, Necessary, and Effective, or "SANE," vaccines through education and information. SaneVax is one of several civil society organizations around the world challenging the safety claims of the HPV vaccine. It also connects families of injured children to support groups and others.[1] Although SaneVax's mission is broad, it has focused almost exclusively on HPV vaccines.

From the beginning, SaneVax argued that the HPV vaccine did not meet SANE criteria: the clinical trials did not prove the vaccines Safe, Affordable, Necessary, or Effective. To SaneVax, until the HPV vaccine is proven safe, it should be taken off the market. They believe that authorities should investigate how such an unsafe vaccine made it onto the market and should pursue redress for those injured.

The board includes Rosemary Mathis, Freda Birrell, Stephen Tunley, and Linda Thompson. Freda is a retired administrator based in Scotland, and she reaches out to every injured family that contacts SaneVax. She talks with them, helps make referrals, and lets them know how to connect with other affected families, who usually are the most helpful source of advice. She is SaneVax's primary liaison in Europe with politicians, medical organizations, and civil society. Rosemary Mathis of North Carolina and Steve Tunley of Australia are both parents of HPV-injured daughters. They want to be sure that no other family is unaware of HPV vaccine risks, as they were. Linda Thompson manages SaneVax's budget, which depends upon donations. Despite SaneVax's limited resources, their work makes a global impact. By 2013, people in 157 countries had already visited their website for the latest news on the HPV vaccine.[2]

A MEDICAL MAVERICK SPEAKS OUT

Early in her work at SaneVax, Norma had the good fortune to meet Dr. Sin Hang Lee, a knowledgeable and experienced pathologist with expertise in cervical screening techniques. She contacted him in 2010 to find out more about his work. Although in his late seventies, Dr. Lee was active and still working in his lab at Milford Hospital in Connecticut. When Norma approached him for advice about curious findings in a lab in Canada, he agreed to help.

Born in Hong Kong and educated as a doctor first in China and then in the US and Canada, Dr. Lee had already trained in some of the world's best hospitals. His professional mission was to provide accurate pathology tests for women's health, specifically related to sexually transmitted infections and diseases. By the early 2000s, he had been reading Pap test samples for more than fifty years, even having worked in a lab established by Dr. Papanicolaou, the namesake of the Pap test.

Dr. Lee's approach to pathology fit perfectly with SaneVax's objective to provide the public with solid science. As a pathologist, Dr. Lee's job is to figure out how and why people got sick or died. He has to decide on the most plausible cause of death or disease, and his accuracy rate has to be almost 100 percent. Otherwise, he could be sued for malpractice. He loves pathology as a discipline that links the rigor of science with the art of medicine.

Dr. Lee is distressed by the recent trend in medicine toward the "healthcare industry." By its becoming an "industry," he worries that pathologists, and doctors and scientists generally, are being pushed to stray from fact and educated interpretations toward decisions based on money and politics. Dr. Lee is averse to such influences—he wants to base his views on scientific evidence alone. Perhaps this is why he agreed to look at the case Norma brought to him.

WHY THOSE PREVIOUSLY INFECTED WITH **HPV 16** AND **18** SHOULD NOT GET THE VACCINE

Before Norma ever connected with Dr. Lee, he already had an interest in the HPV vaccine. Shortly after FDA approved the vaccine, Dr. Lee contacted the FDA to make the case that girls must be tested for HPV infection before getting the vaccine. He believed that there was a real risk that the vaccine itself might trigger a dangerous reaction in HPV-infected girls and women that could accelerate abnormal cervical cell growth. He based this interpretation on Merck's clinical trial data and adverse event reports. We discuss this "negative efficacy" risk in Chapter 9.

Dr. Lee theorized that cancer growth in the cervix may be the result of chronic inflammation. His theory had a strong basis. Chronic inflammation of the liver can lead to liver cancer; of the colon can lead to colon cancer; of the stomach can lead to stomach cancer; and of the skin can lead to skin cancer. In the same way, chronic inflammation of the cervix plausibly can lead to cervical cancer. If a woman already has an HPV 16 cervical infection and then receives HPV 16 in the vaccine, she might have a strong antibody-antigen reaction in the cervix. This reaction would promote inflammation, and possibly abnormal growth. The exact molecular mechanism is not yet clear, but the link between inflammation and cancer is well known.

THE MYSTERY IN TORONTO

In early 2011, Norma contacted Dr. Lee about a 13-year-old girl in Toronto who was sexually naive but who had developed severe juvenile rheumatoid arthritis immediately after Gardasil. In lab tests, the girl was positive for HPV in her blood. The girl's mother contacted Norma to see if perhaps the vaccine had infected her daughter. Although Norma knew that Merck and the FDA confirmed that there was no HPV DNA in the vaccine, Norma decided to ask Dr. Lee for his opinion to see if it was possible that Merck and the FDA were mistaken.

Dr. Lee knew from his research that Merck and the FDA declared no HPV DNA in the vaccines. He couldn't imagine that that representation would be wrong. Norma persisted, though, and convinced him to call the lab in Toronto. After talking to the scientist about his methods, Dr. Lee was convinced that it was quite possible that it was true.

Dr. Lee decided to test a vaccine vial for HPV DNA first. He rationalized that if there was no HPV DNA in the vaccine, there would be no point in retesting the girl's blood sample. Norma used her extensive contacts to obtain a sealed vial of Gardasil. He tested the vial and was astonished to find that it contained HPV L1 DNA, which is specific to the Gardasil vaccine. He thought perhaps this was a fluke. He asked Norma to collect more vials so that he could determine if the first vial was an anomaly.

After reaching out for help from parents and activists around the world, SaneVax collected 16 sealed Gardasil vials from Australia, Bulgaria, France, India, New Zealand, Poland, Russia, Spain, and the United States, representing a cross-section of vaccine lots. Using a very sensitive nested PCR method to detect DNA, Dr. Lee found HPV DNA contamination from HPV 18 or HPV 11, or both, *in each vial.*

Dr. Lee would go on to publish his discovery in the peer-reviewed *Journal of Inorganic Biochemistry*.[3] On behalf of SaneVax, Norma wrote to FDA Commissioner Dr. Margaret Hamburg to alert her to Dr. Lee's findings. She published the letter online.[4]

THE FDA DISTINGUISHES HPV DNA FROM HPV DNA FRAGMENTS

In a matter of weeks, an FDA public relations official, Walter Gardner, responded to SaneVax.[5] The FDA made several remarkable admissions. It acknowledged that the vaccine does contain recombinant HPV L1 DNA fragments. It also asserted that these "DNA fragments" are "not harmful" and that DNA is "not a contaminant." The letter stated that Merck and the FDA had long known of "residual fragments" in the vaccine. Nonetheless, it said that "Gardasil is a safe and effective vaccine,"[6] implying the fragments were not harmful to humans.

Norma and Dr. Lee were surprised at this response. The approval of Gardasil was based in part on the condition that the vaccine did not contain viral DNA.[7] Also, in the Merck patent for the "Process for Purifying Human Papillomavirus Virus-Like Particles," it was clearly stated that a PCR-based assay confirmed "this chromatography method is highly effective in removing contaminating DNA from the final product."[8] In other words, contrasting the FDA's response, HPV or viral DNA residues are considered contaminants, and like other contaminants, these viral DNAs must be removed from the final vaccine product. As Dr. Lee found, that is not the case. Yet, to this day, Gardasil package inserts do not state that DNA fragments remain in the vaccine.[9]

Free DNA does not have to cause infection to cause harm. For example, macrophages, or immune system cells, recognize the difference between foreign DNA and a person's own DNA. Macrophages, literally meaning "big eaters" in Greek, are large white blood cells that perform critical "clean-up" functions—engulfing and removing debris, microbes, foreign substances, and more.[10] When foreign viral DNA invades, macrophages can react violently, potentially causing a person to be sick. When fighting off an infection, the macrophages (like some other cells) secrete cytokines, such as tumor necrosis factor (TNF), so that a person develops enough antibody response to prevent the next viral infection. This is beneficial, but if the cells produce too much TNF, it can be toxic.[11] When a person gets a fever or headache after a vaccine, these symptoms may mean that the macrophages are attacking foreign DNA.

In October 2011, Norma answered the FDA.[12] She listed eight prior Merck statements, including several to the FDA, stating that the vaccine "contains no viral DNA."[13] Norma accused the FDA of playing semantic games to make a false distinction between "viral

DNA" and "viral DNA fragments." Whether the HPV DNA was intact or in pieces, it was still DNA.

Norma cited numerous published studies to support her statement to the FDA that "recombinant HPV DNA does not have to be able to infect cells, or to self-reproduce to cause or to trigger a disease."[14] She accused the FDA of being irresponsible to assert safety without any data to support it. It was "highly disturbing" to find out that the FDA and Merck knew "from the very beginning and withheld such an important material fact from consumers; namely that Gardasil has always been contaminated by residual recombinant HPV DNA."[15]

Norma requested information about the FDA's safety claims and documentation showing precisely what information Merck disclosed. She urged the FDA to immediately appoint a committee of unbiased scientists to review the safety impact of the newly discovered residual recombinant DNA. Norma offered SaneVax's cooperation in putting the FDA in contact with injured girls and their families.[16] The FDA did not respond to Norma directly.

A week later, however, the FDA posted a new advisory on its website: "FDA Information on Gardasil—Presence of DNA Fragments Expected, No Safety Risk."[17] The advisory states that the fragments are "not evidence of contamination." Under "Key Facts," it states that the DNA fragments are "not a risk" and that their presence "is not a safety factor."[18] The advisory reiterates that both Merck and the FDA have known "since the early development of Gardasil" that "small quantities of residual recombinant HPV L1-specific DNA fragments remain in the vaccine." The FDA states, however, that the vaccine "does not contain DNA from other HPV genes or any full-length infectious HPV genomes." It then asserts that "there is no evidence of unusual clinical patterns or high reporting rates of adverse events, including autoimmune diseases" based on VAERS.[19]

Norma wasted no time in responding again.[20] She noted the total lack of scientific justification for the FDA's "Key Facts." She pointed out that the FDA's mission is "helping the public get the accurate, science-based information they need to use medicines," yet their safety proclamation puts forth none.[21] She assailed the FDA's interpretation of VAERS data and asked why the VAERS reports for Gardasil injuries did "not raise a red flag requiring investigation." She challenged the FDA to provide scientific documentation. She concluded, "Anything less than full compliance is a betrayal of the public trust."[22]

SaneVax sent Dr. Lee's findings to the EMA, as well. The EMA's reply was similar: it was aware of certain DNA impurities in the vaccine. Through a Freedom of Information request, the authors obtained an internal EMA memo discussing SaneVax's letter. In meeting minutes, the EMA considered asking Merck to retest the "incriminated 13 batches" to see if the amount of DNA was indeed below the WHO minimum threshold.[23] It decided that this would "finally do more harm than good as it could be interpreted by SaneVax as a sort of control or justification."[24] Like the FDA, the EMA apparently simply accepted Merck's representation that the DNA fragments were harmless. But are they harmless? It appears that there is a body of evidence that shows that they are not totally harmless. Moreover, DNA can even act as an adjuvant in vaccines, something Merck was actively researching at the time, which Dr. Lee later discovered.

Non-B Conformation DNA

Norma and Dr. Lee didn't stop there in their quest to discover the truth about the HPV vaccine. Norma next asked Dr. Lee if he would test the postmortem tissue of an 18-year-old New Zealand girl who died six months after receiving three Gardasil shots. She died in her sleep, and the autopsy report gave no cause of death. The girl's parents contacted SaneVax for assistance. It commissioned Dr. Lee to test tissue samples for a fee not to exceed one dollar, to avoid any perceived conflict of interest if he was paid more. The test would determine if recombinant HPV DNA was in the blood or spleen samples. To Dr. Lee's amazement, it was. He published his findings in a peer-reviewed journal in early December 2012.[25]

Initially, Dr. Lee could not find HPV 16 DNA, but he quickly realized that the standard primers used to detect DNA by PCR might not be sufficiently specific. He had to use very special primers, to be able to detect and sequence this unusual DNA. When he did, he found HPV 16 L1 gene DNA fragments in the macrophages of the tissue samples. They fully matched Merck's HPV 16 L1 found in a gene database. In other words, the only way the girl could have had this type of gene sequence was from Gardasil.

The unusual DNA Dr. Lee found in the tissue was in so-called "non-B conformation." To explain the difference between B and non-B conformation DNA, Dr. Lee urged Norma to think of it as a rope or string. If you have a knot or kink in the line, enzymes can't get through to decompose the DNA. In order for the body to degrade and pass it out, DNA must be in B-conformation, or the natural conformation. Usually in order to prevent foreign DNA from entering cells, the body metabolizes any foreign DNA with enzymes and excretes it. When DNA is in B-conformation, enzymes can break it down.

Having found HPV 16 DNA in non-B conformation in the New Zealand girl's postmortem samples, and knowing that it evaded detection with standard primers, Dr. Lee rechecked the New Zealand Gardasil vials he had previously tested and in which he'd found HPV 11 and 18.[26] Using the special primers, he now found non-B conformation HPV 16 DNA in *each* of these samples, as well.[27] In 2014, a team of French scientists reported that they repeated and confirmed Dr. Lee's findings of DNA in Gardasil vials using a different method than the one Dr. Lee used.[28]

Dr. Lee theorized that HPV DNA fragments in Gardasil attach to residual aluminum-based adjuvant and pass into the macrophages as new compounds. He explained that it is like throwing wool yarn on barbed wire. It is still yarn, but it becomes stuck and cannot become untangled. Thus, the HPV 16 DNA fragments are likely becoming long-term stimulators of the immune system in those unable to degrade the non-B conformation HPV DNA. These complexes may remain in the body a long time, traveling well beyond the injection site.[29] This may explain why some reactions occur weeks or months after vaccination and may last many years.

The FDA has never contested Dr. Lee's discovery of HPV DNA fragments in Gardasil vials or in the autopsy samples. Officials have not claimed he faked the data or that his tests were inaccurate. On the contrary, the FDA acknowledged that the DNA sequencing Dr. Lee provided was correct; they knew that he could not possibly have created the recombinant DNA in his lab. The EMA decided against retesting the "incriminated" batches. Dr. Lee's findings forced the FDA and the EMA to issue statements on the presence of DNA in the vaccine, which Dr. Lee considers a triumph of sorts. The public, though, is still in the dark.

Dr. Lee believed that the FDA was led to believe in 2006 that all HPV DNA contaminants had been removed from the final HPV vaccine product. He understood the FDA's October 21, 2011, advisory as an attempt to save face for the federal agency and for Merck, although one it took at the expense of public safety. He imagined that Merck's methods were probably not sensitive enough to pick up the HPV DNA contaminants in the vaccine product when they checked for it, but he was also confident that Merck could have found it if it had wanted to. The labs at Merck were far better equipped than his own; and his detection methods were certainly available to them.

This is not the first time that Merck may have incorrectly identified vaccine ingredients. For over a decade, Merck identified the adjuvant it used in Recombivax HB, a hepatitis B vaccine, as aluminum hydroxide—a traditional aluminum-based adjuvant. The FDA and CDC also refer to aluminum hydroxide in the vaccine, including in the FDA's "summary basis for approval" of Recombivax HB.[30] In 1999, FDA approved a "supplement" to the Recombivax HB license application "to include the use of a preservative-free . . . bulk alum product" in connection with removing Thimerosal from the vaccine.[31]

Following that approval, Merck, in 2000, disclosed that Recombivax HB was mislabeled and it contained AAHS and not aluminum hydroxide, a completely different compound. It said that the vaccine had purportedly "always" contained AAHS.[32] Was the adjuvant changed in 1999, or was Merck earlier unaware of the consequences of its production process when it claimed that

Recombivax HB used aluminum hydroxide? Unlike Gardasil, in which the VLPs are added to "preformed" AAHS,[33] in Recombivax HB, AAHS appears to be a result of the vaccine production process, but there is no mention of aluminum hydroxide.[34] One has to wonder how the Recombivax HB adjuvant mix-up could have occurred and, if aluminum hydroxide was swapped out for AAHS, a very different adjuvant (see Chapter 20), why FDA did not require Merck to conduct new clinical trials for what amounted to a new vaccine.

The Recombivax HB package insert now reads: "All formulations contain approximately 0.5 mg of aluminum (provided as amorphous aluminum hydroxyphosphate sulfate, previously referred to as aluminum hydroxide) per mL of vaccine."[35] Even that change—by using the phrase "previously referred to"—gives the impression that the two adjuvants are comparable, when they are not. Dr. Lee and Norma still await changes to Gardasil's package insert to reflect the HPV DNA fragments bound to AAHS in the vial.

By the end of 2012, through their collaboration, Dr. Lee and Norma had proven that Gardasil vaccines contained viral HPV DNA fragments and that those fragments appeared to have played a role in a teenager's death. Norma had been able to publicize these findings and even wrest an FDA admission and advisory. But what if the DNA fragments or the non-B conformation wasn't the worst part of this story?

Is Gardasil Using an Undisclosed Adjuvant?

Although Merck touts the immune-boosting properties of AAHS, Dr. Lee's research suggests that AAHS alone is not strong enough to elicit high antibody titers from HPV L1 VLPs. Dr. Lee argues that recombinant HPV vaccines need an additional adjuvant-like component, known as a toll-like receptor (TLR) agonist, to trigger necessary cytokine reactions at the cellular level.[36] In most vaccinations, the host's dying DNA or DAMPs (Damage-Associated Molecular Patterns), which are released at the injection site, activate this TLR process, tripping the biological mechanism to induce immunity.[37]

Unlike with other vaccines, Dr. Lee theorized that with Gardasil, free DNA from the DAMPs is insufficient to activate the body's natural TLR agonists to trigger the intended immune response. Therefore, Gardasil needs an additional adjuvant to work. AAHS needs a specific TLR agonist, such as a phospholipid or a DNA molecule, to cause the host to respond strongly enough against the invading VLPs to create antibodies.[38] In essence, what Dr. Lee is saying is that the vaccine, as it is described by the FDA and Merck, would not produce the desired result. It needs another boost, a TLR 9 agonist, for the body to create the necessary antibodies to work.

Only a few other vaccines use the same VLP technology as Gardasil, and those vaccines have disclosed TLR agonists. Merck's recombinant hepatitis B vaccine Recombivax HB uses the phospholipid component of the hepatitis B surface antigen as a built-in TLR agonist.[39] For Cervarix, GSK combined aluminum hydroxide with a TLR4 agonist known as monophosphoryl lipid A (MPL) to form the AS04 adjuvant "system" to sufficiently enhance the innate immune response. These are all different mechanisms, and they are disclosed in the description of the vaccine.[40]

So what about Gardasil? What is the TLR agonist that enables the HPV VLPs to ignite the chain reaction to mount an immune response? Gardasil does not have a declared phospholipid like Recombivax HB or Cervarix. As we now know, Dr. Lee found recombinant HPV DNA fragments in *every* vial of Gardasil he has tested. Could these DNA fragments be undisclosed TLR9 agonists? Dr. Lee believes they are. The viral DNA and the AAHS may be combining to create the strongest immune-boosting adjuvant in use in any vaccine. Moreover, it's one the FDA has never approved.

Dr. Lee further considers that this TLR9 agonist made up of the viral DNA could be promoting autoimmune illnesses in susceptible people because of its sustained TLR9 stimulation, which is associated with many autoimmune syndromes.[41] He hypothesizes that the DNA fragments may also be in non-B conformation, making them even harder for the host's enzymatic system to degrade.

Is there any evidence that Merck may have known that the DNA fragments in the vaccine could act as a TLR9 agonist? Is it conceivable that Merck chose not to disclose what it knew to the FDA? We know that Merck filed patent number CA2280839A1 in 1997 to develop this kind of vaccine adjuvant technology.[42] The term TLR9 was not widely used at the time and does not appear in the patent, but the language suggests that this was indeed a patent for just such a product. The patent shows that Merck was aware that free DNA could bind in non-B conformation to an adjuvant, resist enzyme-induced degradation, and amplify the immune response.[43] *Business Wire* also published a press release in 2006 announcing the joint venture between Merck and a company called Idera Pharmaceuticals.[44] They formed a collaboration to research, develop, and commercialize TLR agonists for vaccines being developed by Merck for cancer and infectious diseases.

Dr. Lee has submitted this information as expert testimony in a vaccine injury case and to a global online scientific forum.[45] Given Dr. Lee's track record in making new scientific discoveries about Gardasil, the wider scientific community should take note.

20.

ALUMINUM-CONTAINING
ADJUVANTS: FUELING
THE FIRE?

"[T]he toxicology of vaccines, not to mention the toxicology of adjuvants, has been a really neglected area." [1] *Dr. Jesse L. Goodman, former Director of FDA's CBER, 2008*

In Chapter 7, we introduced readers to the aluminum-containing fauxcebos used in the HPV vaccine clinical trials. Now we return for a closer look at the science and health implications of injecting aluminum-containing adjuvants into children and young adults.

Many researchers and parents have questions about aluminum safety. Regulators' assurances about it contrast sharply with an ever-increasing body of science showing the dangers of injected aluminum. Vaccine program stakeholders like the FDA, CDC, and WHO argue that vaccines contain such small amounts of aluminum that they cannot be toxic. [2] Some vaccine proponents point out that we consume far more aluminum in food and medications than we get in vaccines. [3] These statements oversimplify the complex issues surrounding aluminum toxicity, particularly in vaccines.

ALUMINUM IS EVERYWHERE

Aluminum is ubiquitous. Industry continues to mine and refine aluminum to meet demands for its wide-ranging uses. Aluminum is in everything from airplanes to deodorant. It is in makeup and lotions, in drugs, and in food storage and preparation materials like foil and cans. We are living in what some have called "The Age of Aluminum."[4] Abundance, however, is not equivalent to safety.

Dr. Christopher Exley, of the UK's Keele University, is one of the world's foremost aluminum toxicity experts. He has spent more than thirty years researching aluminum and has serious concerns about its health effects. As he describes: "My research career (1984–present) has focused upon an intriguing paradox; 'how come the third most abundant element of the Earth's crust (aluminium) is non-essential and largely inimical to life?'"[5] Bound in the earth's crust with silicon, aluminum may be relatively safe because it is inaccessible—as Dr. Exley says, it is "effectively excluded from the biosphere"[6]—but what happens when it is no longer sequestered?

Aluminum compounds become biologically active when unbound from silicon and removed from the earth's crust. Aluminum accumulates in the environment and does not return to the earth's crust. We are exposed to "an ever increasing burden of potentially biologically available aluminium."[7] Not only does aluminum have no known biological benefit,[8] but a growing body of research recognizes that aluminum is a toxin, impairing many important biological functions and causing adverse effects in humans, as well as plants and animals.[9]

WHY ARE ALUMINUM-CONTAINING ADJUVANTS IN VACCINES?

An adjuvant is the immune reaction kick-starter in a vaccine. It stimulates an immune response[10] when a vaccine does not have a live or attenuated antigen and instead is "killed" or inactivated. Live or attenuated virus vaccines such as the measles-mumps-rubella vaccine do not need an adjuvant because the immune system will already be able to recognize the viral proteins. For vaccines requiring adjuvants, aluminum-based ones are the primary choice today for pediatric vaccines. Antibody levels (or titers) are one way to measure whether the immune system has responded to the vaccine.

In 1989 Dr. Charles A. Janeway, Jr., a noted immunologist, referred to adjuvants as "the immunologist's dirty little secret."[11] He asked the question, "Why do we need to use adjuvants?" and answered it straightforwardly: "To be honest, the answer is not known."[12]

He went on to discuss the likely reasons adjuvants are needed, including the need for "effective antigen uptake into macrophages," white blood cells that clean up debris and other matter from our bodies, and the "provision of co[-]stimulatory activity."[13] Though Dr. Janeway made these comments almost three decades ago, our understanding of the immune system is still far from complete, and new discoveries continue. Given this, it is not surprising that even those with expertise in immunology and adjuvants acknowledge "[t]he adjuvant action of aluminum appears to be complex and is not yet fully understood."[14] So then how can the FDA, WHO, and other regulators be confident aluminum compounds are safe in vaccines when scientists are not even sure how they work?

IS ALUMINUM SAFE?

"Aluminum is considered to be an essential metal with quantities fluctuating naturally during normal cellular activity. It is found in all tissues and is also believed to play an important role in the development of a healthy fetus."[15] *Children's Hospital of Philadelphia Vaccine Education Center, Statement Reviewed by Dr. Paul Offit, April 2013*

Dr. Exley says point blank: "It has never been demonstrated that aluminium is safe," and he has been critical of those who stridently profess that aluminum plays a positive role in health.[16] The case continues to mount that aluminum—even ingested—is dangerous. Aluminum exposure seems to play a role in a number of diseases, including autoimmune diseases.[17] Scientists also have associated aluminum with breast cancer[18] and Alzheimer's disease.[19] Contrary to the statement above, which the Children's Hospital of Philadelphia has since removed from its website, recent studies indicate that aluminum may have negative effects in fetuses and newborns.[20] While not directly related to lower consumer exposures to aluminum, the International Agency for Research on Cancer classifies occupational exposures in aluminum production as cancer-causing.[21]

Dr. Exley is far from alone in his criticism of aluminum. Dr. Suzanne Humphries, a nephrologist (kidney specialist), maintains "aluminum is toxic to all life forms." Drs. Christopher Shaw and Lucija Tomljenovic, researchers who have extensively studied vaccines and aluminum for a number of years, suggest that aluminum is not only neurotoxic—it is toxic to *many* body functions and processes.[22]

Yet the FDA says aluminum salts are "generally regarded as safe" (GRAS status) in food.[23] This seems to further justify their use in vaccines. Those who maintain that aluminum in vaccines is safe point out that in the first six months of life, infants consume more aluminum in breast milk or formula than they get in vaccines.[24] For example, in a widely circulated video, Dr. Paul Offit said, "there is algorithmically so much more aluminum that you ingest that you actually have far more aluminum in your circulation because of what you eat and drink than you would ever get from a vaccine."[25]

Even if aluminum is safe to consume at some level—an assumption that recent research challenges[26]—that doesn't mean that injected aluminum is necessarily safe. Simply comparing the amounts of aluminum in food with the amount in vaccines fails to acknowledge the biological difference between ingesting and injecting.[27] When we eat aluminum, very little is absorbed (.01 percent to 5 percent)[28] into the bloodstream because it passes through the digestive system unabsorbed, gets filtered by the liver and kidneys, and is excreted. When injected, aluminum bypasses the protective processes of the gut, and we essentially absorb 100 percent. The 2013 study by Dr. Tammy Movsas and colleagues, reporting that there was little aluminum in infants' blood or urine following vaccination, hardly exonerates aluminum. Rather, it begs the question of where all the injected aluminum-containing adjuvants went.[29]

Aluminum's toxicity to individuals with low kidney clearance, including dialysis patients and premature babies, is well established. In fact, the FDA mandates that package inserts for certain forms of intravenous nutrition used for premature babies include a warning, that the product "contains aluminum that may be toxic. Aluminum may reach toxic levels with prolonged parenteral administration if kidney function is impaired."[30]

Despite its own toxicity warnings on IV nutrition products, the FDA presumes the safety of aluminum in vaccine adjuvants. Presumption of product safety based on long-term use is dangerous. Still, the FDA contends that aluminum-containing adjuvants are safe because aluminum salts have been used in vaccines since 1926.[31] This presumption does not recognize, among other things, the different, more immune stimulatory aluminum-based adjuvants used today as well as the many more vaccines on today's immunization schedules. Even so, the debate over the safety of aluminum-containing adjuvants is not new.[32] Indeed, going back to the 1920s, scientists knew that injecting aluminum was potentially harmful. Testifying before the Federal Trade Commission in hearings concerning alum in baking powder, Dr. Victor C. Vaughan, a toxicologist from the University of Michigan, stated, "[a]ll salts of aluminum are poisonous when injected subcutaneously or intravenously. . . . My conclusion is that the salts of aluminum are harmful in the human body."[33] At the same hearing, Dr. Harry Gideon Wells, Professor of Pathology, University of Chicago, testified that "[w]hen injected into the tissue so that it comes in contact with living cells, it is found to be a virulent poison" and noted that it caused injury to the nervous system, even when ingested.[34]

A few decades later, in the 1950s and 1960s, the UK and Canada recommended using aluminum-free vaccines, while, conversely, the US began to advise using aluminum-adjuvanted vaccines.[35] The US stance obviously prevailed. In 2000, Dr. John Clements of the WHO explained that because the public did not perceive aluminum to be dangerous, regulators were "in a much more comfortable wicket in terms of defending its presence in vaccines."[36] Since then, as evidence of aluminum's toxicity has mounted, that position should be much less comfortable.

Dr. Derek O'Hagan (then of Novartis Vaccines and Diagnostics and later head of Global Discovery Support and New Technologies at GSK Vaccines) noted in 2008 that adjuvants should be comprised of materials that are "biodegradable and biocompatible."[37] Aluminum-containing adjuvants seem to fail these criteria. Unlike ingested aluminum, most of which healthy people excrete efficiently, injected aluminum persists in the body. While scientists previously thought we quickly excreted injected aluminum,[38] recent research demonstrates the opposite is true. Injected aluminum remains in the body—perhaps for a decade, or longer, following vaccination.[39] Aluminum nanoparticles combine with certain cells, becoming long-lived cells impeding aluminum's ability to dissolve or be excreted.[40] The brain and nervous system seem particularly susceptible to the damaging inflammatory processes of aluminum.[41]

Aluminum has the ability to disrupt many biological systems. It acts on both the immune system and the central nervous system separately and synergistically.[42] By stimulating certain types of immune responses, aluminum-containing adjuvants can even "set up an individual for allergic reactions to vaccine components," and aluminum-adjuvanted vaccines may even induce a contact allergy to aluminum.[43] The extent of aluminum's toxic impact depends on factors including: the form and size of aluminum particles, the method of administration, concentration, duration of exposure, proximity of repeated exposures, age, and genetics.[44] In a peer-reviewed article published in early 2018, Dr. Exley and his colleagues discovered extraordinarily high levels of aluminum in donor brain tissue from five deceased individuals with autism.[45] Particularly for the youngest donors, the levels appear unprecedented.[46] For example, researchers found aluminum levels in a 15-year-old boy's tissue comparable to samples in an individual almost three times as old with familial Alzheimer's disease[47]—a disease in which aluminum and genetic predisposition appear to play a role in etiology.[48]

Are apparently healthy young people with normal kidney function—the children and young adults receiving HPV vaccines—at risk, as well? As we dig deeper, research is mounting that aluminum-containing adjuvants have the potential to do great harm.

ARE ALUMINUM-CONTAINING ADJUVANTS SAFE?

"[P]ervasive uncertainty" . . . is a term that I think describes issues relating to things such as . . . aluminum and trying to assess the potential hazard and risk."[49] Dr. Martin Meyers, acting director of the National Vaccine Program Office, 2000

Researchers in the United States, Canada, the UK, France, Israel, and elsewhere continue to publish groundbreaking results that challenge assumptions about aluminum safety. This research is long overdue.

While aluminum-containing adjuvants have been used in vaccines for decades, no comprehensive safety studies against placebos exist. As Dr. Exley points out, "[t]here are no clinically-approved aluminium adjuvants only clinically approved vaccines which use aluminium adjuvants."[50] Under FDA regulations, manufacturers submit an entire vaccine formulation for licensure, not individual components.[51] The FDA considers the viral antigen to be the only "active" ingredient in vaccines. It treats the adjuvant as an "added" or an "inactive" ingredient, even though its entire purpose is to cause action, i.e., to stimulate the immune system.[52] Adjuvant safety claims are not based on rigorous safety analyses. A purported "good track record"[53] for a few forms of aluminum salts has been generalized to cover all aluminum containing adjuvants, no matter how different these substances may be.

Scientists in and outside the vaccine industry acknowledge "inclusion of an adjuvant in a vaccine must always be justified."[54] Is an adjuvant justified merely because it increases antibody production? Federal regulations require that "[a]n adjuvant shall not be introduced into a product unless there is satisfactory evidence that it does not affect adversely the *safety* or potency of the product."[55] (Emphasis added.) How do manufacturers comply with this regulation in the absence of safety testing?

Under FDA regulations, aluminum-containing vaccines are considered safe with up to 0.85 mg of aluminum per dose.[56] The FDA did not establish its upper limit on aluminum in vaccines on the basis of safety trials, however. In fact, in May 2000, when he was asked how this limit was determined, [the FDA's] Dr. Norman Baylor responded:

> Unfortunately, I could not. I mean, we have been trying to figure that out. We have been trying to figure that out as far as going back in the historical records and determining how they came up with that and going back to the preamble to the regulation. We have just been unsuccessful with that but we are still trying to figure that out.[57]

It is troubling that the FDA could not explain how it determined a supposedly safe level of an adjuvant for injection into newborn infants, among others. But, even more worrisome, it turns out that this limit appears unrelated to safety. A little more than a year after this meeting, Dr. Baylor and his colleagues at the FDA reported that "[t]he amount of 15 mg of alum or 0.85 mg aluminum per dose was selected empirically from data that demonstrated that this amount of aluminum enhanced the antigenicity and effectiveness of the vaccine."[58] In short, it appears that FDA put in place the 0.85 limit because data demonstrated that it enhanced the ability of the vaccine antigen to stimulate the production of antibodies, not safety.[59] The upper limit is also an estimate based on an average daily dosage over time and not doses administered at key points in time, such as the dose intervals CDC recommends in its vaccine schedule. Finally, the upper limit also does not take into consideration any aluminum buildup potentially remaining in the body from previous aluminum-containing vaccines or other exposures.

In 2004, the WHO recognized that "[a]djuvant safety is an important and neglected field."[60] What have regulators done in the interim? Instead of conducting safety testing of adjuvants—especially newer ones—the FDA, EMA and other regulators approved Gardasil and Cervarix with potent adjuvants lacking evidence of safety in humans.

In December 2008, two years after the FDA approved Gardasil, the US government convened a "Workshop on Adjuvants and Adjuvanted Preventive and Therapeutic Vaccines for Infectious Disease Indications."[61] The Workshop brought together experts from the FDA, CDC, WHO, the pharmaceutical industry, research institutions, and the Gates Foundation, among others, to discuss the then-current state of affairs on adjuvant research, including safety issues. Despite the experience of those gathered, they admitted that adjuvants' mechanisms to produce immunity are not well understood and that researchers have been "relatively negligent" about adjuvant toxicity.[62]

During that workshop, the FDA's Dr. Jesse Goodman acknowledged that it did not have evidence on correlation between vaccines that caused symptoms such as fever or a site-specific reaction, like soreness, and serious adverse events, including neurological ones.[63] In fact, he noted that it would be difficult to find that correlate. Just because there is no evidence of a link, however, one cannot assume it doesn't exist. He noted that "there are very few of these studies with adequate numbers of controls with long-term follow up or with children."[64] As vaccine manufactures use increasingly immunogenic adjuvants, it is also important to understand more about the interaction between how adjuvants combined with antigens stimulate the immune system and mechanisms that may cause adverse outcomes.[65]

What is aluminum adjuvant safety based on? The answer is, surprisingly little. A recent review article by Masson et al. analyzed the three main studies upon which many aluminum adjuvant proponents rely to support the safety of aluminum-containing adjuvants.[66] This analysis, funded partially by French government agencies, along with a US nonprofit, demonstrates again the paucity of sound toxicokinetic research supporting the use of aluminum-containing adjuvants. Toxicokinetics studies absorption, distribution, metabo-lization, and excretion of chemicals and toxins, mostly in animal models.[67] The authors of the review detail the shortcomings of each of the three studies analyzed and reach the inevitable conclusion that toxicokinetic research to date has failed to appropriately assess the "real life" risks of aluminum-containing adjuvants to humans.[68] As such, the authors called for new and better studies of both tradi-tional and newer aluminum-based adjuvants.[69]

Proponents of aluminum-containing adjuvants often argue that the dose of aluminum in any vaccine is too low to cause damage. They should take note of important recent research from a global co-alition of scientific experts on aluminum (some of whom authored the above discussed critique) that challenges the toxicology adage that "the dose makes the poison," the very foundations of the argu-ment made by the FDA and other vaccine proponents that "low" doses of aluminum-containing adjuvants are safe. In "Non-linear dose-response of aluminum hydroxide adjuvant particles: Selective low dose neurotoxicity," published in 2017, Guillemette Crépeaux and others examined a number of outcomes in mice to assess the toxicity and transport of aluminum hydroxide.[70] While not used in any of the HPV vaccines and thus not directly applicable, it is a common adjuvant in other vaccines. The results of this study sug-gest that all aluminum-containing adjuvant should receive rigorous examination.[71]

The researchers injected dosages of 200, 400, and 800 mcg/kg (micrograms per kilogram of body weight) of the adjuvant, which translates to the mice receiving the equivalent "of 2, 4 and 8 human doses of Al-containing vaccine" using a recommended conversion method.[72] They injected the mice three times with a four-day inter-val between doses.[73] The researchers found that the *lowest* dosages (i.e., those closer to human vaccine doses) were most toxic because that aluminum traveled most readily away from the injection site.[74] At higher dosages, mice formed what are called granulomas at the injection site. Granulomas are nodules composed of macrophages that effectively "wall off" a toxin or infection, thus stopping at least some of the adjuvant from migrating to the brain or elsewhere.

The potential implications of this study are tremendous for childhood vaccination. The researchers concluded that comparing injected aluminum exposure to other routes of exposure (e.g., oral) or types of aluminum (e.g., soluble) may not be valid and noted that "[in] the context of massive development of vaccine-based strategies worldwide, the present study may suggest that aluminium adjuvant toxicokinetics and safety require reevaluation."[75] This should have been a wake-up call to public health agencies concerning the safety of aluminum in vaccines. More recently, another peer-reviewed study challenges the foundation upon which aluminum safety is based and identifies a number of missteps by US regulatory authorities that raise serious safety questions.[76]

Dr. Romain Gherardi is the former director of the Neuromuscular Pathology Expert Centre at the Université Paris-Est and remains a professor there. He is a world-recognized expert in aluminum toxicity and aluminum-containing adjuvants. Dr. Gherardi also was one of the authors of the study on nonlinear dose-response. Faced with mounting evidence concerning aluminum safety, he wrote to the heads of US Health & Human Services, the NIH, the FDA, and the CDC in June 2017.[77] In his letter, he stated: "I solemnly declare that more research on the role of aluminum adjuvant in vaccines and neurological disorders . . . is essential and urgently required."[78] From all available indications, a year later—with even more studies demonstrating aluminum's neurotoxicity—these regulatory agencies, instead of acknowledging and investigating Dr. Gherardi's concerns and those raised by numerous peer-reviewed studies, continue to conduct business as usual with respect to aluminum-containing adjuvants.

So why do the FDA and other regulatory agencies still allow these adjuvants—particularly new, more powerful aluminum-based adjuvants or adjuvant systems containing aluminum—despite evidence raising concerns about safety?

In a 2004 review of aluminum adjuvants and DTP vaccines, Cochrane Vaccine Field researchers Tom Jefferson and colleagues concluded, despite acknowledging "a lack of good-quality evidence," that further research on aluminum-adjuvanted vaccines was unwarranted: "We doubt whether there is sufficient evidence to support further research on the topic or a potentially far-reaching decision such as the replacement of aluminum salt in vaccines."[79] The authors acknowledged that "[e]vidence on the adverse effects of aluminum salts is not plentiful, despite their ubiquitous and long-standing use as adjuvants."[80] Jefferson acknowledged in the conflicts of interest statement at the end of the review that he owned "shares in GlaxoSmithKline, manufacturer of some aluminium-containing vaccines" but stated that GSK had no role in the review.[81]

Based on the authors' own recognition of the limited scope of available evidence, it is puzzling that they suggested that further research was unwarranted. Were researchers concerned about the potential implications of what they might discover? They acknowledged:

> Assessment of the safety of aluminium in vaccines is important because replacement of aluminium compounds in currently licensed vaccines would necessitate the introduction of a completely new compound that would have to be investigated before licensing. No obvious candidates to replace aluminium are available, so withdrawal for safety reasons would severely affect the immunogenicity and protective effect of some currently licensed vaccines and threaten immunization programmes worldwide.[82]

Dr. Christopher Exley, criticizing this review, pointed out more than a decade ago[83] that it should be obvious that the mere fact that aluminum has been in longtime use in vaccines does not necessarily prove that it is safe. Only well-designed safety studies can prove this. In addition, researcher Elizabeth Hart from Australia has been one of the more vocal critics of the 2004 study, calling repeatedly for its retraction.[84] While, as she notes,[85] Jefferson has since acknowledged the potential neurotoxicity of aluminum,[86] defenders of aluminum adjuvants still rely on this review to exonerate the adjuvants.

Even at the Cochrane Collaboration, the door may remain open on the issue. Cochrane recently released a protocol for its forthcoming review of "[a]luminum adjuvants used in vaccines versus placebo or no intervention."[87] This new review purports to be a comprehensive review of aluminum-containing adjuvants used in vaccines. Indeed, the protocol recognizes specific concerns about HPV vaccines.[88] It remains to be seen if this review will answer questions left open by the 2004 review. Given that HPV vaccines have shed new light on aluminum concerns, we await results. The US and EU have approved few adjuvants, and even then only as part of the vaccine, not separately.[89] The review protocol again raises concerns about "the lack of suitable alternatives" if evidence demonstrates that aluminum adjuvants are unsafe.[90]

Both the 2004 review and the protocol for the forthcoming review highlight real-world implications for vaccine manufacturers and public health authorities if some or all aluminum adjuvants are determined to be unsafe. The question must be asked, Can we ignore questions about the safety of injected aluminum to protect immunization programs rather than ask those questions to protect those who receive vaccines? This issue echoes the FDA's concerns with protecting the US vaccine program when questions were raised about the polio vaccine in the mid-1980s: "any possible doubts, whether or not well founded, about the safety of the vaccine cannot be allowed to exist in view of the need to assure that that vaccine will continue to be used to the maximum extent consistent with the nation's public health."[91]

Almost a decade after the WHO's statement, Dr. Exley and fellow aluminum experts Romain Gherardi, François-Jérôme Authier, and others concluded in a 2013 study that aluminum "has high neurotoxic potential, and planning administration of continuously escalating doses of this poorly biodegradable adjuvant in the population should be carefully evaluated by regulatory agencies since the compound may be insidiously unsafe."[92] The WHO's safety rhetoric seems at odds with the continued absence of adjuvant safety studies. Dr. Exley was spot-on when he said, "[i]t is a sobering thought that aluminum adjuvants have not had to pass any of the safety trials that would be expected of any drug or treatment . . . .until the requisite research is carried out it is misleading to conclude that aluminum adjuvants are safe for all to use."[93]

ALL ALUMINUM-CONTAINING ADJUVANTS ARE NOT CREATED EQUAL

"Toxicity increases with potency. If you want a better adjuvant, you can expect to get some more toxicities with it."[94] *Dr. Robert Hunter (University of Texas at Houston), 2000.*

The FDA appears to base its safety presumption on the false premise that all aluminum-containing adjuvants are the same. This is not the case at all. Different adjuvants have different chemical formulations and unique physical and functional attributes. To that point, the adjuvants in the Gardasil variants and Cervarix have different formulations with different properties. Unlike many older adjuvants, the adjuvants from the two manufacturers are highly immunogenic,[95] which also suggests they may be likely to cause local and systemic adverse events by provoking long-term immune responses.[96] Even vaccine proponents like Dr. Baylor acknowledge that adjuvants lack "universality."[97] Scientists, and regulators like the EMA, recognize that different aluminum-containing adjuvants have varying physical properties and antigen-binding characteristics.[98] Studies on one won't necessarily translate to others.[99] So too an adjuvant that appears to be safe and effective with one antigen may not necessarily be safe or effective with a different one.[100]

Thus, regulators should not impute the apparent safety of one aluminum-containing adjuvant to others. Nor should the safety of a vaccine containing a unique antigen/adjuvant combination be presumed, even if the adjuvant appeared safe in combination with other antigens.[101] In other words, adjuvant safety assessment should be a two-step process: the adjuvant should be safe on its own, and it should then be demonstrated to be safe when combined with the specific antigen at issue. Neither Merck's AAHS nor GSK's AS04 meets these criteria.

Merck and GSK chose the adjuvants for their HPV vaccines because they purportedly elicited greater immune response than traditional aluminum-based adjuvants. For example, research led by Merck employees demonstrated in a mouse model that, for HPV 16 L1 VLPs, immunogenicity of the antigen was greatly affected by the type of aluminum-containing adjuvant used. AAHS was the most immunogenic of the three aluminum-based adjuvants researchers compared.[102] Moreover, AAHS is a nanoscale adjuvant with higher surface area to volume ratio than the traditional aluminum-based adjuvants with larger-sized particles.[103] The nanoparticles make AAHS more potent and also potentially more able to cross the blood-brain barrier.[104] Additionally, as discussed in Chapter 19, the DNA fragments in Gardasil may act as a TLR9 agonist to create a stronger adjuvant when bonding to AAHS.

Yet research concerning the safety of AAHS and AS04 appears lacking, both for the adjuvants separately and in combination with the HPV antigens—as demonstrated by the problematic safety data collection and assessment during the clinical trials, as we discuss in Part I. As the EMA recognizes: "Unpredictability of adjuvant effects in humans results from a complex interplay between such factors as route of administration, antigen dose and the nature of the antigen. For this reason, a final safety evaluation of the newly developed vaccine formulation can only be conducted on the basis of clinical trials."[105] In that regard, the failure of the clinical trials for these vaccines to adequately assess safety is significant.

Cervarix was the first vaccine approved in the US using "AS04," an adjuvant system based on combining two adjuvants: aluminum hydroxide and MPL, a lipid derived from a salmonella strain.[106] Still, the FDA did not require GSK to provide human safety studies showing that this supposedly "novel" adjuvant was safe. In fact, the researchers who carried out preclinical animal testing of AS04 in rabbits and rats admitted that evaluating autoimmune response—a known potential issue with adjuvanted vaccines—in particular was difficult in an animal model.[107] With no demonstrated safety for the various forms of aluminum-containing adjuvants used, the FDA allows these substances to be injected into infants, children, and adults.

Similarly, Merck claims that AAHS is proprietary.[108] The scientific literature describes AAHS as "a proprietary aluminum hydroxyphosphate sulfate formulation that is both physically and functionally distinct from traditional aluminum phosphate and aluminum hydroxide adjuvants."[109] Some sources even refer to it as "Merck Aluminum Adjuvant," or MAA.[110] We and others have been unable to find a patent for AAHS, and human safety testing data are not readily available, despite Merck's Dr. Patrick Brill-Edwards telling the FDA's VRBPAC that AAHS "has a well-established safety record."[111]

The FDA gives manufacturers an option to submit what is known as a "drug master file" for the adjuvant only, which typically includes, among other things, toxicology assessments for the adjuvant alone.[112] However, even where a master file is submitted, the the FDA apparently only refers to it when the product's sponsor makes reference to material contained in the drug master file.[113] When we asked the FDA to provide safety data concerning AAHS and AS04, it did not direct us to information from any master file. Instead, the FDA told us that its "evaluation of safety and effectiveness for both vaccines is available on FDA's website."[114] It then provided links to the approval documents for the vaccines but provided no information regarding safety studies for the adjuvants themselves. Similarly, the EMA, citing its own guidelines, approved Gardasil with no additional safety testing of the AAHS adjuvant required, apparently on the basis of AAHS's use in other earlier approved vaccines.[115]

Raising further questions about the purported proprietary nature of AAHS and its safety, researchers have found that some non-Merck vaccines were adjuvanted with AAHS or a very similar formulation, despite labeling to the contrary.[116] In particular, DTP vaccines have a long history of serious adverse events attributed to them, many of which were blamed on the whole cell pertussis endotoxins used in the vaccines.[117] Certain of these vaccines appear to have contained AAHS or a similar adjuvant, though undisclosed, which Dr. Suzanne Humphries posits could be at least partially responsible for some adverse events that continued to occur in some children even after the whole cell pertussis component was removed.[118] Dr. Humphries supports her theory with evidence that there still were severe reactions in some children who received only diphtheria and tetanus vaccines, containing the above adjuvants, without the pertussis component.[119]

Those who support continued use of aluminum-containing adjuvants in vaccines often rely on animal and epidemiological studies (frequently industry-funded) as "proof" of the safety of these adjuvants. These studies, whether animal or human, purporting to absolve aluminum adjuvants or vaccines (HPV vaccines in particular), especially for rarer conditions, such as autoimmune diseases, often are simply too small or poorly designed to detect a signal.[120] For example, many of these studies look at extremely short time frames, which will miss diseases or conditions that may not be symptomatic immediately following vaccination. A 2018 analysis of aluminum adjuvant toxicokinetic studies by Jean-Daniel Masson, Guillemette Crépeaux, François-Jérôme Authier, Christopher Exley, and Romain K. Gherardi emphasized the importance of finding "biological plausibility of a causal link."[121] As we have shown, the work of many scientists now provides mounting evidence of that biological plausibility, but a randomized and controlled trial on the safety aluminum adjuvants (and particularly on the adjuvants used in HPV vaccines) has yet to be done.[122]

The long-term health consequences of aluminum—and particularly of aluminum-containing adjuvants—are potentially devastating. Moreover, accepting aluminum as safe and allowing the use of aluminum-containing adjuvants as "controls" in the HPV vaccine clinical trials may have resulted in "an underestimation of the true rate of adverse outcomes associated with aluminum-adjuvanted vaccines."[123] As Drs. Tomljenovic and Shaw have stated: "a comprehensive evaluation of the overall impact of aluminum on human health is overdue."[124]

21.

WHAT ELSE IS IN THE VIAL?

Aluminum-containing adjuvants feature prominently in the HPV vaccine debate, as we learned in the last chapter and in Chapter 7. With Gardasil as the main focus, we must look more closely at what is actually in the vial, as the aluminum-containing adjuvant is not the only ingredient critics are concerned about. Gardasil and Gardasil 9 also contain polysorbate 80, sodium borate, L-histidine, and genetically modified yeast—ingredients that were included in all of the so-called "placebo" formulations in the Gardasil clinical trials. As is the case with VLPs, there is insufficient research on these substances, particular as used and injected into humans, in vaccines. In assessing the safety of vaccines, we must consider the potential health risks of all components of the vaccine.

Governmental agencies that should be protecting us seem to have bypassed safety requirements for these other ingredients. For example, the FDA does not mention safety on ingredients other than adjuvants: "All ingredients used in a licensed product, and any diluent provided as an aid in the administration of the product, shall meet generally accepted standards of purity and quality."[1] Purity and quality certainly are important, but where is the requirement that vaccine manufacturers demonstrate the safety of these injected ingredients? Vaccine manufacturers are permitted to use ingredients in vaccines without evidence that they are safe to inject into humans and are only required to study the vaccine as a whole during clinical trials.

Regarding Gardasil 9, there are even more questions. The EMA commented on certain "adventitious agents" used during the fermentation process and questioned their source in its preclinical review. For example, the EMA asked the manufacturers to provide the source for L-galactose and L-tyrosine because they were derived from animal or human sources.[2] The public may be surprised to learn that the L-tyrosine "is extracted from human hair sourced from China or from poultry feathers."[3] These are not ingredients one would expect during the vaccine's manufacturing process, but if the EMA is seeking clarification that these agents come from a reputable source to rule out the risk of transmitting spongiform encephalopathy (mad cow disease), then should the public be concerned, as well?

Given the dearth of research on these ingredients as vaccine components, out of necessity we rely on research about other routes of exposure (such as ingesting) and doses, and research in animals, recognizing that there are obvious shortcomings with such comparisons. Given the limited research available, regulators and manufacturers should redouble efforts to demonstrate the safety of these ingredients independent of the vaccine as well as in the vaccine.

POLYSORBATE 80

Gardasil and Gardasil 9 (but not Cervarix) contain a substance called polysorbate 80. You may never have heard of polysorbate 80, but you likely have regular exposure to this multipurpose chemical compound. Polysorbate 80 is used primarily in food, cosmetics, and pharmaceuticals—including vaccines.[4] There are several ways in which polysorbate 80 could potentially be problematic in vaccines.

What is Polysorbate 80?

In food, polysorbate 80 acts as a binder and emulsifier, lessening separation and giving food a creamy, smooth texture. It even slows down ice cream from melting. Polysorbate 80 is approved by the FDA and is "generally regarded as safe" for many food uses—everything from frozen desserts to spiced canned green beans and a great deal in between—in varying amounts depending on the specific food product.[5] If you eat a diet emphasizing prepared foods, you likely consume polysorbate 80 regularly.

The "food" approval for polysorbate 80 also extends beyond what you might expect. Pursuant to FDA regulations, polysorbate 80 can be added to herbicides to treat crops.[6] In cosmetics, other personal care products, and cleaners, polysorbate 80 (and other polysorbates) help disperse oil in water and help dissolve and blend ingredients. Polysorbate 80 is added to some drugs to aid delivery of active ingredients to the brain.[7] In vaccines like Gardasil and Gardasil 9, polysorbate 80 serves as a stabilizer, surfactant, and emulsifier—it keeps the various components of the vaccine evenly distributed in the liquid.

Opening the Blood-Brain Barrier

The blood-brain barrier (BBB) is a membrane that serves to separate the brain and central nervous system from the circulating blood system. The BBB stops or restricts passage of substances from our bloodstream to our brain and CNS. Polysorbate 80 is well known to breach the blood-brain barrier. In fact, polysorbate 80 is added to some drugs for the very purpose of opening up the blood-brain barrier to allow the active ingredients to cross into the brain and elicit the desired response or reaction.[8] If polysorbate 80 eases access across the BBB for drugs, it stands to reason that the same may be true for vaccine components, including VLPs and aluminum, which could then cross from the bloodstream into the brain. Researchers have found HPV L1 particles in brain tissue of girls who died following the vaccine.[9] Further, research has shown that macrophages may act as a kind of "Trojan Horse" mechanism, engulfing aluminum nanoparticles and carrying them into the brain across the BBB.[10] Cancer research concerning drug delivery systems also suggests that macrophages may be able to bypass the BBB to reach the brain.[11] The interplay between these two potential delivery mechanisms needs more research.

How Well Studied Is Polysorbate 80?

The bottom line is that polysorbate 80 is not well studied for toxicity or other harms in humans; and, in particular, no safety studies that we have found report on the effects of injecting polysorbate 80 into humans—though reports hint at potential problems.

The current safety data sheet for polysorbate 80 from manufacturer Sigma Aldrich describes it as "[n]ot a hazardous substance or mixture" but goes on to bluntly state: "[t]o the best of our knowledge, the chemical, physical, and toxicological properties have not been thoroughly investigated."[12] Similarly, the International Agency for Research on Cancer and other agencies and governmental oversight organizations do not recognize polysorbate 80 as a carcinogen. Yet the safety data sheet reports "equivocal" data concerning carcinogenicity and tumorigenic effects of polysorbate 80 in rodents.[13] In other words, the data aren't clear on whether polysorbate 80 is cancer-causing or not. The safety data sheet further notes that there are no data on reproductive toxicity.

Little is known about its potential to harm—especially when injected (versus ingested in food or applied topically in a cosmetic)—yet there are several biologically plausible ways that polysorbate 80 could cause or exacerbate harm.

Potential Pathways to Harm?

Cardiac Depressant

The drug amiodarone, a heart rhythm regulator, has long been known to result in hypotension (abnormally low blood pressure) in both humans and dogs, an effect that has been attributed to polysorbate 80, which is a component of IV amiodarone.[14] More than 30 years ago, researchers experimented with dogs to see if polysorbate 80 alone produced the same effects seen when patients were administered amiodarone.[15] In the polysorbate-only dosed dogs, they saw effects similar to those seen in humans and dogs treated with amiodarone, thus concluding that polysorbate 80 acts as a "potent depressant of the cardiac conduction system in the dog," causing steep blood pressure drops and decreased heart rate, among other effects.[16]

Reproductive Effects

There are a few studies on polysorbate 80 and rats, which may give clues as to a possible explanation of some reproductive adverse events in humans. Little research in humans is available, however.

While the data on the effects of polysorbate 80 on ovaries are limited, in at least two animal studies,[17] scientists demonstrated that injecting it into female rats caused ovarian damage, and feeding rats diets high (20 percent of the diet) in polysorbate 80 was ovary toxic. While available animal studies have significant limitations, including the strength of the solution injected and the dose of polysorbate 80 fed, they nonetheless suggest that we need to pay more attention to the reports of premature ovarian failure in young women who receive Gardasil.[18] Until scientists undertake more studies, we cannot dismiss the possibility of a biologically plausible link.

Proinflammatory

Recent studies have shown that in a mouse model, ingested polysorbate 80 is proinflammatory to the gut, alters the gut microbiota, and may potentially contribute to a rise in colon cancer, to metabolic syndrome, and to colitis, among other things.[19] While these studies were in rodents and the polysorbate 80 was dosed orally, the proinflammatory nature of polysorbate 80, particularly where it is given with another proinflammatory agent (aluminum), also calls for closer examination. If polysorbate 80 can cause inflammation in the gastrointestinal tract, can it also cause inflammation elsewhere in the body, including in the brain?

Sensitization and Anaphylaxis

We have found three published reports concerning potential polysorbate 80 hypersensitivity reactions to Gardasil. In 2012, Italian researchers published what they say is the first case of polysorbate 80 hypersensitivity causing a vaccine adverse reaction.[20] In this case study, skin tests confirmed that polysorbate 80 played a role in a seventeen-year-old girl's hypersensitivity reaction following her third Gardasil shot.[21] She experienced a variety of symptoms including hives, shortness of breath, wheezing, red eyes, swollen eyelids, and allergy-like nasal symptoms.[22] Notably, this young woman also had a significant medical history, including autoimmune thyroiditis, Type I diabetes, and seasonal rhinitis.[23] In concluding their case study presentation, the researchers noted that doctors "may be unaware of the ubiquitous presence of polysorbate 80 or of its potential biological and pharmacologic activity. Therefore, in cases of unclear hypersensitivity reactions, especially after [non-oral] administration of drugs," clinicians should consider the possibility of reactions to polysorbates.[24]

Two other reports come out of Australia. Shortly after school-based Gardasil programs were introduced, polysorbate 80 was implicated as a potential cause for anaphylactic reactions following vaccination.[25] Researchers identified seven cases of anaphylaxis. While still considered low, the rate of anaphylaxis following HPV vaccination (2.6/100,000) was substantially higher than that for other vaccines given in a school setting. Gardasil and Gardasil 9 inserts now caution providers to be prepared in case of an anaphylactic reaction.[26] In an accompanying commentary, Dr. Neal Halsey discounted the potential role of polysorbate 80 in causing such reactions but acknowledged further investigation was warranted.[27]

Similarly, the second Australian report, examining twenty-five girls with potential hypersensitivity reactions, found one case of anaphylaxis and another of delayed anaphylactic reaction (suggesting a non-IgE mediated reaction).[28] None of the girls studied was positive for an IgE allergy to polysorbate 80, but the investigators noted that other mechanisms of reactivity to polysorbate 80 and other components should be explored.[29]

Most recently, a 2014 case study implicated polysorbate 80 as a possible cause of anaphylaxis in a 64-year-old patient receiving IV amiodarone, the cardiac drug mentioned above.[30]

Given the ubiquitous presence of polysorbate 80 in prepared foods and medicines, sensitization to polysorbate 80 through vaccination is a plausible mechanism for such a reaction. Simply because there are no studies of injected polysorbate 80 in humans does not mean we can ignore the research available. At a minimum, the FDA should be able to point to research to show that injecting polysorbate 80 is safe. It has not done so.

SODIUM BORATE

Sodium borate, also known as borax, is a common ingredient in household cleaning products (such as laundry products), pest control products, and many industrial applications (including gold mining). It is not generally found in pediatric vaccines—with the exceptions of Gardasil, Gardasil 9, and VAQTA (a Hepatitis A vaccine also manufactured by Merck).[31] Gardasil and Gardasil 9 contain 25 mcg of this ingredient per dose. In the vaccines, sodium borate is added as a buffer, an ingredient added to maintain the pH of the vaccine.[32] We called Merck to ask about sodium borate's safety profile. Merck told us that that it can only provide a package insert for the vaccine and not safety information on each ingredient. No one at Merck could tell us why sodium borate was in the vaccine, at least not over the phone, and Merck has not responded to our written requests for information following up the telephone call.

Digging deeper, it turns out that not much seems to be known about sodium borate safety generally, let alone as a vaccine component for injection into humans. But what is known—and unknown—is concerning. The European Chemicals Agency hazard classification and labeling requires a "DANGER!" warning on borax and states that borax "may damage fertility or the unborn child."[33] Below is an example of a warning label on a European Borax product (99 percent pure):[34]

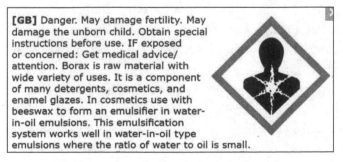

[GB] Danger. May damage fertility. May damage the unborn child. Obtain special instructions before use. IF exposed or concerned: Get medical advice/ attention. Borax is raw material with wide variety of uses. It is a component of many detergents, cosmetics, and enamel glazes. In cosmetics use with beeswax to form an emulsifier in water-in-oil emulsions. This emulsification system works well in water-in-oil type emulsions where the ratio of water to oil is small.

Source: see note 34 above.

Earlier we discussed the differences between ingesting and injecting aluminum and how ingested aluminum clears the body in a very different, quicker way than injected aluminum, which can be retained for extended periods of time in critical organs. Despite these differences, we noted broad (but troubling) assumptions that if aluminum is "safe" to ingest, it is safe to inject. Recent aluminum research shows these assumptions to be false, but, for the moment, let's just pretend they are true.

Would the converse also hold true? If a substance was not safe to ingest, should we still inject it without any further proof of safety? Not in the United States. A real-life example shows the absurdity of the FDA allowing injectable sodium borate. Borax is banned as a food additive in the United States.[35] In Europe, borax is allowed as an additive only in caviar, but not in any other food.[36] When asked about borax in caviar, the FDA responded to an inquiry as follows:

> The FDA has not evaluated the safe use of borax as direct additive in caviar or any food, nor have we evaluated its GRAS status for use in caviar. There is no allowed amount of borax that may be used in caviar sold in U.S. interstate commerce, regardless of where it is produced.[37]

So the FDA says we can inject borax without evaluating its safety, but we cannot eat borax without evaluation.

While we don't know if this small amount of borax can do any damage when injected into the human body, neither does anyone else, including the FDA. Symptoms of overdose or sodium borate toxicity, however, are quite similar to some reported Gardasil reactions: collapsing, fainting or loss of consciousness, convulsions or seizures, nausea, fever, dizziness, and skin irritations.[38] While oral toxicities occur at doses much higher than the amounts in Gardasil, the route of exposure needs to be considered, as well. Is it possible that a lower injected dose may cause an adverse reaction? The Material Data Safety Sheet for Sodium Borate states that information concerning carcinogenic effects, mutagenic effects, teratogenic effects, and developmental toxicity data is unavailable.[39]

As data from the European Food Safety Authority shows, there is evidence that sodium borate has adverse effects on male reproductive systems in rats, mice, and dogs.[40] Similarly, a report from the US Forest Service issued shortly before the FDA approved Gardasil found that "[r]esults of developmental, subchronic and chronic toxicity studies show that the primary targets for borate toxicity are the developing fetus and the male reproductive system. Regarding developmental effects, gestational exposure of rats, mice, and rabbits to boric acid resulted in increased fetal deaths, decreased in fetal weight, and increased fetal malformations."[41]

In short, we do not know the effects of injecting sodium borate in humans. This ingredient requires a warning label in Europe and is banned from food in the United States, yet the FDA approved a vaccine allowing it to be injected into millions of children and young adults. It points to a certain lack of oversight for vaccine ingredients. Out of an abundance of caution, until more research has been done, the FDA should not allow injectable sodium borate, in the same way that it bans ingestible sodium borate.

L-HISTIDINE

Gardasil is the first vaccine to contain L-histidine. Currently, Gardasil, Gardasil 9, and Bexsero (GSK's Meningococcal B vaccine) are the only vaccines licensed for use in the United States containing L-histidine or histidine. We know that L-Histidine is a vasodilator—it widens blood vessels in the body—but it's unclear what its role is in the vaccine.

L-histidine is an essential amino acid but is usually not produced in sufficient quantities by the human body.[42] Instead, we get L-histidine from our diets.[43] L-histidine is important in many bodily functions, including tissue repair and growth, blood cell production, and others, and appears to play a role in the development of embryos and organs in animal models.[44]

While there is scant data on L-histidine and vaccines, some have posited that L-histidine in Gardasil or Gardasil 9 may cause the immune system to malfunction, attacking the L-histidine in the body as if it were a foreign substance.[45] Notably, low L-histidine levels have been associated with autoimmune disease, particularly rheumatoid arthritis.[46]

L-histidine is a precursor of histamine, which is necessary to trigger inflammation to fight infections. However, histamine in excess can cause negative reactions; think of inflammation in allergic reactions. Excess histamine may also be involved in the development of some autoimmune diseases. Histamine has the potential to impact many different organs and systems in the body, including the nervous, respiratory, cardiac, and reproductive systems.[47] Here, where the vaccines are engineered to promote a high immune response, an allergy or hypersensitivity, for example, other components of the vaccine could result in a histamine release. A person then may develop or exacerbate histamine intolerance, the symptoms of which are similar to many experienced postvaccination with Gardasil, such as headache, fatigue, hives, dizziness, nausea, anxiety, and even menstrual and digestive issues.[48] L-histidine can cause a drop in blood pressure and has been associated with irregular heart rhythms and tachycardia (an excessively fast heartbeat). In short, there are a number of mechanisms by which L-histidine and histamine could potentially be associated with adverse outcomes.

YEAST

Gardasil is fermented in *Saccharomyces cerevisiae* (brewer's yeast). Merck excluded from the FUTURE II protocol anyone allergic to yeast.[49] Concerns about *Saccharomyces cerevisiae* go beyond allergies and include autoimmune illnesses, however. High levels of anti-*Saccharomyces cerevisiae* autoantibodies (ASCAs) are associated with Crohn's disease. There is a growing body of research associating ASCAs with other autoimmune conditions, including "antiphospholipid syndrome, systematic lupus erythematosus, type 1 diabetes mellitus, and rheumatoid arthritis."[50] Of particular interest, since autoimmune illnesses can take so long to diagnose, ASCAs may be present many years before a person finally obtains an autoimmune diagnosis.[51]

BENZONASE™

In the original protocol for FUTURE II, Merck included in its exclusion criteria "Individuals allergic to any vaccine component, including aluminum, yeast, or BENZONASE™ (nuclease, Nycomed [used to remove residual nucleic acids from this and other vaccines])."[52] This section—and the entire protocol—fails to mention known Gardasil ingredients such as polysorbate 80, sodium borate, and L-histidine. By contrast, Benzonase—an ingredient that does not appear (at least not easily locatable) in most documents concerning Gardasil and does not appear on the package insert as an ingredient—was listed as an allergen of concern.

Benzonase is, however, mentioned in a Merck patent for the purification of VLPs.[53] It is an enzyme that can break down, among other things, DNA fragments in a vaccine.[54] Benzonase is prepared using an E. coli expression system and contains trace amounts of "aerobic bacteria, yeasts, and molds."[55] If Benzonase is added early in the manufacturing process, any residual Benzonase should be purified out of the vaccine. If it is added later, does it totally degrade, and, if not, why is it not listed on the package insert? Or is Benzonase even used in Gardasil as marketed?

There is no evidence that we could locate concerning Benzonase toxicity, but apparently Merck was concerned about Benzonase allergies in the clinical trials and, for unknown reasons, apparently is not sufficiently concerned to list it in its package inserts.

GENETICALLY MODIFIED VACCINES

Many people have concerns about genetically modified (GM) foods and their effects on health. Foods at the grocery store have "non-GMO" labels because of this concern. Several legislatures have considered laws to require labeling of GMO ingredients, but what about GM vaccines? Some also use the term *genetically engineered* to describe these products, and the two are often used interchangeably. HPV vaccines are genetically modified or recombinant, meaning that they contain organisms that scientists have genetically recombined and manipulated.

Gardasil is not Merck's first genetically modified vaccine. Its hepatitis B vaccine, aptly named Recombivax HB, has been in use for decades and contains the same aluminum-based adjuvant as the HPV vaccine (though, as noted earlier in Chapter 19, there is some dispute concerning when AAHS first was used in the HepB vaccine). Approved in July 1986, Recombivax HB was the first genetically modified vaccine approved by FDA for use in humans.[56] Doctors routinely administer Recombivax HB to newborn babies, although little clinical trial data support its safety, and some studies suggest its association with neurodevelopmental harms.[57] Merck cultivates the hepatitis B and HPV VLPs in genetically modified yeast. Cervarix is cultivated on insect cells. And HPV vaccines won't be the last GM vaccines. Vaccine manufacturers have in the pipeline GM vaccines for malaria, Ebola, West Nile virus, and HIV, among others.[58]

Frankly, no one yet knows the long-term effects of GM vaccines. Vaccine advocates suggest there are no problems with genetic modification.[59] By contrast, Dr. Lee and others think there are many unanswered questions about recombinant DNA in vaccines.[60] He points out that genetically engineered DNA is known to behave differently from natural DNA. He believes that once recombinant DNA inserts itself into a human cell, the consequences are hard to predict.

The aluminum-containing adjuvants in Gardasil and Cervarix have garnered much-deserved attention, with concerns over aluminum mounting from both experts and the public. Many of the other components of the HPV vaccines need to be studied much more closely, as well. The assumed safety of these ingredients is troubling and potentially dangerous.

22.

HPV Vaccines, Autoimmunity, and Molecular Mimicry

"The number of viral matches and their locations makes the occurrence of side autoimmune cross-reactions in the human host following HPV16-based vaccination almost unavoidable."[1]
DR. DARJA KANDUC, UNIVERSITY OF BARI, ITALY (2009)

Many people, including scientists, are describing autoimmune diseases devastating once-healthy young people after HPV vaccination. We are learning of new syndromes and disorders we had never heard of before. Could these conditions be related to aluminum-containing adjuvants?

While the HPV vaccine clinical trials showed little difference in adverse outcomes between vaccine recipients and those who received aluminum-containing adjuvants as controls, this says nothing about the safety of injected aluminum. When aluminum-containing adjuvants bind with antigens, like HPV types—desirable from an antigenicity standpoint—it is more difficult for the body to excrete the aluminum.[2] AAHS, Merck's adjuvant, forms a chemical bond to antigens (unlike some aluminum-based adjuvants that form an electrostatic bond) and appears to have an "enhanced binding capacity."[3] Macrophages can engulf injected nanoparticles of the adjuvant and carry them across the blood-brain barrier and blood-cerebral spinal fluid barrier, inciting inflammatory responses and a cascade of neurological and other effects.[4] Dr. Humphries described AAHS as provoking an "immune system bonfire."[5] Repeated exposure to adjuvants and persistence of aluminum from adjuvants may lead to immune system hyperactivation and chronic inflammation.

Scientists worldwide are devoting themselves to the study of aluminum's deleterious effects. Dr. Romain Gherardi and his colleagues in France have studied aluminum-containing adjuvants related to a condition known as macrophagic myofasciitis (MMF), which causes a variety of debilitating symptoms including chronic fatigue and cognitive decline.[6] In 2011, Drs. Yehuda Shoenfeld and Nancy Agmon-Levin coined the acronym ASIA, Autoimmune Inflammatory Syndrome Induced by Adjuvants,[7] describing autoimmune symptoms recognized for some time.[8] ASIA encompasses a broad spectrum of neurological and autoimmune conditions following vaccination with aluminum-adjuvanted vaccines. Many of these conditions correspond to the "new medical conditions" reported after HPV vaccination.[9] The overlap is substantial: muscle weakness, joint pain, chronic fatigue and sleep disturbances, neurological symptoms, cognitive impairments, and fever, among others.[10]

The extensive independent research of Dr. Gherardi, Dr. Shoenfeld, and others into autoimmune disease and aluminum-containing adjuvants contrasts sharply with the work of industry-sponsored scientists. For example, in 2008, GSK's Thomas Verstraeten concluded that there was no increase in relative risk of autoimmune diseases after GSK AS04-adjuvanted vaccines.[11] "Controls" in this study received either aluminum hydroxide, a different aluminum-adjuvanted vaccine, or a nonadjuvanted vaccine, rather than an inert saline placebo.[12] The GSK-affiliated authors admit that their analysis was "not set up primarily to study autoimmune disorders, but mainly to evaluate the general safety profile of the vaccines, as well as their immunogenicity and/or efficacy."[13] But how can one really evaluate a general safety profile with a study design that lacks an inert control group? Furthermore, the industry-associated authors followed trial participants most closely for only fifteen days after each dose using self-reporting tools or "spontaneous reporting." Symptoms of autoimmune disorders may not manifest immediately, and autoimmune illnesses can take years to diagnose. The industry-sponsored trials were not designed to fully capture autoimmune signals.[14] On the contrary, one could argue that they were designed to hide potential autoimmune impacts.

Why do only some people develop autoimmune conditions while others seem fine? If the vaccines can cause autoimmune disease, why isn't everyone susceptible? Many researchers believe there is a genetically vulnerable subset of people who develop autoimmune conditions following exposure to an adjuvant, causing chronic immune system stimulation.[15] We are all vulnerable to environmental toxins, many of which interact synergistically with aluminum and some of which can promote aluminum uptake to the brain. Pervasive environmental chemicals of concern include fluoride, pesticides, glyphosate, some drugs, and mercury.

Doctors need to be aware that vaccines may be able to trigger autoimmune diseases in a genetically susceptible population.[16] If doctors are not trained to recognize the potential connections to vaccination, injuries will continue to go unreported and untracked. In 2017, Drs. Jill R. Schofield of the University of Colorado and Jeanne E. Hendrickson of Yale University published an important article that included a case report of an 11-year-old girl diagnosed with POTS and neurocardiogenic syncope, among other problems, following her first dose of Gardasil.[17] Intravenous immunoglobulin and other treatments led to some improvement in her health. In discussing "HPV vaccination syndrome," Drs. Schofield and Hendrickson report that they "believe that this is the first reported case of biopsy-proven autonomic neuropathy developing within days of HPV vaccination."[18] Independent investigators and public health authorities debate HPV vaccination syndrome[19] but some experts and clinicians urge caution in vaccinating. Drs. Schofield and Hendrickson suggest, in particular, that medical personnel consider not vaccinating patients with "personal or family history of autoimmune disease and/or autonomic disorders" and that primary care medical providers learn to recognize the potential side effects, including neurological ones, following HPV vaccination.[20] Patients are reporting HPV vaccination syndrome, POTS, CRPS, and a myriad of other conditions associated with HPV vaccination. Doctors' failure to recognize symptoms potentially related to HPV vaccination may explain, at least in part, the profound disconnect between injured individuals and mainstream medical opinion.

POTENTIAL MECHANISMS FOR VACCINE-INDUCED AUTOIMMUNITY

Researchers offer a few possible explanations for vaccine-induced autoimmunity. First, researchers are exploring whether a person who has had a first exposure to HPV itself or the vaccine might, on subsequent exposures, experience a stronger immune system response, called an anamnestic response.[21] That heightened immune response could result in the "sudden onset of autoimmunity."[22] The body's immune response, based on antibody levels, to a natural HPV infection is fairly weak. But HPV vaccines use adjuvants whose very purpose is to cause a heightened immune response. It makes sense that the vaccine might trigger a more aggressive immune response than natural infection.[23] Ian Frazer, one of the vaccine developers, has described the vaccine antibody response as *80 to 100 times* stronger than natural infection.[24] Further, the antibody response is much higher in preteens and young teens than in young women in their late teens to midtwenties.[25] Another possible mechanism explaining autoimmunity is called "bystander activation." Unlike molecular mimicry, discussed below, bystander activation involves the activation of nonspecific cells or processes that can begin a cascade of events leading to autoimmunity.[26]

HPV VACCINES AND MOLECULAR MIMICRY

Another possible explanation for autoimmunity following HPV vaccination—perhaps the one garnering the most attention—is based on the theory of molecular mimicry, which focuses on a vaccine's VLPs, either alone or in combination with the adjuvant.[27] At the heart of molecular mimicry are proteins and peptides, found in both our bodies and the vaccines. Our bodies are made up of proteins and peptides, both of which are made up of amino acids. Distinguishing them from peptides, proteins have longer amino acid chains and carry out specific biological functions.

Molecular mimicry occurs when a foreign antigen, such as a viral protein or peptide, looks like human proteins or peptides. In other words, it mimics the human protein or peptide, confusing the immune system. Instead of just attacking the foreign invader as "the other," the immune system targets the actual protein or peptide sequence in the body because of its similarity to the invading antigen. The immune system then mounts a continuous inflammatory immune response, resulting in an autoimmune disease.[28]

Drs. Tomljenovic and Shaw's work on the brain tissue of two young women who died after Gardasil vaccination supports the molecular mimicry theory.[29] The two women suffered from cerebral vasculitis symptoms, which resemble other reported adverse events after Gardasil vaccination.[30] Drs. Shaw and Tomljenovic stated that the brain tissue samples showed:

> [S]trong evidence of an autoimmune vasculitis triggered by the cross-reactive HPV-16 L1 antibodies binding to the wall of the cerebral blood vessels. . . . In addition, there was clear evidence of the presence of HPV-16 L1 particles within the cerebral vasculature with some HPV-16 L1 particles adhering to the blood vessel walls. . . . In contrast, HPV-18 L1 antibodies did not bind to the cerebral blood vessels or any other neural tissues.[31]

They found the vaccine-type HPV16 virus antibodies that the macrophages most likely carried to brain and spleen tissues, where they remained even after death. The brain tissue samples also showed signs of "pathogenic immune processes."[32] In other words, the scientists discovered that the anti-HPV16 antibodies breached the blood-brain barrier, enabling the autoimmune responses.

TRYING TO ASSUAGE PUBLIC CONCERN ABOUT MOLECULAR MIMICRY

Controversy connecting molecular mimicry, autoimmune disease, and HPV vaccines is heating up. In late summer 2017, apparently in response to media attention, Children's Hospital of Philadelphia posted a video featuring Dr. Paul Offit,[33] a vaccinologist with ties to industry and government. Dismissing concerns about molecular mimicry, Dr. Offit stated that the HPV vaccine has been:

> . . . formally studied in more than a million people, and it's been shown not to cause any of the side effects that people were worried about. Specifically, the autoimmune diseases, which I think has gotten the most media attention. So, let me explain why it is not only that we've shown it hasn't, but why it doesn't make sense that it would have caused those problems.[34]

In the video, Dr. Offit explains that molecular mimicry occurs when "there is a protein in that vaccine that mimics a protein on the surface of your cells."[35] He claims "the HPV vaccine doesn't mimic any sort of protein that exists in the human body, so it doesn't make sense that it would have ever caused a problem."[36] Dr. Offit admits here that molecular mimicry is theoretically possible but not with the HPV vaccine, however. He appears to be at odds with published research on molecular mimicry, the human papillomavirus itself, and HPV vaccines.

Researchers in the past several years have demonstrated that there are *many* matches between HPV and human proteins, including dozens of sites on the HPV 16 L1 protein alone.[37] The HPV 16 L1 protein is in all HPV vaccines currently on the market. Furthermore, many of these matches are found in areas of the proteins involved in regulating functions that, if disrupted, could lead to autoimmune[38] as well as cardiac disturbances.[39]

Research also shows an association in human and HPV peptides—particularly for many of the HPV types in Gardasil 9.[40] In a 2017 study, researchers attempted to determine whether HPV may be a contributing factor to the development of lupus due to molecular mimicry.[41] They concluded that there was enough evidence to support this hypothesis and recommended that future vaccines be designed to avoid cross-reactivity with vaccine peptides that could potentially cause lupus in the host.[42]

Dr. Offit continues that "the human papillomavirus itself, the wild-type virus, the natural virus, doesn't cause autoimmunity, therefore it doesn't make sense that the vaccine would cause autoimmunity."[43] He adds that since the natural infection "where the virus replicates thousands of times would cause a higher burden on your immune system than the vaccine, it doesn't make sense the vaccine would cause an autoimmune response."[44] Dr. Offit does not mention the recent scientific research that contradicts him.

The natural HPV infection may be a factor in developing autoimmune diseases, such as lupus.[45] As a general rule, natural infections from HPV produce a weak antibody response; the vaccines elicit a much stronger response. Not only are Dr. Offit's statements incompatible with peer-reviewed research, they fail to address whether the overwhelming HPV vaccine-induced antibody response might trigger immune responses that could lead to autoimmunity and other adverse events.[46] Many scientists now believe we should be concerned about the long-term effects of the extraordinarily potent antibody responses evoked, especially in preteens. Certainly much more research remains to be done, but adopting a reductionist approach, as Dr. Offit seems to do, can give the impression that this is settled science, when in fact the opposite is true.

HPV Vaccine Researchers Are Asking, Can We Build A Better Vaccine?

In December 2008, the several US federal agencies including the FDA and NIH convened an adjuvant workshop where the FDA's Dr. Jesse Goodman discussed whether scientists could develop vaccines that would reduce dependence on adjuvants.[47] In the future, this may be possible with HPV and other DNA vaccines. New research is seeking to develop vaccines with no overlap between human and viral proteins, thus reducing the risk of cross-reactivity and possibly eliminating the need for any adjuvant. If the peptides in the vaccine are entirely foreign to the human body, they would evoke a strong immunologic response on their own.[48]

In 2017, the German Cancer Research Center (DKFZ) announced that it had developed a heat-stable HPV vaccine, primarily for use in the lower-resource countries. It is based on HPV envelope proteins, using the L2 protein rather than VLPs. This vaccine is purportedly less expensive and more protective than existing vaccines because, according to the researchers, L2 is identical in all oncogenic HPV types. Available information is based on preclinical results. Clinical trials are planned but have yet to be conducted; it is not clear what the outcome will be or if this new vaccine will eliminate any of the cross-reactivity risk of existing vaccines.[49]

Autoimmune diseases remain among the most serious problems reportedly related to HPV vaccines. Research is elucidating the role of the HPV vaccine in autoimmune and other serious conditions and identifying those who may be most susceptible to injury. It is imperative that doctors learn how to identify and treat autoimmune reactions from HPV vaccines.

23.

THE OVERLOOKED FALLOUT
FROM THE HPV VACCINE

"The Devil is in the details," goes the old adage, and this is surely true in the debate about HPV vaccines. Their safety and effectiveness depend not only good clinical trials, as we've explored above, but on accurate information about HPV testing, transmission, prevalence, type replacement, and causation. So in this science-heavy chapter, we review current information on these dimensions of the virus and the vaccine. This information shows just how complicated the human ecosystem is, and how uncertain the benefits and risks of the HPV vaccine.

NEW SCREENING GUIDELINES: LESS FREQUENT SCREENING AND ELIMINATING PAP TESTS?

In Chapter 4, we discussed cervical screening generally, including concerns about whether women would continue to screen after HPV vaccination. Here, we discuss changing guidelines that may impact health outcomes. Current cervical screening guidelines are in flux. Some readers will remember the days of annual Pap tests. No one liked them, but they were an accepted part of annual gynecological care. Those times are gone. For the average woman, annual Pap tests have given way to testing every three to five years, depending on age and other factors, with initial screening at age 21, regardless of sexual activity.[1] Today, newer DNA and RNA HPV tests are replacing or being used together with Pap tests.[2] These newer tests, which still require swabbing the cervix like Pap tests, detect the HPV virus. Pap tests detect abnormal cervical cell growth, whether HPV-related or not.

Some experts favor less frequent screening because of the risk of excessive invasive treatment, like biopsies or the removal of abnormal growths, when most would likely resolve on their own. They argue that not only is overdiagnosis and overtreatment emotionally difficult, but invasive treatments might cause unnecessary harm to the cervix and risk future pregnancy complications.[3] While these experts argue that screenings every three to five years are sufficient to detect and treat any serious problems, other doctors and patients disagree and screen more frequently, believing the true rationale behind these policy changes is cost cutting, not health.[4]

Controversy surrounds these newer HPV DNA and RNA testing. While acknowledging pluses and minuses for Pap tests and HPV DNA testing, a recent Cochrane Collaboration review favors the HPV DNA testing overall. Still, the report recognizes that "[e]vidence from prospective longitudinal studies is needed to establish the relative clinical implications of these tests."[5] Critics of the newer HPV tests believe that they are not adequately sensitive and may lead to false negative results. As cervical abnormal cell growth progresses, it may contain less and less viral material. This means that an HPV test needs to be extremely sensitive to detect only a few DNA copies of HPV in a cell, particularly in late-stage lesions.[6] A 2015 article analyzed the screening results from over 250,000 women. It concluded that almost 20 percent of women with cervical cancer may receive false negative results from HPV DNA testing alone. Cotesting with Pap and HPV testing is most effective.[7]

Doing away with Pap tests altogether thus seems to create the risk of missing some precancerous and cancerous conditions, particularly those not related to HPV. As discussed in a 2014 article by Zhao et al., studies have confirmed that HPV-negative cervical cancers do exist.[8] These findings support continued cotesting to reduce the potential to miss cervical disease that HPV DNA or RNA testing alone would not detect.

Because only persistent HPV infections seem to lead to abnormal cell growth and possible cervical cancer, HPV DNA tests ideally would provide accurate, type-specific results to track persistence. While these HPV DNA tests usually provide type-specific results for HPV 16 and 18, the results for other types are nonspecific "pooled" results of several other high-risk HPV types, some of which are in Gardasil 9 and others of which are not.[9] This may mean that if a doctor sees an HPV-vaccinated patient with a positive HPV DNA test from the "pooled" results, she will not know if the patient suffered possible vaccine failure (i.e., the patient is infected with a type found in the vaccine) and if repeated positive HPV tests for the pooled types represent serial infections with different types or a persistent infection with one type. Given that some of the types in the pooled results are more common in African American women and some pooled types are not even included in HPV vaccines, this lack of specificity may pose serious risks.

Nonetheless, despite the lack of long-term data on the use of the newer DNA and RNA tests and their limitations, many national health regulatory bodies, including in the US, the UK, Australia, and Ireland, are pushing either to fully replace Pap tests with HPV DNA testing or at least to make it the primary cervical cancer screening tool.[10]

In September 2017, the US Preventive Services Task Force issued draft recommendations for women ages 30 to 64 (they left recommendations for younger and older women unchanged). They recommended eliminating the five-year cotesting option and that women 30 to 64 get either a Pap test every three years or HPV DNA testing every five years.[11] A number of organizations pushed back, arguing that cotesting is important and that medically underserved women, particularly Latina and African American women, may not receive adequate testing and treatment if insurance does not reimburse cotesting.[12] Critics pointed out that the Task Force's recommendations seem racially biased, relying on information from countries with primarily white populations. These recommendations may leave minority women at particular risk.[13]

Taking a strong stand in favor of DNA tests over Pap tests, Australia eliminated Pap tests as part of the first-line screening process in December 2017. Instead, Australian women 25 to 74 years old will be screened every five years using HPV DNA testing alone.[14] Only if a DNA test returns a positive result will a lab perform a Pap test looking for abnormal cells from the same sample.[15]

SCREENING IN LOW-RESOURCE COUNTRIES

What about screening and treatment in low-resource countries without access to even basic gynecologic care? While women in these countries face many barriers, innovative, low-tech options are proliferating. While Pap tests are not expensive, the medical infrastructure in some areas is so weak that getting samples to a lab is not feasible. In many countries, there are not enough qualified pathologists to interpret samples.

One of the most promising options in low-resource countries is called visual inspection with acetic acid, or vinegar, called VIA. The WHO ran a VIA demonstration project in several low-resource countries from 2005 to 2009, and a number of countries have now adopted VIA programs.[16] VIA is inexpensive and easy, allowing general practitioners, nurses, midwives, and others to perform cervical screening.[17] Even cell phone apps and accessories allow clinicians to take high-quality photos of cervical lesions and seek expert advice.[18]

If a clinic has cryotherapy, healthcare professionals can freeze off lesions the same day. Cryotherapy does not require expensive equipment, and general practitioners can perform the procedure, unlike many of the specialized treatment methods in high-resource countries.[19] Other screening methods allow women to collect cervical samples at home for DNA testing, using a swab kit.[20] This option may help overcome barriers, such as distance to a clinic, shortages of medical providers, and cultural barriers.[21] In Australia, self-collection is an option for certain never-screened and under-screened populations. Information from this new screening program notes, however, that self-collection is about 70 percent as effective as medical sampling.[22] Still, low-cost innovations are making it possible for more women to receive screening than ever before.

Late-stage identification of cancer in low-resource countries remains a serious problem and contributes to higher mortality rates. Treatment, even where available, may not be as effective in late-identified cancers. Programs like one created in Tanzania to train lay health aides to take health histories and recognize signs and symptoms of various cancers, including cervical cancer, are important. A pilot program in rural villages in Tanzania demonstrated that, with a modest financial and training investment, these aides could "downstage" cancers, i.e., identify cancer at an earlier stage, and thus increase potential for a positive outcome even with existing treatment resources.[23] In this pilot program, cervical and breast cancer had the greatest downstaging, even though potential cervical cancer was identified initially on medical history, not examination.[24]

There may be natural solutions to speed recovery from HPV infections and to treat cervical cancer, as well. Several studies have shown that curcumin has a beneficial impact on cervical cancer cells and even downregulates the primary oncoproteins E6 and E7 in HPV cancer cell lines.[25] Scientists are exploring how to deliver adequate doses of curcumin in an appropriate way. A compound in shiitake mushrooms is also promising. Investigators at the University of Texas Health Science Center have been conducting preclinical studies and clinical trials[26] on this natural substance. In a small study of HPV-positive women, the compound reduces or resolves HPV infections after three to six months of treatment.[27] Further, researchers are studying a compound in nigella sativa, also known as black seed, as a treatment for cervical cancer.[28] Finally, as we noted in Chapter 4, poor nutrition is a risk factor for cervical cancer, as may be certain genetic changes like MTHFR polymorphisms that affect how your body metabolizes particular nutrients.[29] Scientists are studying whether some key nutrients, including folate or folic acid, vitamin B12, and selenium, may do more than reduce risk and also may be associated with regression of CINs.[30] Scientists should continue to explore these and other similar low-cost, low-tech options to prevent or reverse cervical disease.

REVACCINATING WITH GARDASIL 9 IF YOU HAD GARDASIL?

Gardasil 9 has replaced Gardasil in the US and is likely to be rolled out in many other countries in the coming years. Should those who already have received Gardasil revaccinate with Gardasil 9 to receive protection against the five additional high-risk HPV types in the newer vaccine? While this may have superficial appeal to some,[31] to do so would go beyond CDC recommendations. Moreover, in the Gardasil 9 clinical trials, girls and young women who had received Gardasil and were then vaccinated again with Gardasil 9 had *lower* antibody levels to the new HPV types in Gardasil 9 compared to those who only received Gardasil 9.[32] Because there is no established antibody level associated with protection from HPV infection,[33] it's not clear whether those who get both vaccine series will be protected against the new types. Those considering revaccinating must also keep in mind that they will get either 2 or 3 doses of the new vaccine with more than twice the AAHS as in original Gardasil. The evidence suggests that revaccinating girls and boys who previously received Gardasil may have little medical benefit and may carry potential risks.

IS HPV ONLY SEXUALLY TRANSMITTED?

Many doctors and public health authorities recommend vaccinating children at age eleven or twelve, and even as young as nine, because children at that age presumably are not sexually active. But all people, including children, can get HPV infections in other ways. What if many children who are not sexually active still have HPV infections at the time of vaccination? Sexual transmission may be the most likely route to HPV infection and one that has been the focus of research since the mid-1800s.[34] But that is not the whole story.[35]

Nonsexual transmission of HPV is an important concern. As we discussed in Chapter 9, some women may be at higher risk for CIN2 or 3 lesions or worse after vaccination if they had antibodies to HPV or an ongoing HPV infection at the time of vaccination. Merck and the FDA seem to presume that because the target population of 9-to-12-year-olds is generally sexually naive that they are thus HPV naive. They seem to assume that the negative efficacy issue in 16-to-23-years-olds in the clinical trials is irrelevant. But this assumption is flawed.

There are no baseline Pap or DNA testing data for the few 9-to-12-year-old girls in the Gardasil clinical trials, only blood tests for antibodies. This makes sense, as those girls were too young for gynecological exams. However, blood tests indicated that some children in the clinical trials already had HPV antibodies before vaccination.[36] No one at Merck or the FDA seemed concerned during the prelicensing discussions about these positive antibody results. We simply don't know if children who are HPV positive at the time of vaccination or who may have had a prior infection are now at increased risk for serious disease progression. In particular, these children may be going through hormonal changes, the impact of which is poorly understood. Yet, as we described in Chapter 9, the FDA did not recommend prescreening, and some organizations went further to specifically advise against it. Parents cannot even opt to check for HPV antibodies before vaccinating because no commercial HPV antibody blood test is available. We simply do not know the long-term effects of HPV negative efficacy in children.

TRANSMISSION TO INFANTS AND CHILDREN

Perhaps the most widely recognized nonsexual HPV transmission route is "vertical transmission," from infected mothers to infants during childbirth. While this type of transmission is clearly possible, some studies find transmission from infected mothers rare (1–5 percent), while others suggest it is common (40–80 percent).[37] Some children born to infected mothers even have persistent HPV infections.[38] Scientists have detected HPV in both breast milk and amniotic fluid, as well.[39]

HPV infections in fact may be common among children and adolescents. In 2016, Bacopoulou and colleagues reported results of a study of 95 children and young adults aged 2 to 21. They found that 37.9 *percent* of children and adolescents had a genital HPV infection, including 28.6 percent of non-sexually active 11-to-19-year-olds and 34.5 percent of 2-to-10-year-olds. The authors concluded: "[t]he significant percentage of sexually inexperienced women genitally infected with HPV indicates a substantial nonsexual method of transmission because genital low and high risk HPV infections were common in girls without any history of sexual abuse or sexual activity."[40] They suggested many possible nonsexual ways children might have acquired HPV, including autoinoculation (transferring, for example, from one's own hands to genitals) and nonsexual transfer between individuals (e.g., from caretaker to child).[41] The study authors acknowledge the many unanswered questions about these infections in early life on future cancer risk. Scientists do not yet know how long infections last, whether early infections protect individuals in later life, and what these data mean for cervical health.

Public health officials endorse HPV vaccination of preteens because this age group exhibited a more robust antibody response than older subjects in the clinical trials did. This recommendation also seems based on the belief that sexual intercourse is essentially the only vector for HPV infection. That premise is flawed in light of studies evidencing HPV infection in young children.[42]

HPV PREVALENCE

What HPV types a woman might acquire depends on where she lives and her race, among other factors.[43] Since HPV types have been coexisting with humans for thousands of years, it makes sense that different patterns developed in different places. Because type prevalence can have a huge impact on how well vaccines work, ideally vaccines should fit the population receiving it. HPV vaccines, however, are one-size-fits-all. Of the at least two hundred identified HPV types, scientists have found that twelve to eighteen are potentially oncogenic in humans.[44] In particular, scientists estimate that HPV types 16 and 18 are associated with about 70 percent of cervical cancer globally, though HPV prevalence and the burden of HPV-related cancers differ around the world.[45] But the focus on types 16 and 18 may leaving some women at risk of infection from other types.

Even within the US, the HPV prevalence and the types of HPV associated with cervical cancer vary by race, ethnicity, and location.[46] Latina women are the most likely to receive cervical cancer diagnoses and to die from cervical cancer in the US, followed by African American women.[47] Cervical cancer deaths are twice as high among African American women in the US compared to Caucasian women, even though some sources report that they have about the same Pap screening rates.[48]

At least one study[49] has challenged the assumption that non-HPV infection risk factors (all those factors identified in Chapter 4) explain the differences in cervical cancer rates among women of different races and ethnicities. While those factors undoubtedly play a role, differences in HPV types found in lesions of women of different races may provide important new clues. Researchers are questioning why these differences in HPV types exist among different populations and what they mean for one-size-fits-all HPV vaccination.[50]

A small study at Duke University showed that African American women have a much lower prevalence of HPV 16 and 18 in precancerous lesions compared to Caucasian women.[51] In fact, the two groups have very different HPV types in early precancerous lesions as well as in later stage lesions.[52] These different patterns may help explain why African American women are at higher risk. Researchers are exploring several theories. No matter the explanation for these differences, it remains that three of the six HPV types most common in African American women with late stage precancerous legions, HPV types 35, 66, and 68, are not in any HPV vaccines.[53]

In 2008, Spanish researchers published results showing the real-life implications of one-size-fits-all HPV vaccines.[54] They found HPV 16 or 18 present in 42.7 percent of women examined with CIN2 or CIN3. However, HPV 16 and 18 types alone were present in only 28.2 percent of cases without coinfection with other high-risk or probable high-risk types.[55] In 55.8 percent of cases, high-risk or probable high-risk HPV types other than 16 or 18 were found in CIN2 or CIN3. The researchers pointed out that high-risk types besides HPV 16 and 18 were more frequent and that the difference was statistically significant.[56] Furthermore, several of the lesions tested negative for *any* HPV type.[57]

These differences in type prevalence likely make a difference in how well HPV vaccines work for different women around the globe and raise the issue of whether manufacturers should customize them. At the time the vaccines were developed, proponents like Professor Margaret Stanley, a British virologist, acknowledged that they had "no answer" about customization.[58] While tailoring the vaccine to specific groups may be cost-prohibitive, it is important to at least acknowledge and monitor the varying effectiveness of the vaccines in different populations.

Scientists still have a lot of work to do: learning how HPV types exist in diverse populations and in diverse precancerous and cancerous growths and even the exact mechanism whereby HPV is associated with cancer.

HPV TYPE REPLACEMENT

HPV vaccines target a limited number of HPV types associated with cervical cancer and other cancers. Yet many mistakenly believe that HPV vaccines protect against all cervical cancer and HPV-related cancers.

It is critical to understand that HPV infection can come from nonvaccine HPV types. Further, coinfections with many HPV types are common.[59] For instance, a woman may have an infection with both vaccine and nonvaccine HPV types. The relationships between types, both of the same HPV species and among species, is complex. For example, certain combinations of coinfections with different HPV types may have greater carcinogenic potential than others.[60] Moreover, the relationships among different types and subtypes of HPV need to be studied further, since the elimination or significant reduction of vaccine-targeted types may impact the balance of HPV ecology with unknown consequences.[61]

Because HPV vaccines protect against only limited HPV types, some scientists are concerned about "type replacement." This means that when a vaccine protects against infection from a particular type of the virus, infections caused by other types may become more common. And these less-common types potentially could be more menacing. In other words, perhaps they are less prevalent because they are more lethal, destroying the host more quickly, thereby limiting transmission. When Merck introduced Gardasil, Professor Stanley acknowledged that type replacement "is another unanswerable question at the present and should be addressed by long-term studies in vaccinated populations."[62]

In 2006, Thomas R. Broker, then-president of the International Papillomavirus Society, articulated this concern about HPV type replacement and the quandary about how to develop a vaccine:

> Nature abhors the vacuum and these ecological niches are going to be vacant when HPV 16 and 18 and 6 and 11 are minimized, and I'm deeply concerned that there'll be back-fill of those ecologic niches by these very, very similar types. I think it's imperative to expand the coverage in the vaccines. We don't know, however, because the studies have never been done, whether a cocktail with 14 types would be equally effective against all 14 or whether they might actually conflict with each other. We simply don't know. We don't suspect that there's much cross protection of one type to any other even similar type. So far the evidence doesn't suggest that.[63]

Clearly, leading experts were concerned about type replacement even before the launch of the first HPV vaccine. While there is some limited evidence of cross-protection, a bigger concern is that more rare and potentially more deadly types, not targeted by the vaccine, may increase in prevalence.

The FDA did express concerns about type replacement before licensing Gardasil.[64] It was an "item for discussion" in a May 2006 VRBPAC meeting; the FDA described it as an "important concern" during its evaluation.[65] VRBPAC participants noted that cases of disease due to other HPV types observed in the clinical trials had the potential to "counter the efficacy results of Gardasil™ for the

HPV types found in the vaccine."[66] As a condition for FDA fast-track approval, in a letter dated June 8, 2006, Merck agreed to follow up on the type replacement issue in a fourteen-year study on the cohort enrolled in study protocol 015, in the Nordic countries in Europe. Merck's final report on Protocol 015 is due to the FDA on December 31, 2018.[67] While some researchers argue that type replacement will not occur because HPV types are stable, several studies now suggest that it may be occurring and warrants further research. Recent research also suggests that there are thousands of HPV 16 genomes, and few women infected with "HPV 16" share identical HPV 16 DNA sequences.[68] This may further challenge the theory that HPVs are invulnerable to evolutionary changes.

A 2016 German study by Fischer et al. notes that the "proportion of [high risk]-HPV types not covered by vaccination may increase in the near future" but does not predict whether this increase will cause more precancerous lesions and cervical cancer.[69] Additionally, a 2015 study using data from the US National Health and Nutrition Examination Survey (NHANES) 2007–2012 found that vaccinated women had a higher prevalence of high-risk nonvaccine types than women who had not been vaccinated.[70] Both of these studies note that vaccines covering additional types may diminish the type replacement,[71] but there is no vaccine that covers all types of high-risk HPV.

In 2016, the CDC concluded: "[T]here is no clear indication that type placement is occurring."[72] Yet the data in that very study suggest that type replacement in fact may be occurring. For example, CDC researchers found that the overall prevalence of HPV in the "prevaccine" era (2003–2006) was 54.4 percent and actually increased to 58.1 percent overall (56.7 percent for those vaccinated) in the vaccine era (2009–2012).[73] Researchers also reported significant drops in Gardasil-targeted HPV types from the prevaccine era to the vaccine era—from 18.6 percent down to 2.1 percent for the four types in original Gardasil.[74] Given that there was not a corresponding drop in overall infection rates even among the vaccinated, it is fair to wonder what fills the gaps. HPV type replacement certainly is one possibility.

Independent researchers at the Institute for Pure and Applied Knowledge (IPAK) recently analyzed the data from this 2016 CDC study using "Fisher's Exact Test," a test of statistical significance, and asserted that the CDC study shows type replacement. IPAK's graph below demonstrates that in the postvaccine period, the percentage of infections decreased for the HPV types in original Gardasil (data collection was before Gardasil 9) but increased for infections from other HPV types:[75]

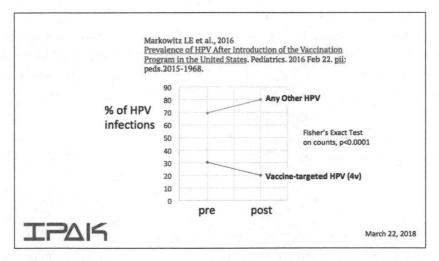

Source: Institute for Pure and Applied Knowledge, see note 75 above.

In short, evidence suggests that HPV type replacement may be occurring. Scientists need to study further if it's occurring and what that means for women's health. While studies fall on both sides of this question, the controversy over HPV type replacement from the vaccine is only increasing.

In addition to type replacement, scientists have raised concerns about recombination of HPV within each HPV type. Each HPV type has variants within it (i.e., not all type 16 HPV is identical). Changes to the various proteins, including the oncoproteins E6 and E7, and the major capsid proteins L1 and L2 in variants of the same type could, over time, have many impacts. They could influence how infections spread, how HPV types might respond to treatment, how virulent HPV types might become, as well as how effective HPV vaccines might be in the future.[76] With enough differences, novel types may emerge. This recombination is essentially evolution of the virus. While scientists have uncovered evidence of HPV recombination, particularly in HPV 16, the evolution of the virus and the impact of recombinant HPV variants warrant significant further study.

ORIGINAL ANTIGENIC SIN

Another potential concern about HPV vaccines arises from the theory of "Original Antigenic Sin" (or OAS). In 1960, Dr. Thomas Francis, Jr., a doctor and epidemiologist, first raised the problem of OAS with influenza, although others had raised it before for other infectious diseases.[77] OAS explains that the immune system "remembers" past viruses or bacteria and fights back against these or similar invaders when it encounters them again. When the body confronts a virus or bacterium, it produces antibodies and forms memory B and T cells against it.[78] When OAS occurs, if the body then encounters a similar but nonidentical pathogen, the body may respond as if it were again encountering the first invader, not the second. In relying on its memory of the first infection, it may not fully protect against the new, second invader. Thus, the body might not mount an adequate response to the second infection because of its memory of the first.

This phenomenon occurs with vaccines, particularly those against influenza (both seasonal and, for example, H1N1), so that a vaccine against one type of flu may not protect someone from other types. This theory is one of the ways some scientists explain flu vaccines' high failure rates. In fact, a vaccine against one type may actually prejudice a person encountering a different, but similar, type. With pertussis, for example, recovering from the infection naturally provides broader protection against reinfection with other types of the bacterium than the pertussis vaccine does.[79] Given the large number of HPV types identified to date (over 200 with more than a dozen currently considered carcinogenic) and the limited type protection from HPV vaccines, original antigenic sin may be a problem.[80]

Could OAS already be at play with Gardasil 9? In a clinical trial study in which girls who had received the full Gardasil series were revaccinated with Gardasil 9, the revaccinated girls had lower, and not necessarily protective, titers to the new HPV types in Gardasil 9 compared to girls who had not previously been vaccinated with Gardasil and received only Gardasil 9. As researchers wrote recently about Gardasil 9, "[T]here are not studies about 'original antigenic sin' that could be generated by the previous vaccine. It is not known if this vaccine could be used as a booster for young people already vaccinated."[81]

Does HPV Cause All Cervical Cancer?

The Generally Accepted Theory of HPV Infection to Cervical Cancer Progression

When a person has an HPV infection, the immune system recognizes the infected cells and may destroy them. If the immune system does not destroy the infected cells, persistent infection occurs and may lead to precancerous lesions, which still may resolve on their own or eventually progress to cancer. The process is complicated, and scientists do not yet fully understand it.[82] When there is persistent infection, the HPV-infected cells begin to make cancer proteins that allow for viruses to replicate and for the infected cells to avoid cell death.[83] In particular, two of the so-called oncoproteins found in HPV, E6 and E7 interfere with normal cell functions, leading to cancerous cell growth. E6 and E7 each target certain tumor-suppression proteins in a healthy cell to deactivate or destroy them.[84] Recent research is suggesting that a polymorphism of p53 (the tumor-suppressor protein against which E6 acts) may impact cervical cancer development. There are certain other genetic mutations that may be associated with cervical cancer susceptibility as well, further demonstrating the individuality of cancer risk and progression.[85]

So is HPV the cause of all cervical cancer, as the rhetoric suggests? While, as discussed below, there is debate over the association between HPV and cervical cancer or the extent of non-HPV related cervical cancer, at a minimum, at least some cervical cancers are not associated with HPV.[86] The CDC, for example, states "about 90 percent of cervical . . . cancers are attributable to HPV."[87] Even Dr. Harald zur Hausen, who first isolated high-risk HPV in cervical cancer cells, points out that, while more than 95 percent of cervical cancer biopsies contain high risk HPV types, this does not necessarily mean that HPV infections *caused* the cervical tumors.[88] Dr. zur Hausen acknowledged that only more research can provide more accurate estimates concerning HPV and cervical cancer.[89]

Another Theory Challenges the Orthodoxy

Is the generally accepted theory of HPV infection the only plausible route for a woman to develop cervical cancer? Is it possible that other factors are at work, at least in some cases? Why do so few women with HPV infections develop cervical cancer? Why does cervical cancer develop so slowly, 20 to 40 years after infection? Why is there so much variation in lesions and cervical tumors caused by the same family of viruses?[90] It is known that chronic inflammation could lead to cancer.[91] Is it possible that chronic inflammation from persistent, untreated infections leads to cervical cancer?

In a report from Egypt, researchers looked into the association between HPV and cervical cancer, examining 100 cervical specimens from premalignant and malignant lesions. They found HPV in only 39.5 percent of the precancerous lesions and in only 33.5 percent of the cancerous lesions.[92] If HPV wasn't causing cervical cancer in the majority of these women, what was it? Recall as well the Spanish research discussed earlier in which some of the lesions tested were negative for HPV.[93]

Harking back to research by Dr. Papanicolaou, the namesake of the Pap test, scientists at University of California at Berkeley recently challenged the accepted viral theory of cervical cancer causation.[94] They questioned the notion that a virus could lead to cancer twenty or more years after infection.[95] Their new line of research centers on cervical cancers with unique cancer-specific characteristics or karyotypes. A karyotype depicts the number, size, and shape of chromosomes in an organism or species.

These researchers theorize that other cancer-causing agents catalyze normal cells to mutate, eventually creating karyotypes. In a small study, they examined nine cervical cancer samples and found HPV DNA (though incomplete) in seven samples. In two samples, they detected none.

The scientists found cancer-specific karyotypes in all the cancerous tissue they tested.[96] To the Berkeley researchers, the genetic makeup of these karyotypes suggests that the cervical cancers they examined originated not with HPVs but with these karyotypes, which mutated from the women's own cells.[97] They argue that any HPV DNA is an incomplete latent artifact of prior infections and cannot cause cancer cells to form.[98] Even Merck acknowledges that HPV DNA integrates in late-stage CIN lesions and tumors as part of the progression from HPV infection to cancer. Merck recognizes that little viral DNA or L1 or L2 proteins are found in some cervical tumors. However, E6 and E7 oncoproteins are prevalent in tumors.[99] Recall, too, that HPV DNA testing in late-stage lesions and cancerous tumors can yield false negative results because of the lack of viral material in the cells.

The Berkeley research team hypothesized that, among other things, the long lag time between HPV infection and cervical cancer likely means that HPV is not the cause of cervical cancer.[100] Karyotypes, which are triggered by different carcinogenic agents, are the more likely culprits.[101] Cigarette smoke is a well-established carcinogenic agent associated with many cancers, including cervical cancer. When smoking rates dropped in the US, so did cervical cancer rates.[102] Smokers are at least twice as likely to develop cervical cancer as nonsmokers.[103] While smoking doesn't explain all cervical cancers, could it be a more central factor than scientists generally think?

Even if the karyotype theory does not hold up to scrutiny, it begs the question why smoking is not more central to recommendations for preventing cervical cancer, especially in low-resource countries where women often cook over fires or in areas with poor ventilation, escalating their cervical cancer risks.[104] Even though other scientists have put forward similar theories, the scientific community has largely ignored them.[105] One of the lead researchers of the Berkeley team, Dr. Duesberg, a professor of molecular and cell biology, is not afraid of controversy. He contacted Norma Erickson of SaneVax and explained his theory to her. He saw the value in getting this information out to SaneVax followers. Norma studied his paper and published a readable explanation of it with Dr. Duesberg on the SaneVax website in 2015.[106] To Norma, this karyotype hypothesis is worth exploring, as the HPV theory of cancer causation seems incomplete.

If even a small percentage of cervical cancers are not related to HPV, the move toward primary HPV DNA and RNA screening is troubling because it may miss some cervical disease and leave some women at higher risk.

CONCLUSION

At a deep level, almost everything about HPV and the vaccine to prevent it is uncertain: how to best test for HPV infection; how and when people transmit the infection; how common the infections are; and even whether HPV infections lead directly to cancer. Yet despite these uncertainties, prominent medical institutions are encouraging and even mandating that all preteens get these vaccines. Part IV explores how this dialectic between vaccine promotion and reservations based on uncertainty and apparent harm has played out in five distinct countries around the world.

PART IV

THE ASCENT OF DISSENT

24.

JAPAN: PULLING THE PLUG

Every year, about 9,400 women in Japan are diagnosed with cervical cancer and about 3,600 of them die.[1] Cervical screening is available in Japan, but participation rates languish around 30 percent, contributing to the relatively high death rate from cervical cancer.[2] Attitudes toward gynecological care in Japan differ from those in the US. In Japan, cervical screening usually takes place in a women's hospital setting, where women usually go only when they are pregnant or ill. Gynecologists, mostly men, do not promote Pap tests, and insurance rarely covers it.[3] The Japanese Health Ministry has long recognized that it needs to do more to encourage Japanese women to get Pap tests, something that is needed even with an HPV vaccination program.

Japan licensed Cervarix and Gardasil in 2009 and 2011, respectively.[4] By 2010, most local governments subsidized the cost of this expensive vaccine to ensure availability. In April 2013, the Japanese Ministry of Health, Labor, and Welfare added the vaccine to the recommended schedule, thus ensuring it would be available free of charge to all eligible girls.[5] The newspaper *Japan Times* estimated that by June 2013, 8.3 million girls had received the HPV vaccine, or 70 percent of those girls born between 1994 and 1998.[6] Despite giving the impression of a successful program initially, the Ministry abruptly suspended its proactive recommendation on June 14, 2013, less than three months after it had added the vaccine to the immunization schedule, due to "an undeniable causal relationship between persistent pain and the vaccination."[7] This announcement came one day after the WHO issued a press release declaring the vaccine safe.[8]

Since then, despite significant tensions around reinstatement of the recommendation, the Ministry continues to make the vaccine available in its national immunization program but does not proactively recommend it. The result has been that uptake among girls dropped from over 70 percent in 2013 to around 1 percent in 2018, destroying corporate sales projections for Japan but, perhaps more important, undermining confidence in the vaccine in other markets.[9] Headlines like "HPV Vaccination Crisis in Japan" in the *Lancet* epitomized scientists' and world health officials' surprise.[10]

More than many other countries, Japan has previously questioned the safety and efficacy of vaccines on a national level. In 1993, Japan suspended a measles-mumps-rubella vaccine that it introduced in 1989 after observing high rates of meningitis associated with the mumps component.[11] After that, the government recommended that the measlesmumps-rubella vaccines be administered separately for several years. Furthermore, the government declared all childhood immunizations voluntary as of 1994.[12] Uptake is high, but it is based on the Ministry's recommendations, not mandates.

Another national vaccine incident occurred in 2011, when the Ministry temporarily suspended Pfizer's Prevnar vaccine against meningitis and pneumonia and Sanofi's HiB vaccine against Haemophilus influenza type b following reports of four infant deaths. The vaccines were reintroduced after evidence seemed to clear the vaccines of a causal role in the deaths.[13] Despite reintroduction of those vaccines, Japan's history suggests greater caution when it comes to vaccines than in many other countries.

As early as March 2010, some HPV-vaccinated girls complained to the media of complex regional pain syndrome (CRPS) after vaccination.[14] In March 2013, a month before the Ministry approved the vaccine to be added to the national program, the *Asahi* newspaper reported on 50 girls suffering from CRPS and 100 unable to attend school after getting the HPV vaccine. Television also covered the HPV-vaccinated girls. Shortly after, a group of victims and their families held a press conference to show videos of girls with seizures and balance problems.[15]

Why the Ministry approved the HPV vaccine amid growing injury concerns is unclear. On June 14, the day the Ministry announced the suspension of the program, the Vaccine Adverse Reactions Review Committee (VARRC), a civil society group, held a press conference, featuring girls who claimed to have been injured by the vaccine. The girls said they experienced a range of symptoms including seizures, severe headaches, and partial paralysis.[16]

Critics of Japan's vaccination program do not appreciate this cautious approach, however. A letter published in *Lancet* in August 2013 after the suspension of the HPV vaccination program suggested that Japan's vaccination program suffers from a "failure of governance" and argued that "reform . . . is essential."[17] The authors suggest that Japan's vaccine program should more closely model the US program, stating: "Decisions should be made by an independent advisory committee, such as the Advisory Committee on Immunization Practices in the U.S.A., rather than a committee organized by government bureaucrats."[18]

The Ministry discovered that the adverse events reported after Gardasil and Cervarix were many times higher than other vaccines on the recommended schedule.[19] The Ministry said it wanted more time to assess HPV side effects before its next recommendation. Newspapers reported that a government task force had analyzed 1,968 reported adverse events following HPV vaccination and had found 106 of them to be serious.[20] The Ministry intended to decide about reinstatement of its recommendation by the following December.

In October 2013, Dr. Tetsuya Miyamoto, director of the Office of Vaccination Policy at the Ministry's Health Policy Bureau, together with other Japanese medical professionals, embarked on a six-month HPV vaccine fact-finding mission. The delegation travelled to London to meet with health officials and scientists to gather more information on the vaccines. SaneVax, which had been keeping a close eye on developments, heard of this meeting from a Japanese victim support group and a journalist with *Kyodo News*, Mr. Mutsuo Fukushima. SaneVax wanted to meet with the delegation so that it could hear the international concerns on safety and not just the government and industry perspective. SaneVax contacted Dr. Miyamoto, and he graciously agreed to meet with SaneVax's experts to listen to their concerns.[21]

SaneVax gathered an international team of doctors and scientists, including Dr. Sin Hang Lee and others.[22] SaneVax's Freda Birrell also attended. While one cannot know the effect Dr. Lee and others had on Dr. Miyamoto and his team, the December deadline to reinstate the vaccine came and went without a decision, punting reinstatement to the following year.

In January 2014, the Japanese advisory committee on immunization policy released an official report, dismissing the diverse pain and motor dysfunction girls were experiencing as psychogenic and noting that the government should "provide counseling" to the affected girls for these "psychosomatic reactions."[23] This was in direct contrast to the reports from doctors and researchers who had examined the girls, who could not explain away their conditions as "psychosomatic" in nature.[24]

Due in large part to the efforts of Japanese Senators Yamatani and Nakagawa, *Kyodo News* journalist Mr. Fukushima, and SaneVax, Japan hosted a closed International Symposium on Adverse Reactions to HPV Vaccines on February 25–26, 2014, for physicians and scientists.[25] Experts from Canada, the US, the UK, France, and Japan presented, including Drs. Lee, Authier, Tomljenovic, Sasaki, Shiozawa, Kiyoshi, Hama, and Fukushima.[26] A public hearing was held the following day, when the Ministry of Health addressed public concerns. Dr. Lee also spoke at this meeting, and the Ministry published the minutes online.[27]

The symposium and the public hearing were forums for dialogue between scientists critical of the HPV vaccine and those supporting its reintroduction in Japan. To date, such scientific forums with proponents and critics of the vaccine together discussing it have been exceptionally rare. They explored the plausible mechanisms whereby the vaccine is causing injury, including problems with residual HPV DNA and its combination with aluminum, causing cytokine storms and tumor necrosis factor release, leading to reported injuries and deaths.[28] Dr. Harumi Sakai, a Japanese researcher and organizer of the event, suggested that the adverse event rate for HPV vaccine may be 9 percent and that women who become pregnant within two years after vaccination abort or miscarry 30 percent of their babies.[29]

Industry-friendly presentations at the Symposium emphasized what they saw as methodological flaws in the critics' research that overstated safety concerns and injuries were just psychosomatic reactions. Dr. Lee, after presenting data from an autopsy on a girl who reportedly died from the HPV vaccine, asked the audience to raise their hands if they thought that a psychosomatic reaction could cause brain inflammation. No one did.[30] On February 27, 2014, the day after the Symposium and the press conference, doctors from around Japan started writing the Ministry, saying that they did not accept that the girls' symptoms were psychosomatic.

A few weeks later, on March 12, Dr. Robert Pless, chairman of the Global Advisory Committee on Vaccine Safety (GACVS), issued a statement reassuring the public of the HPV vaccine's safety; he said that its "benefit-risk profile remains favorable."[31] As we learned in Chapter 17, this statement was planned ahead of the symposium in cooperation with the Ministry for Health. Dr. Pless attempted to refute the scientific evidence presented by Dr. Lee at the February symposium. Dr. Lee later complained to the WHO as to what he considered collusion between the Japanese Ministry and GACVS, to discredit him prior to the symposium, as discussed in Chapter 17.[32] The WHO never acknowledged Dr. Lee's complaint.

At the end of March 2014, the relevant Japanese Ministry committee met again to decide whether to reinstate the HPV vaccine recommendation in its national vaccine schedule. They voted no, and the deadline passed once again.

GUIDELINES FOR MANAGING SYMPTOMS

In August 2015, despite being in the middle of an international firestorm, the Japan Medical Association and the Japanese Association of Medical Sciences issued official guidelines for managing symptoms post vaccination.[33] The Japanese Health Ministry also published a list of medical institutions where those who needed help could go to see trained staff. There was even a helpline. The guidelines were published in Japanese and not reported widely outside Japan, until *Medscape Medical News* translated the document and published it on its website.[34] Incredibly, there was no coverage in medical journals or in Western mainstream media. Not only was the Japanese government refusing to reinstate the vaccination program, the Medical Association was doubling down by acknowledging that reactions were medical. Contrary to the official 2014 report that determined that reactions were psychogenic,[35] the guidelines specifically caution against referring to a patient's symptoms as psychogenic. Instead, doctors should refer to symptoms as a "syndrome characterized by pain of unknown etiology."[36]

According to *Medscape*, the guidelines lay out specific instructions for medical professionals to follow when people report reactions to the vaccine.[37] Those include obtaining medical histories, conducting a physical exam, and evaluating severity of pain in three categories: (1) pain due to inflammation; (2) neuropathic pain; and (3) psychological pain. It also recommends blood and urine tests and referrals to specialists. The guidelines stress the importance of mental and physical care of the family, as well.[38] The Japan Society of Obstetrics and Gynecology acknowledged the guidelines as important but hastened to add its continued support for the reinstatement of the HPV vaccine, as it considered such adverse events rare.[39]

At a press briefing announcing the guidelines, *Medscape* reported, the president of the Japan Medical Association recommended waiting to reinstate the vaccine.[40] The president of the Japan Association of Medical Sciences went a step further and stated that there is no proof that the vaccine prevents cancer, acknowledging, however, reports that precancerous conditions had declined.[41] In other words, they recommended a "wait and see" approach while taking care of those who reacted adversely. Japan stands alone in the world for now, for taking such a cautious approach. The research group that authored the HPV vaccine injury guidelines is made up of doctors and scientists from universities and medical schools all over Japan. One of the authors is Dr. Shuichi Ikeda, who had already studied approximately 200 girls who had suffered post-HPV vaccination illnesses. He is considered an expert in diagnosing and treating their multiple symptoms.[42]

Dr. Ikeda may be better known in Japan for his controversial public disagreement with medical journalist Dr. Riko Muranaka, a former WHO infectious disease doctor who specialized in avian flu pandemics. In March 2016, Dr. Ikeda and his team published a research paper on a mouse experiment whereby a mouse injected with the vaccine suffered brain damage. His findings were announced in a press conference and further cemented the fears of the Japanese people over the vaccine. At around this time, Dr. Muranaka began taking an interest in the HPV controversy and wrote a series of articles in support of the vaccine.[43]

Dr. Muranaka, criticized Dr. Ikeda's mouse study in *Wedge*, a major business magazine in Japan, and made allegations of scientific misconduct in his work. Dr. Ikeda's university conducted its own investigation and cleared him of this serious charge but did ask that he clarify his findings.[44] Soon after, Dr. Ikeda sued Dr. Muranaka for defamation, based on her statements that he falsified data in his experiment. The Ministry for Health apologized publicly if Dr. Ikeda's study had caused confusion for the Japanese people and denied that the vaccine was associated with reported symptoms.[45]

Dr. Muranaka's criticism of Dr. Ikeda's findings in the mouse study made its way to the *Wall Street Journal*, where she described his study as "highly misleading," a slightly lesser charge of falsifying data and scientific misconduct.[46] Dr. Muranaka was quoted in the *Financial Times* about why she made the accusations: "It is about the consequences it [the study] has for 10,000 women and their families who get cervical cancer each year in Japan and the 3,000 who die from it."[47] Dr. Ikeda's libel lawsuit against Dr. Muranaka is ongoing at the time of writing and is not expected to conclude until late 2018. Dr. Muranaka is funding her own legal fees, although according to an article on the case, she is accepting donations from a "support group."[48] In 2017, Dr. Muranaka earned the prestigious John Maddox prize in the UK for her part in fighting HPV vaccine "misinformation," and for "championing evidence in the face of hostility and threats."[49]

This controversy did not stop Dr. Ikeda's work. He was quoted in the *Financial Times* saying, "I am relieved that University proved it was not fabrication or manipulation. I will do my best for the girls suffering from adverse reactions to HPV vaccine as before."[50]

There was good reason that the Medical Association and the Association of Medical Sciences were cautious about reinstating the vaccine. Dr. Shuichi Ikeda and his colleagues published clinical findings in 2017 in an article titled, "Suspected Adverse Effects After Human Papillomavirus Vaccination: A Temporal Relationship Between Vaccine Administration and the Appearance of Symptoms in Japan."[51] Much like Dr. Louise Brinth's study of 53 cases in Denmark, the Japanese study comprised clinical cases referred to Dr. Ikeda at the Shinshu University Hospital in Matsumoto. This groundbreaking analysis of 120 female patients goes into great detail as to diagnostic techniques and clinical evidence of harm. The study clarifies the temporal relationship between the vaccine and postvaccination symptoms. According to the study, "the vast majority of [cases] have been ascribed to chronic regional pain syndrome, orthostatic intolerance, and/or cognitive dysfunction."[52]

INDUSTRY PUSHES BACK

Pharmaceutical industry executives would not like to see the events in Japan repeat themselves; they fear that Japan's decision not to recommend the HPV vaccine could influence other national immunization programs to reject the vaccine. Heidi Larson, a UK anthropologist and leading proponent for the HPV vaccine, coauthored an article in a scientific journal on the "global response to Japan's suspension of its HPV vaccine recommendation."[53] Dr. Larson heads up the newly formed "Vaccine Confidence Project" at the London School of Hygiene and Tropical Medicine, funded by the WHO and the Bill and Melinda Gates Foundation. The project's mission is to track vaccine hesitancy worldwide by "building an information surveillance system" to monitor social media for "false" information and quickly stem bad press associated with vaccines.[54]

Another industry-sponsored response, coauthored by Heidi Larson, came from the US Center for Strategic and International Studies, a Washington, DC, think tank. It issued a report in April 2015, "HPV Vaccination in Japan: The Continuing Debate and Global Impacts," after having received "generous support" from Merck.[55] This was a follow-up report to one published in May, 2014, by the same authors.[56] The Center is better known for public policy studies in cyber security, foreign policy, defense policy, and climate change but has recently started working in the area of global health to advance US interests.[57]

The Center's study suggests that the accounts of adverse events from Japan are "unverified" and that the girls merely "claim" to have suffered adverse events.[58] The report states that Japan's failure in "not actively promoting HPV vaccination is putting the Japanese population at long-term unnecessary risk."[59] The authors recommend that "high-level Japanese political leadership [restore] an active recommendation for HPV vaccination."[60]

The report references "antivaccine" groups that gain media attention and those who have suffered adverse events as "victims," in quotation marks to question the authenticity of their claims. SaneVax is one of the "antivaccine" groups that the report references, although it fails to mention that SaneVax supported the Ministry of Health's public hearing on February 26, 2014.[61] In its commentary on the girls' conditions, the report offers no other explanation for the adverse events than psychogenesis. It notes that "members of the public may perceive this label, 'psychogenic' and the term 'mass hysteria' as patronizing and dismissive of real concerns and actual physical suffering."[62] Despite acknowledging this concern, the report sticks by its psychogenic explanation for injuries.

The report highlights India and Japan as having failed to counter negative messages about the vaccine quickly. It points to a direct correlation between immediate responses to negative media stories and public confidence. The authors showcase Japan and India as examples of what governments should not do. The authors conclude that there have been "serious spillover effects" outside Japan and that senior members of the Japanese government should step up to find a "lasting resolution," presumably reinstating the national recommendation to use the HPV vaccine.[63]

Furthermore, the authors blame social media for the controversy and refer to victim groups pejoratively as "antivaccine," which is not a term that the advocacy groups accept as accurate. The report dwells on the role of social media and how "antivaccine groups have strengthened their control of the narrative,"[64] suggesting a kind of standoff between the Japanese Ministry of Health and the advocacy groups. The authors never seriously consider the possibility that the girls' accounts of injury are true or that such reactions are even possible. With a central theme to dismiss all reported claims of adverse events as false, the report blames bad publicity worldwide on the Japanese Ministry for failing to reintroduce its proactive HPV vaccine recommendation.

HPV Vaccine Activists Advance in Court

In July 2016, a victims' group in Japan filed a class action lawsuit against the government, Merck, and GSK for injuries from HPV vaccines.[65] The group of 119 plaintiffs, which may expand, seeks damages of 15 million yen for each injured person (around $135,000) and access to a network of medical specialists to address their chronic health issues. Japan has a vaccine injury compensation program, and some victims may have already received some compensation at the state level. One of the claims is that the vaccine program was implemented illegally. Scientists and lawyers involved in the case published an article in 2017 about the case, saying:

> Today's diagnostics and therapeutics were created by listening to patients' voices and conducting careful examinations. It is irresponsible to dismiss a patient's complaint as a psychogenic reaction or a general phenomenon among young women without conducting a thorough examination.[66]

Just as in India, this lawsuit is pending at the time of writing.

SaneVax has attempted to analyze why Japan dropped its proactive recommendation for the HPV vaccine. It identified three meaningful factors: (1) mobilization of the families of those who suffered adverse events; (2) engagement of medical professionals to assess the adverse events in an unbiased way; and (3) the engagement of Japanese politicians to hear both sides of the HPV vaccine debate. SaneVax, Dr. Lee, and others fully understood the power of Japan's example, as did the industry. If one country could reject the vaccine despite industry pressure, surely others could, too. Japan continues to be a center of influence in the HPV vaccine debate. Both its attention to the girls' medical needs and its refusal to recommend the vaccine to its citizens means that the world will continue to monitor what happens next.

25.

DENMARK: PUSHING BACK IN EUROPE

The epicenter of the HPV vaccine controversy in continental Europe is the Kingdom of Denmark. A small country with a population of approximately 6 million people, it is the smallest of the Scandinavian countries. Unfortunately, around 100 Danish women die from cervical cancer annually.[1]

Denmark, as we know from Kesia and Sesilje's story in Chapter 2, was a clinical trial center during the development stages of both Gardasil and Cervarix and continues to support an "extension study" location at Frederiksberg Hospital under the supervision of Dr. Jesper Mehlsen. Schools do not administer the vaccine as in Ireland and the UK, but the National Medicines Agency recommends it, as does the Danish National Cancer Society. The vaccine is available in drugstores and fitness centers around the country.[2]

Kesia's and Sesilje's stories start later in the Danish chronicles. They made the connection between their illnesses and the clinical trials in 2016, long after the vaccine was introduced in Denmark. Before this, many families had begun to report injuries following the vaccine in Denmark. One such family was the Viborg family.

Karsten Viborg was a typical family man enjoying life with his wife and two teenage children. He had no idea when he and his wife consented to the Gardasil vaccine for their 12-year-old daughter in 2010 that their lives would never be the same. Their daughter Rikke did not react immediately to the vaccine. Her symptoms crept up on her over time. First she experienced headaches, pain, and flu-like symptoms. As time went on, and with each subsequent vaccine dose, her symptoms became more severe. Following the third dose in 2011, she had severe and chronic headaches, frequent fainting without any warning, paralysis from her hips down, and insomnia. She experienced more than 30 different symptoms in all, although she was only twelve years old. When she was healthy, she was an active scuba diver, played handball, and was very athletic. Following the vaccine, she was absent from school 70 percent of the time from 2011 to 2014. A few doctors were starting to admit to Karsten that his daughter's symptoms were related to the Gardasil vaccine, but they said there was nothing they could do.

That didn't sit well with Karsten, since he could not accept that his young daughter would be sick for the foreseeable future. She needed medical help. He began researching Gardasil side effects and came across stories of other girls with similar symptoms. He became aware of the work of Drs. Chris Shaw and Lucija Tomljenovic rather quickly. Karsten wrote to Dr. Shaw, and to his surprise, Dr. Shaw wrote back right away. Dr. Shaw could not help with treatment protocols but put Karsten in touch with Dr. Yehuda Shoenfeld in Israel, a world-renowned autoimmune disease specialist.

Dr. Shoenfeld kindly put Karsten in touch with a doctor in Scandinavia, Professor Vera Stejskal in Stockholm. Little did Karsten know at the time that, in his first toe-dipping into the world of HPV vaccines, he had just made contact with some of the most prominent trailblazers in this controversial arena. Professor Stejskal suggested Karsten travel to an autism conference in Edinburgh, Scotland, where she would be speaking.[3] He was confused as to why this would be relevant to his daughter's case, but he went because he trusted Professor Stejskal's perspective.

Despite the conference's focus on recovery from autism, Karsten quickly understood its relevance to his daughter's plight. He learned all he could about biomedical healing and what the body can do to heal once one addresses root causes of illness. This was profoundly inspiring to Karsten. As an engineer, he was not familiar with such ideas, but he saw the value in using natural approaches to rebuild Rikke's immune system and to change her diet to lower inflammation. It couldn't hurt, and she was so sick that he had to try. Professor Stejskal died on September 27, 2017, to the sadness of the Viborg family. Karsten knew that without her guidance, his daughter would never have gotten the help she needed.

Karsten was motivated and began to see significant improvements in Rikke as soon as he made the changes he learned about in Edinburgh. Karsten began studying and reading journals to learn all he could about autoimmune disorders and recovery. He read over 700 scientific papers and became an expert in HPV vaccine injury, specifically side effects from Gardasil. He travelled to Germany, Switzerland, France, and Scotland to find answers and treatment protocols. With the help of an enormous team of doctors and specialists, Rikke gradually recovered from her illnesses and resumed a relatively normal life. It wasn't easy, and without the hundreds of scientific tests and treatment protocols, it would not have happened. And the cost was great. Karsten discovered that Rikke's treatment in local hospitals cost around DKK250,000 (about $40,000), which is a large sum of money, especially when there is no clear diagnosis. And this doesn't include the personal expenses Karsten incurred to travel to doctors and clinics around Europe. Recovery from autoimmune illness is expensive and time-consuming, he learned.

Through this journey, Karsten discovered that there were many more "Rikkes" in Denmark. He formed the patient group "HPV Victims Denmark" in early 2015 with other parents of children with similar issues. As in other countries, Danish families were thrown into this controversy because they could not receive the help they needed for their sick children. Doctors could find no medical explanation for their conditions and routinely recommended psychological testing. The government repeatedly denied any association with the vaccine. If there was no diagnosis and doctors believed the symptoms were psychosomatic, then families held out little hope for their children's recovery. Karsten shared his daughter's story to inspire others that recovery was possible. Soon he became more directly involved in advocacy as people began sharing this information on social media.

As social media stories were shared widely, media attention grew. It wasn't long before a TV station, TV2 Denmark, approached some injured girls and their families about taking part in a documentary called *The Vaccinated Girls*. It would be about the controversy brewing around the vaccine. The documentary featured many of the girls in Karsten's patient support group and raised the alarm about the side effects of the vaccine, in particular in athletic girls. The documentary screened on March 26, 2015, and quickly took off on social media.[4]

The documentary featured Dr. Louise Brinth, a physician at the Danish Syncope Unit in Frederiksberg Hospital, known as the Syncope Centre. Dr. Brinth voiced her concerns that most of the girls at the Centre reported that their symptoms started shortly after receiving Gardasil. She said in the film that in 1997, the Centre saw two POTS cases; in 2014, there were 57. By 2017, the Centre had seen over 400 girls who sought treatment after receiving Gardasil. It has become one of the only specialist clinics in the world, specializing in diagnosing and treating girls with symptoms potentially linked to HPV vaccines.

Dr. Brinth's colleague Dr. Jesper Mehlsen, with 30 years' experience of diagnosing and treating autonomic dysfunction and POTS, also appeared in the film, saying that the girls had virtually the same spontaneous stories and didn't know one another before they arrived at the Centre. Throughout his career, Dr. Mehlsen has published 125 scientific papers in peer-reviewed journals; six of those focus on HPV vaccination. Ironically, he was a principal investigator in some early clinical trials on HPV vaccines in Denmark. He is regarded as an expert in his field.

Both doctors would become pivotal to the HPV vaccine controversy in Denmark. Together they published three peer-reviewed scientific articles relating to the HPV vaccine and its side effects.[5] They began to report all cases of suspected vaccine reactions to the Danish Health and Medicines Authority, as they were legally required to do. The first case was referred to their Center in 2011, over a year after the vaccine was introduced. By 2013, they had seven more cases. Word spread in Denmark that their Center was not dismissing the girls' reactions as psychosomatic, and they were one of the few places that offered a treatment plan, at least for some of the symptoms related to a POTS diagnosis.

Over the next few years, they received more and more case referrals. The Danish Health Authority cooperated with Dr. Brinth and her colleagues and took the situation seriously. By 2013, as more cases kept coming in, the Health Authority requested Drs. Brinth and Mehlsen to draft a formal report on their findings. Their report to the Health Authority was the first such report, detailing 35 post-HPV vaccine cases. The Health Authority immediately forwarded the report to the EMA for review.[6] Of the 35 cases, the report noted:

> Twenty-five had a high level of physical activity before vaccination and irregular periods were reported by all patients not on treatment with oral contraception. Serum bilirubin was below the lower detection limit in 17 patients. Twenty-one of the referred patients fulfilled the criteria for a diagnosis of POTS (60 percent, 95 percent CI 43-77 percent). All patients had orthostatic intolerance, 94 percent nausea, 82 percent chronic headache, 82 percent fatigue, 77 percent cognitive dysfunction, 72 percent segmental dystonia, 68 percent neuropathic pain.[7]

Since Dr. Brinth was a POTS specialist and 60 percent of the girls had this diagnosis, POTS became the focus. Dr. Brinth repeatedly asked the EMA and other health authorities to note the significance of other symptoms in their report. The EMA did not take these into consideration, however, and concluded in December 2014 that the relationship between POTS and Gardasil could be "neither confirmed nor denied."[8] The Danish Health Authority posted a statement on their websites following the EMA decision, saying that even if POTS was classified as an adverse reaction to the vaccine, they would not withdraw it from the vaccine schedule, as the benefit of preventing hundreds of cases of cancer each year would still outweigh the suspected reported adverse reactions.[9]

Despite their continued support of the HPV vaccine program following the EMA review, the Health Authority responded to

increased media and public pressure to look into the growing number of girls who were becoming ill, whatever the cause. There was
also some political pressure. The HPV Victims group, including
Karsten Viborg, met with members of Parliament throughout this
time to try to obtain support and recognition for their girls' chronic
illnesses.

From this grassroots advocacy effort, an unlikely ally appeared.
Liselott Blixt of the Danish People's Party was one of the first politicians to push for Denmark to adopt the HPV vaccine. Ironically, she
became the first to seek its removal from the national recommended
vaccine schedule. After her own daughter fell ill following the vaccine,
she campaigned strenuously for the vaccine to be removed. Blixt is
the chairperson of Parliament's Health Committee;[10] her opponents
criticize her stance on the vaccine as "grossly irresponsible."[11]

Despite opposition, Blixt eventually secured 7 million Danish
kroner (around $1 million) for an independent investigation into
the vaccine's side effects in October 2015. The funds have gone
to three institutions: 4 million Kroner to Frederiksberg Hospital
under the direction of Dr. Jesper Mehlsen, 1.5 million Kroner to
the Statens Serum Institut, and the remaining 1.5million to Aarhus
University under the direction of Dr. Kim Varming.[12] The world
eagerly awaits the outcome of these studies.

In March 2015, amid growing pressure, the health departments
of the five "regions," or states, in Denmark announced that they
would open five new "HPV Clinics," in addition to the one in
Frederiksberg Hospital. This would help alleviate Drs. Brinth and
Mehlsen of their growing caseload. Over 1,300 cases flooded the
HPV clinics shortly after opening.[13] The response was much higher
than expected; waiting lists of six to nine months were normal.[14]
Each clinic was to institute an intake process to collect data on
the girls' symptoms, and some medical tests were to be performed.
From a request on social media, we were able to gather from those
that sought treatment that the clinics did not actually perform even
basic laboratory work and they mostly referred girls for psychological examination. We cannot confirm these reports, but to date, no

official information has been published on any data collected at these clinics.

Over 2,300 adverse events from the HPV vaccine have been reported officially in Denmark; over 1,000 of those reports were considered *severe*.[15] The Statens Serum Institute reported 150 adverse events per 100,000 shots sold in 2015, including POTS, CRPS, and "medically unexplained physical symptoms."[16]

Many HPV vaccine proponents blame the publicity around the documentary for the spike in reported adverse events. Danish health authorities implied that the reports were not related to the HPV vaccine and that the girls who would have succumbed to autonomic disorders anyway may have been swayed by what they saw on TV.[17] They attributed the mistaken association with the vaccine as unfortunate yet mere coincidence. In 2018, both the English subtitled version and TV2's Danish version of the documentary have been removed from the Internet.

The documentary may well have raised awareness about HPV vaccine injury and may have alerted people who experienced similar temporal reactions following the HPV vaccine to report them. This does not explain away, however, the physical pain girls are reporting to the centers after HPV vaccination. Danish psychologist Dr. Peter La Cour saw many girls who suspected their reactions were from the vaccine. He believes that they experience both physical and psychological pain, with the latter made worse by the "blame the victim" phenomenon. In a presentation he gave to the Danish Society for Medical Philosophy, Ethics and Method in November 2016 (a presentation Karsten Viborg attended),[18] Dr. La Cour explains that while they have no diagnosis in psychiatry for what the girls are experiencing, and there are no biomarkers to look for, they must adopt a more modern model in approaching their diagnosis and treatment. He believes that the unfiltered debate in the media and online does not go unnoticed by the girls, which is harmful to their rehabilitation. He does not believe that social media has had an impact on the proliferation of their symptoms. In other words, he does not believe that social media is responsible for a kind of mass hysteria or reaction to vaccination. In his experience with Facebook groups for all kinds of illnesses, HPV vaccine patient groups on social media are not different. Patients want acknowledgement, support, and help in coping with their daily symptoms. Dr. La Cour believes that patient groups online "reflect the level of symptom burden, they do not invent symptom burden."[19]

In 2015, Drs. Brinth and Mehlsen published their second article on 53 patients, entitled "Suspected side effects to the quadrivalent human papilloma vaccine."[20] The results were alarming:

> 52 out of 53 patients (98 percent) reported that their activities of daily living were seriously affected, and 40 (75 percent) had to quit school or work for more than two months due to their symptoms.
>
> Headache: 53 (100 percent)
>
> Orthostatic intolerance: 51 (96 percent)
>
> Syncope: 24 (45 percent)
>
> POTS: 28 (53 percent)
>
> Fatigue: 51 (96 percent)
>
> Cognitive dysfunction: 47 (89 percent)
>
> Disordered sleep: 45 (85 percent)
>
> Visual symptoms: 37 (70 percent)
>
> Blurring of vision: 44 (83 percent)
>
> Gastrointestinal symptoms: 48 (91 percent)
>
> Neuropathic pain: 35 patients (66 percent)
>
> Motor symptoms: 35 (66 percent)
>
> Dyspnoea: 35 (66 percent)
>
> Skin disorders: 34 (64 percent)

Voiding dysfunction: 31 (59 percent)

Limb weakness: 30 (57 percent)

Vascular abnormalities: 27 (51 percent)

Irregular periods: 15/31 not on pill (48 percent)

Sicca symptoms: 21 (40 percent)

Hyperventilation: 18 (34 percent)

Dr. Brinth and her colleagues sent this new information to the Health Authority once again, and again, Denmark requested the EMA to conduct a safety review. Despite Dr. Brinth's objections, the EMA again focused its review on POTS and, unexpectedly, CRPS, even though CRPS was not part of Dr. Brinth's research. Nevertheless, the EMA issued a draft assessment report a few months later, on November 29, 2015.[21] The EMA dismissed Dr. Brinth's findings and now rejected their previous conclusion that they could not "confirm or deny" a causal link and replaced it with a more resolute position that there is no causal link with the vaccine, which we discussed in Chapter 17. Immediately issuing a detailed 50-page response, Dr. Brinth harshly criticized the Agency's assessment of her cases.[22] She asserted that the EMA unfairly criticized her work, clinical expertise, and judgment.[23]

The EMA also criticized a 2015 pharmacovigilance study from the Uppsala Monitoring Centre in Uppsala, Sweden.[24] The Danish Medicines Agency contacted the Uppsala Centre in 2014 for assistance so that it could compare Dr. Brinth's data to those from Uppsala.[25] The Health Authority wanted to understand if this was a true signal using Uppsala's passive adverse event reporting system Vigibase, which the WHO sponsors. The Uppsala Centre is the most highly respected pharmacovigilance center in the world.[26] Uppsala agreed to look at Dr. Brinth's data, specifically related to POTS, and Uppsala published its findings.[27] Dr. Rebecca Chandler, a physician and research scientist originally from the US, headed up the Uppsala team.

Dr. Chandler's research identified gaps in the monitoring and reporting of adverse events following the HPV vaccine due to inconsistent diagnostic criteria for conditions such as POTS, CRPS, and fatigue-related symptoms. Her analysis also found inconsistencies in the way doctors categorize clusters of symptoms as serious or nonserious. Dr. Chandler's team used a new technique called "cluster analysis" to delve deeper into the data to achieve a better understanding. They found cases in four small clusters, which they analyzed further. All the cases they analyzed were from before January 2015, so any possible reporting bias following the release of the "Vaccinated Girls" documentary in March 2015 could not affect the study.[28]

Dr. Chandler concluded that a disproportionate number of adverse events, both expected adverse events and unconfirmed ones, followed HPV vaccination compared to other vaccinations. Her article hypothesized that the adverse event reports suggested an association with fatigue-like symptoms, which could include POTS and other disorders. The article described this "signal":

> A causal association with the HPV vaccine remains uncertain; however, we believe that a more thorough investigation of this signal is required to ensure continued public trust in both vaccination programmes and regulatory authorities.

The EMA did not agree with Dr. Chandler's findings or the call for further investigation, however. Ignoring Dr. Chandler's observations based on data from the WHO database, it stated that no link existed between the HPV vaccine with POTS and CRPS.[29] Dr. Chandler criticized the EMA's assessment of her work. In an interview with Medscape she said, "I was disappointed by the poor quality of the document."[30]

The Danish Health Authority embraced the EMA decision and continues to recommend the HPV vaccine. The EMA report coincided, however, with the Health Authority's unexpected decision in January 2016 to replace Gardasil with GSK's Cervarix.[31] The government tender for HPV vaccine supply included criteria for "efficacy, adverse reactions, additional effects . . . and price."[32] Unfortunately, no international media covered this major supplier switch given the controversial association between Gardasil and adverse events over the previous three years. Despite reassurance from the EMA and the Danish Health Authority, uptake of the HPV vaccine declined from the high of 80 percent when the vaccine was first introduced in 2009 to 15 percent in 2016.[33] Uptake is currently on the rise, however, due to a public awareness campaign by the Health Authority called "Stop HPV, Stop Cervical Cancer."[34]

THE CONTROVERSY CONTINUES

The controversy with the EMA and the Cochrane Nordic Centre has only increased the public's resistance to the vaccine. Despite this, there is still a push to give the HPV vaccine to as many girls, and now boys, as possible. Cervarix was indicated by the EMA to prevent anal cancer in 2016, and this paved the way for promotion of this vaccine to boys in Denmark.[35]

The Danish Cancer Society, Kræftens Bekæmpelse, joined the Danish Medicines Agency in a joint information campaign to improve uptake rates. Merck Sharp and Dohme entered into several partnership agreements with the Cancer Society until 2024, worth almost 17 million Kroner (about $2.6 million) for follow-up research relating to the FUTURE II and FUTURE 9 (Gardasil 9) studies.[36]

Since parent groups like Karsten's are still seeking answers about what happened to their daughters, the controversy is unlikely to end anytime soon. Vaccine promotion campaigns will do little to ease 2,500 girls' suffering. Demark is the only European country to date where the HPV vaccine program has essentially collapsed. Therefore, like Japan, the spotlight will remain on Denmark for some time as to what happened and why. Also like Japan, Denmark has a group of doctors studying the suspected side effects of the HPV vaccine. The scientific community eagerly awaits the outcome of Dr. Mehlsen's study on more than 800 girls in his clinic at Frederiksberg Hospital, the goal of which is to examine the "biological and pathophysiological factors in girls/women experiencing symptoms suspected to be adverse reactions from HPV vaccination."[37]

Whatever the outcome, the work of Drs. Brinth and Mehlsen and their colleagues deserves close examination, as does Vigibase data on adverse events. Epidemiological studies, currently cited to dispel associations with side effects, are alone insufficient. More basic science research is needed. Dr. Chandler has criticized the usefulness of epidemiological studies that rely on a single-diagnosis concept to detect safety signals.[38] The HPV controversy has become an "elephant in the room" in Denmark and elsewhere. But as long as Drs. Brinth, Mehlsen, and Chandler can continue their research in this area, there is hope to unlock this scientific mystery.

26.

IRELAND: INJECTED AND NEGLECTED

"Some of the tactics employed [by campaigners] can only be equated to a form of emotional terrorism. As a result the uptake of the HPV vaccine in this country has dropped to an all-time low." Tony O'Brien, director general, Health Service Executive Ireland, Irish Examiner August 31, 2017[1]

ABBEY'S STORY

On September 22, 2014, at just twelve years old, Abbey Colohan received her first shot of Gardasil in a small office in her school with a friend by her side. She was nervous about it, but no more than other girls. It hurt a lot, but she put on a brave face. She was sitting down for the prescribed fifteen minutes after the shot, when she immediately felt incapacitated and could not speak. When the fifteen minutes were up, she tried to get up to go back to class but fell backward. The doctor present in the room told her to lie down on the mats they had ready. She began to jerk uncontrollably, and the doctor told her she was just having a panic attack and it would be over soon.

Lorraine, Abbey's mother, got a call from the school saying that Abbey was unwell and she should pick her up. The school didn't tell Lorraine what happened; she presumed Abbey was just feeling ill after the vaccine that day. She sent her husband, Martin, to get her. When he got to the school, he saw Abbey completely "out of it" on the mat and asked why the doctor hadn't called an ambulance. It had been an hour and twenty minutes since Abbey had had the vaccine and she appeared to be having a seizure. She was twitching and couldn't speak or walk unassisted, with pupils dilated.

The health service staff dismissed Martin's concerns and said it was just a normal reaction to the vaccine and that Abbey was having a panic attack. Nurses asked what Abbey had for breakfast that day and if perhaps her reaction was to that. Martin said she had had Cocopops but wasn't allergic to anything. The nurses concluded, however, that it must have been the Cocopops, since they had never seen anything like this before. Incredulous, Martin knew it was not a simple food reaction or a standard effect of a vaccine, the way one would expect. By this time, Abbey's condition had stabilized, and he brought her home.

When her mother saw Abbey arrive home with Martin, she was in shock. She had never seen her daughter look so unwell. Abbey was gray-purple in color, and she still couldn't speak. Her pupils were dilated, and her joints were red and swollen. Abbey pointed to her chest as the only way she could tell her mother where she felt pain. Lorraine felt that a completely different child came home from school that day from the perfectly healthy and happy one who left that morning.

The next day Abbey stayed home, and Lorraine called the school to see what had happened and if they had filed a school incident report. She spoke to the school principal, who did not know anything about Abbey convulsing after the vaccine, despite many students having witnessed it. Lorraine tracked down the "flying" vaccination staff, as they had moved on to another school, and spoke with the doctor who had administered the vaccine to Abbey. The doctor recalled "the jerking child" but suggested to Lorraine that Abbey must have had an underlying condition and that it wasn't due to the vaccine. The doctor said she had never seen such a reaction before. Lorraine wondered how this was somehow justification for not filing an adverse event report with the Department of Health. Something didn't add up. Later, Lorraine would learn that the FDA knew that "jerking," or "tonic-clonic movements" indicative of seizures, were common reactions to the vaccine as far back as 2009.[2] It was indicated as a "warning" on the front page of the package insert she found online.[3] So why didn't the doctor at the school know about this?

Abbey went back to school after taking a day to rest, as Lorraine thought she had recovered and that her convulsions would not recur. She was wrong. A few hours later, Abbey collapsed at school again. This time, a trained emergency responder came to Abbey's aid and recorded in a school incident report that Abbey was "incoherent, confused, had rapid breathing, her body was shaking, and she had no control over her movement. She was hot, and her eyes were rolling back." The medic observed that Abbey was having a brief epileptic fit or a staring episode, or a seizure. This time, the school called an ambulance, which rushed Abbey to the hospital, where she spent the next six days.

Doctors at the hospital did all kinds of tests but found no abnormalities. They referred Abbey to a psychologist, thinking that her condition was psychosomatic. Lorraine could not accept this diagnosis given Abbey's immediate reaction to the vaccine.

Abbey's life has never been the same since 2014. It now revolves around doctors and specialists who are trying to ease her pain. She now suffers from recurring seizures and cannot predict when she will have a good day or a bad one. She is still constantly fatigued and in a lot of pain throughout her body almost three years after the first dose of the vaccine. According to Ireland's health service, they were not notified of Abbey's reaction. In a letter Lorraine received, they stated that they "do not recall any child that had an anaphylactic reaction" and that "there was no evidence that Abbey had an anaphylactic reaction to the HPV vaccine." But many people witnessed Abbey's collapse. There are also hospital records and three school incident reports from when Abbey collapsed two days following the vaccine. There is no doubt in the Colohans' minds as to what happened, and they have vowed to fight for more answers.

VACCINE APPROVAL AMID CONTROVERSY

Ireland has one of the most aggressive infant vaccine schedules outside of the United States and has relatively high uptake rates even though vaccinations are not a requirement to attend school. Despite the public's overwhelming trust in the vaccination program, the introduction of the HPV vaccine was fraught with political controversy from the outset.

Ireland is demographically similar to Denmark and has similar cervical cancer rates at around 300 cases per year or 11 per 100,000 women. Tragically, around 90 women—or 3.7 per 100,000—lose their lives each year.[4]

In August 2008, the Irish Minister for Health Mary Harney announced that Ireland would be introducing the HPV vaccine Gardasil's 3-dose program. The high cost of the vaccine was a major hurdle to overcome for the minister, in the midst of one of Ireland's biggest housing collapses and recession. It would take another two years for Minister Harney to finally approve the vaccine after Merck offered the health service a reduced cost per vaccine.[5] The political and public pressure to adopt a program was intensifying. This politically charged emotional campaign, along with the price reduction, led to the start of Ireland's school-based HPV vaccination program in September 2010.[6]

Upon hearing the news, Mothers' Alliance Ireland (MAI), a parent advocacy group, immediately wrote a detailed open letter to the Ministers for Health and Education and the Irish Medicines Board, criticizing the health assessment report.[7] The group also wrote to every school principal in the country with the same concerns. Critics were quick to cite MAI's conservative religious leanings and concerns that the vaccine would increase promiscuity, in order to dismiss their complaints. The letter from MAI, however, pointed to more serious concerns expressed by the Health Assessment group (HIQA) who recommended the vaccine in 2008, regarding the lack of duration of protection, the side effects, and the risk of disease enhancement for those already infected with HPV.[8] MAI's concerns went unanswered.

Right before the program began, the *Irish Examiner* published an article with balanced information, outlining the risks of the vaccine.[9] However, highlighting the questions around the safety gaps in the vaccine's history had no real impact, and vaccination rates among preteen girls would reach over 80 percent in the first year. This high uptake rate stood to reason because the vaccine was offered directly in the schools.[10]

The vaccination packet that children received in the school consent packet in 2010 contained a bright pink, glossy, easy-to-read HPV brochure.[11] Parents had a few days to return the consent forms, which did not contain the manufacturer's Patient Information Leaflet (PIL), which is given with all drugs distributed in Ireland. This denied parents prior, free, and informed consent.[12] The parents were directed to do their own research on the Health Service's website,[13] but with so little time and assurances on the brochure that there were few side effects, there is little incentive to do so.

The health agency specifically instructs the schools not to provide any nongovernment-approved information in the packets going home to parents.[14] The Health Service rationalizes its failure to provide information essential to informed consent by relying on an industry-funded study of medical literacy, which states that Ireland has high levels of illiteracy and needs simplified language.[15] The HSE informed staff in their 2015 guidelines for immunization that 1 in 4 Irish adults have literacy problems and would have difficulty understanding the patient information leaflet.[16] The manufacturer's leaflet cites many more warnings about side effects and also includes reported adverse events from the postlicensing period.[17] By contrast, the Health Service leaflet contains enticing graphics aimed at teenagers and makes expansive claims like "the HPV vaccine protects against cervical cancer."[18]

An Irish website, Comelook.org, served as an early monitor and critical commentator on Ireland's decision to adopt the HPV vaccine. It requested and analyzed adverse event reports from the relevant state regulatory body, the Irish Medicines Board (IMB), and published the alarming assertion that in its first year, medical personnel observed almost 25 times the maximum anaphylaxis rate they expected from the HPV vaccine.[19] Yet no one at the Irish Medicines Board (later renamed the Health Products Regulatory Authority) or the media reported on these reactions. Comelook.org published information and analyses of the situation as it unfolded, which the mainstream media neglected to do. Although written in a somewhat sardonic tone, the articles had copious citations and revealed a level of detail about the HPV vaccine's immediate impact on Irish children that was not being reported elsewhere.

REGRET

Kiva Murphy is a native of Dublin who unwittingly found herself in the middle of this controversy, all because she followed the recommendations and vaccinated her daughter Kelly with three doses of the HPV vaccine in the 2012–13 school year. Kelly's health got progressively worse with each dose. Kiva was unwavering in her dedication to healing her daughter and finding out the truth about what happened to her once vibrant, athletic daughter. Like many mothers in this situation, Kiva began searching for answers on the Internet. She had started to suspect that it was related to the HPV vaccine and suggested this to Kelly's doctors. After running many blood tests, they told her that there was nothing wrong with Kelly and that it is normal for teenagers to have the painful symptoms Kelly was experiencing.

In May 2015, while searching for answers, Kiva clicked on SaneVax's website. Kiva read the story of Katie Robinson from Red Hill, Pennsylvania, and realized that her daughter had reacted to Gardasil in precisely the same way.[20] She wasn't sure before reading someone else's story that this really could have happened after a vaccine. It was the same timing, the same reactions, and the same gradual decline into chronic, unexplained ill health. She felt punched in the stomach, realizing for the first time what had happened to her daughter. There was one Irish story on SaneVax at that time. Karen Smyth from County Louth had written her daughter's story just a few months before.[21] Karen was the first Irish mother to brave any public backlash and point to a connection.

Kiva quickly came across other stories in Facebook groups. After describing Kelly's symptoms, she nervously asked in one of these groups about the HPV vaccine and if other girls had experienced these symptoms shortly after getting it, too. Up to this point, Kelly was experiencing chronic "all over pain," especially in her back and extremities. She had thyroid problems, anxiety, insomnia, and heart palpitations and was on multiple medications from the time she woke up to the time she tried, in vain, to sleep at night. She also received intensive physical, hydro, and occupational therapy in an in-patient treatment center to refacilitate some mobility. This was a difficult journey for a child who had only just entered her teens.

To Kiva's surprise and relief, many people responded to her Facebook post. They all had similar stories, specifically following the HPV vaccine, and some of them even saw the same doctors and specialists. They shared information and agreed to keep the conversation going, as there was so much they wanted to learn from one another's experiences. They eventually decided to meet.

This small group of parents met on May 23, 2015, at a coffeehouse in Dublin, where Kiva worked as a manager. Karen Smyth, whose story inspired Kiva to bring everyone together, joined her. Together with their families, the parents shared medical records, information on various specialists, and medical tests. There were few places to get help in Ireland. With socialized medical care, unless parents could pay out of pocket, waiting lists for specialists were years long. Their daughters' medical treatment was becoming increasingly more expensive and out of reach. They wanted their daughters to get better first and foremost. But ultimately, they agreed that something needed to be done to share what they now knew about the risks associated with the vaccine, which the Irish Health Service never shared with them. They didn't want this to happen to anyone else. REGRET, or Reactions and Effects of Gardasil Resulting in Extreme Trauma, was born.

Within a few months of forming, some REGRET parents began sharing their stories with local media outlets and talking to their local politicians. Ann Fitzpatrick from County Carlow was also at that first REGRET meeting. She wrote up her daughter Carol's story and sent it to Norma at SaneVax.[22] Ann worked tirelessly to get the word out; her voice could be heard frequently on local radio in the early days of campaigning for awareness. Parents from all over the country began contacting REGRET via their website because their daughters had similar stories.[23]

ADVOCACY BEGINS IN IRELAND

REGRET's first official meeting took place in August 2015. The group had been engaging favorably with the media, appearing on radio and TV. Open-minded journalists reported some of the girls' compelling stories.[24] At this point, the parents assumed it would just be a matter of time before the minister of health met with them to discuss the issue. Because this was a state-sponsored vaccination program under a state-funded medical system, REGRET parents needed to engage the minister for health to get help for their daughters because they were not getting adequate help from their doctors. Waiting lists for health consultants were sometimes years long, and many of the girls didn't qualify for state help in order to cover the cost of private care. Consultations from private specialists had shorter waiting lists, but unless you had a diagnosis or a referral, insurance was an issue. And not all the families had private health insurance. The REGRET parents couldn't comprehend why the minister was stonewalling them.

Later in August, Karen Smyth, Kiva Murphy, and other parents met with Dr. Kevin Connolly, chairman of the National Immunisation Advisory Committee, who did agree to meet with them and listen to their concerns. Kiva asked Dr. Connolly if he believed that it was the vaccine that caused their daughters' illnesses, and he agreed that it was possible. However, he still believed that the program was an important government policy in the fight against cervical cancer.[25] Dr. Connolly said in a documentary on the REGRET girls that he was sure that the girls would have become ill anyway, as "600 young people develop chronic fatigue every year in any event."[26] There are no published statistics available in Ireland to corroborate Dr. Connolly's statement, and chronic fatigue does not describe the chronic illnesses reported by REGRET daughters.

They claim that they are suffering from clusters of many symptoms, similar to Dr. Chandler's research discussed in the previous chapter. Yet Dr. Connolly did not address this anomaly and continues to tell the public that the girls suffer from "CFS" in numbers they would expect to see in this age group.

In September 2015, Karen and Kiva traveled to London to meet with staff at the European Medicines Agency who were interviewing those who suspected the vaccine had caused their children to become ill.[27] At Denmark's request, the EMA was conducting an investigation into the vaccine and its association with Postural Orthostatic Tachycardia Syndrome (POTS) and Complex Regional Pain Syndrome (CRPS) discussed in earlier chapters. Karen was carrying 77 detailed case histories, which she had solicited from families and compiled into a report. This was no small task to organize, and given subsequent events, she wondered if it was worth the effort or if anyone at the EMA even looked at them. The EMA came to the conclusion only two months later that there was no association between the vaccine and POTS or CRPS.[28]

In 2015 Merck, or Sanofi Pasteur MSD in Europe, changed its recommended dose schedule from three doses to two. It is unclear why Sanofi would rush ahead of countries like the US in recommending such a dramatic change, but it was based on some credible data. Sanofi Pasteur MSD's statement cited a Canadian study, which concluded:

> Responses to HPV-16 and HPV-18 one month after the last dose were non-inferior to those among young women who received 3 doses of the vaccine within 6 months. . . .[29]

A concerned parent, who claimed the vaccine harmed her daughter, emailed the Irish National Immunisation Office, requesting clarification on the new policy, as other countries like the United States were still recommending three doses. A senior medical officer wrote back and confirmed why the policy was changing, stating:

> An effective two-dose schedule reduces the number of vaccinations

needed by each girl and also the incidence of the adverse events.

A two-dose schedule should be more acceptable to students, parents and health care providers. This ultimately may lead to higher uptake of the vaccine, and better overall prevention of cervical cancer and other HPV-related disease outcomes.[30]

The Office was saying that the third dose was no longer needed and furthermore that removing it would reduce the number of reactions. The REGRET parents were left wondering why this new policy change was not making headlines all over the world, if the reason for implementing it was to remove the risk of third-dose reactions. Many of their daughters were most affected after the third dose. They felt a sense of outrage. If the third dose was considered superfluous and indeed dangerous to some, why were doctors in the United States not immediately notified to make this change also? The United States did not fully adopt the change until 2017, after an announcement by the CDC in December 2016.[31]

On December 3, 2015, Kiva's local district senator, Darragh O'Brien, invited Kiva and Karen to present the issue to the Joint Committee on Health and Children in Parliament.[32] By this time, Anna Cannon became REGRET's media spokesperson. Anna had an injured daughter and wanted to help in any way she could. Anna joined Kiva and Karen that day; they all made statements.[33] They came face-to-face for the first time with the Health Service managers of the national HPV vaccination program, who were also invited to make presentations. After the parents' speeches voicing their concerns, the health agency managers reemphasized their position that the vaccine is very safe and effective, citing the EMA's recent assessment as evidence. The assessment they cited was released ahead of schedule, without supporting documentation.[34] Nevertheless, the Health Service managers relied on this preemptive publication to endorse the vaccine's safety and to reject a causal link between the vaccine and the girls' illnesses and the need for an investigation.

The parents argued that their children not only presented with POTS and CRPS, but with many other cluster symptoms, including seizures, chronic pain, syncope, sleep disorders, menstrual disorders, ovarian cysts, pancreatitis, and premature ovarian failure. They arrived at an impasse with the Health Service, as they could neither offer proof nor did they have doctors willing to speak out and validate that the vaccine was causing their daughters' health problems. Anna, Kiva, and Karen would hear no more from the Health Service on the matter.

THE DOCUMENTARY

Despite continued media pressure, some families in REGRET agreed to film a documentary with a national TV station, TV3. The show would feature testimony from Abbey Colohan, Kelly Power, and Laura Smyth. The producers assured the families that they were sincere in wanting to do a fair and balanced report on the controversy.[35] They kept their word. Abbey Colohan's story was finally being told. There was a lot of positive press about the documentary, "Cervical Cancer Vaccine, Is It Safe?" which aired on December 14, 2015.[36] Interest was high, and social media propelled the documentary all over the world. Immediately after the documentary aired, REGRET was inundated with requests for information. However, despite the increased public support, the positive media tide was beginning to turn. In a presentation to professionals in 2017, Dr. Brenda Corcoran of the National Immunisation Office cites both the Danish and the Irish documentaries as reasons for the rapid decline in Ireland's uptake of the vaccine.[37]

THE IRISH CANCER SOCIETY

At the end of August 2016, the Irish Cancer Society began a campaign in partnership with the Health Service to endorse the HPV vaccine.[38] Due to the mounting adverse reports, especially online, from various advocacy and patient groups around the world, vaccine uptake rates in Ireland dropped from 87 percent to 72 percent the previous year.[39] The media began to blame this downturn on REGRET's awareness campaign, specifically the TV3 documentary. To respond, the Cancer Society planned to host two town hall–style meetings in two different cities a few days apart to promote the vaccine.[40] Dr. Margaret Stanley, a scientist from Cambridge University and a consultant for Merck and other pharmaceutical companies, was the guest speaker.[41] The meetings would turn out to be a public relations disaster for the Irish Cancer Society.

After much publicity, the first meeting was held in Galway on August 23, 2016. It was a spirited meeting with a few parents interrupting with questions and raising their voices. The Cancer Society was live-streaming the event on Facebook, which proved problematic when, during the Q&A, 16-year-old Rebecca Hollidge took the microphone to ask a question. Rebecca was relying on a wheelchair for most of her mobility needs, after having received the vaccine. Rebecca challenged Dr. Stanley's claim that the vaccine was safe. The Cancer Society immediately cut the live streaming, but someone in the audience continued to film the exchange anyways. Rebecca asked Dr. Stanley if she ever felt guilty that the vaccine had made so many girls sick, leaving them in wheelchairs and, like her, unable to go to school. While Dr. Stanley initially avoided answering the question, an emotional Rebecca demanded a "yes or no" response. On the spot, Dr. Stanley finally said no, she did not feel guilty.[42] In that moment, a 16-year-old girl in a wheelchair threw down the gauntlet on one of the biggest charities in Ireland and completely turned the intention of the meeting—to promote the vaccine—on its head.

The next day, the video of the exchange went viral on Facebook and had over a million views by the end of the week. The Cancer Society hired security for the second meeting in Cork a few days later. The Q&A following the meeting was cut short at the first sign of Dr. Stanley being challenged by parents. In a radio interview shortly after the event, Robert O'Connor of the Irish Cancer Society referred to the parents confronting Dr. Stanley as "extremist, antivaccine campaigners" who "made explicit threats . . ."[43]

INJECTED AND NEGLECTED, REGRET's WORK IN 2016–17

Just before school began in September 2016, REGRET produced and released another video on Facebook and YouTube as a public service.[44] The aim was to make parents aware of the adverse events listed on the vaccine package insert, which the Health Service had failed to provide for parents in the school consent packets. This video went viral, gaining almost two million views in a short time and served to solidify public support for REGRET. Despite this, however, it did not stop attempts to malign REGRET parents by some proponents of the vaccine.

The fact that these parents' children were fully vaccinated didn't seem to make a difference to their critics, whether it was the Irish Cancer Society, the Health Service management, or prominent media personalities. As the first wave of vaccines was delivered to schools in fall 2016, the Health Service was surprised that uptake was now under 50 percent in most counties.[45]

As the winter months rolled in, REGRET was still no closer to securing an official meeting with the minister for health over the untenable situation in which they and their daughters found themselves. Members of the support group had grown to 350, and some of the girls were becoming quite ill. Neglected by the government and bullied by the media, REGRET started using the tagline "Injected and Neglected" to get more attention for their plight. The media attacks stepped up, and many outlets now referred to REGRET as "antivaccine activists" and continued to blame them for cancer deaths, despite the lack of logic to such an accusation.[46]

The media presented these deaths as a fact in the present rather than as a future hypothesis with many unknown variables. Journalists and broadcasters routinely diagnosed girls' conditions over the airwaves as psychosomatic or as chronic fatigue—reiterating the Health Service's narrative—and suggested that parents were refusing the vaccine based on puritanical fears of teenage sex.[47] Mainstream media compared parents who questioned the HPV vaccine with flat-earthers and climate change deniers, which incited mockery in online forums.[48]

In 2017, the media continued to attack parents relentlessly, some even calling to criminalize the spread of "misinformation" and "fake news." Well-known national radio host Niall Boylan tweeted, "Is it time to start criminally charging these Anti-HPV nut jobs for spreading misinformation & putting young women's lives at risk. #Idiots."[49]

Another outspoken critic was Dr. Ruairi Hanley, a member of the Irish Medical Council, who wrote an article in the *Irish Medical Times* with the title "Fighting The Anti-Vaxxers." In it he wrote, "[A]ny parent who fails to complete the childhood immunization schedule [should lose] 50 percent of their children's allowance payment until the child reaches 18."[50] In Ireland, the "children's allowance" is an age-old tax rebate, originally given to mothers to help pay for their children's basic needs. Any suggestion to withhold this payment from parents, in an effort similar to Australia's "no jab, no pay" policy, would elicit an emotional response from the public, and it did. Even Dr. Hanley's own community of doctors did not support the idea. Dr. Hanley expressed his disappointment at this to the *Irish Times* and referred to the backlash he received from the "lunatic fringe" who disagreed with him as "a sustained attack from antivaccination campaigners online."[51] He likened hesitant parents to "paranoid conspiracy theorists" and "fanatical believers in the pseudoscientific drivel of alternative medicine."[52]

The director general of the Health Service, Tony O'Brien, publicly accused those opposed to the vaccine of using tactics akin to "emotional terrorism" and of "playing God" with other people's lives.[53] Mr. O'Brien was forced to resign in May 2018 over a scandal involving the national cervical screening program, Cervical Check. Following an audit of Pap test results in 2014, Cervical Check realized that over two hundred women had received a false negative result since the program began in 2010. A decision was made not to notify the women or even call them back in for repeat testing. Consequently, some women went on to develop cervical cancer and some died. The scandal is ongoing, with many lawsuits filed and millions of Euros already paid in settlements. In resigning, Mr. O'Brien never admitted fault for his part in the controversy, nor did he apologize for the remarks he made about parents in the HPV vaccine controversy, before leaving the Health Service on a full pension. His remarks about "playing God" with other people's lives seemed hypocritical to parents in REGRET.

The new minister for health, Simon Harris, publicly called on doctors to "come out fighting" against people who pass on "uninformed nonsense" coming from "scaremongers."[54] He publicly called for censorship of any opposition to the vaccine program and for parents to "butt out," stating:

> If you want to give medical advice on vaccinations, become a doctor. If not, get out of the way and stay away from our public health policy.[55]

The parents of REGRET were left dumbfounded when they read this in the media. The window of opportunity for civil discourse clearly had passed, although neither the previous nor current ministers for health ever agreed to meet with the group to discuss the issue and publicly stated that there will never be an investigation.

Attacks also came from the Irish Cancer Society, labeling the parents as "antivaccine activists" and blaming them for the future deaths of 40 young girls then being reported in the media. The focus on girls dying and not middle-aged women seemed deliberately provocative. The Cancer Society branded any critical comments about the vaccine as "misinformation."[56]

It was around this time that it became known that the Irish Cancer Society was the recipient of $200,000 in contributions from Merck.[57] The first payment of exactly $100,000 was made shortly after REGRET formed in July 2015, and the second $100,000 payment was made shortly after the historic "David and Goliath" moment between Rebecca Hollidge and Dr. Stanley at the Irish Cancer Society meeting in August 2016. The timing is coincidental to those events, but it highlights specific points in time relevant to the decline in HPV vaccine uptake. Robert O'Connor, spokesperson for the Cancer Society, denied receiving any funds from Merck when confronted by a parent at the now infamous Galway meeting, by

saying any allegations they had received any money from the manufacturer "is a lie."[58]

With the September 2017 vaccination program looming, and reports of falling uptake rates, the Irish Cancer Society along with the
Health Service launched a new program called the "HPV Vaccine
Alliance," which brought together 30 health, education, and wom-
en's groups to promote the vaccine and stave off the so-called "targeted misinformation" from activist groups.[59] The *Irish Independent*
reported at the time:

> A coalition of more than 30 health, children's and women's
> groups is urging parents to disregard the "fake news" about
> the virtually non-existent side-effects to the HPV vaccine
> that can save hundreds of Irish women a year from develop-
> ing cancer.[60]

PARENTS SPEAK UP

Ireland, unlike the UK and the US, does not have a vaccine injury compensation program. Neither is it possible to bring a class action lawsuit. The threat of hundreds of individual lawsuits remains
a possibility, although it may be cost-prohibitive for most families.

One mother did take on the agency responsible for drug approval
and safety in Ireland. She petitioned the Health Products Regulatory
Agency to revoke MSD's license for its HPV vaccine in Ireland.[61]
Fiona Kirby, a nurse, brought the case on behalf of her daughter,
whom she said suffered "horrendous" consequences from the vaccine.[62] The *Irish Times* reported that Ms. Kirby claimed her daughter
"became extremely fatigued and suffered severe nausea which led to
weight loss and muscle wastage. Her daughter also missed days at
school, was hospitalized with bilateral pneumonia in March 2012
and was on antibiotics for six weeks. Her daughter is now disabled to
the point she needs to be cared for on a permanent basis, she claims."

The High Court eventually dismissed the case, as the court agreed
with the Agency's argument that it did not have jurisdiction to

revoke Gardasil's license, since the EMA had approved it.[63] While the Regulatory Agency cannot revoke a vaccine's European license granted by the EMA, it can remove it from the Irish vaccine schedule. The HSE's website states that the HPRA "has when appropriate withdrawn products from the Irish market where there have been public safety concerns."[64] Likewise, the EMA does not dictate to member countries which vaccines to put on their schedules; each country's health agency decides that. It is unclear, therefore, why the High Court dismissed the case for lack of jurisdiction, but Ms. Kirby has not yet appealed.

In May 2017, Jonathan Irwin, founder of the Jack & Jill Foundation and a prominent Irish citizen, came forward to announce publicly that his daughter had become seriously ill and missed a year of school since she received the Gardasil vaccine.[65] Mr. Irwin is well known for his charitable work and as a former racetrack executive and racing horse breeder. The Jack & Jill Foundation, which he founded with his wife, Mary Ann, provides in-home nursing care for severely disabled children and babies born with life-threatening, debilitating conditions, whose parents would otherwise be unable to afford such services.[66] Following his announcement, he urged Minister for Health Simon Harris to take action. Mr. Irwin is determined to help his daughter and others like her and to find out why she became ill so soon after the vaccine. Mr. Irwin has fought for children's rights for twenty years with the Jack & Jill Foundation and is no stranger to controversy.

THE BOYS ARE NEXT

The Health Service and the minister for health raised the question of vaccinating boys in 2017, despite the conclusion in the original HPV vaccine health assessment ten years prior that it would not be cost-effective.[67] Minister Harris called for a new report on whether to introduce the vaccine for boys[68] and indicated his full support for such a program by saying that his department will roll it out as quickly as possible if the assessment is positive.[69] In July 2018, the assessment committee, the Health Information and Quality Authority (HIQA), announced its favorable opinion that boys should be added to the schedule.[70] The Minister's formal announcement is expected later in 2018. Around the same time, the UK's approval committee announced its recommendation to add boys to its national program and is also expected to expand the program once the minister for health approves the measure.

The vaccine's coinventor, Professor Ian Frazer, gave a talk at a Royal College of Physicians of Ireland (RCPI) conference on July 9, 2018, titled "The opportunity To Eliminate HPV Cancers."[71] A few days ahead of the conference, the RCPI called for the vaccination of boys in a published statement.[72] Professional support for such a move will guarantee that the vaccine program will be extended to boys without delay. The conference was broadcast to doctors all over Ireland, which is an enormous endorsement of just how important the Irish market is to the vaccine's sponsors.

The presence of Gardasil's coinventor in Ireland was too much to bear for many parents, however. While the conference was going on inside the RCPI building, over a hundred REGRET parents protested outside. Three young girls collapsed at the scene, suffering seizures, and were treated by paramedics.[73] It had little effect on those attending the conference. Professor Frazer was earlier awarded highest honor the RCPI could bestow on its guest, an Honorary Fellowship of the Royal College of Physicians of Ireland.[74] The award is given to world leaders in medical science and those who have made an exceptional contribution to society. For the parents of REGRET, this was another blow to their efforts at being heard by medical professionals in Ireland.

It remains to be seen if Ireland will follow other countries where the vaccine uptake has fallen to exceedingly low levels. Uptake has risen to 62 percent from 50 percent, following an aggressive campaign by the government-sponsored "HPV Vaccine Alliance."[75] Given that Ireland is an English-speaking country, should the government not succeed in getting uptake numbers back to where they were, the potential public relations fallout could reverberate globally. Perhaps this is the reason for the intense government-backed campaign?

The future of the vaccine program in Ireland is still uncertain. What we do know is that the controversy is not going away for the parents of Inform Parents and REGRET or families and individuals like the Colohans and Jonathan Irwin. What's clear is that the government is firmly backing the vaccine program for the foreseeable future and will not agree to investigate families' claims. In the worldwide stage of the HPV vaccine controversy, Ireland remains at the center of the storm.

27.

THE UNITED KINGDOM: MEDIA MAGIC

HERALDING THE NEW VACCINE

The United Kingdom introduced Cervarix in the fall of 2008, only a year after the European Commission granted approval and one year before FDA approval.[1] Every girl in the UK aged 12 to 18 was eligible to receive the vaccine at school. Rates of cervical cancer are relatively low in the UK, accounting for less than 1 percent of all cancers, but tragically almost 900 women lose their lives to the disease each year.[2]

Cervical cancer was already at the forefront of mainstream conversation in 2008 because reality TV celebrity Jade Goody was dying from the disease. Goody was best known for her brash appearances on the TV show *Big Brother*, which was popular in the early 2000s.[3] She was often featured in tabloid newspapers and gossip magazines. Diagnosed with advanced stage cervical cancer in September 2008, she became an important story in the rollout of the vaccine. News that Jade Goody was dying of cervical cancer came as a surprise because of her young age. Tabloids reported on her condition daily, which some critics described as intrusive.[4] As a result of Goody's illness, public awareness about cervical cancer increased, causing an uptick in Pap tests and great interest in the HPV vaccine.

THE "JADE GOODY EFFECT"

Sadly, Jade Goody died on March 22, 2009, at the age of 27, leaving behind two children. Before she passed away, she publicly requested that the National Health Service (NHS) reduce the age at which Pap tests start, from 25 to 20 years old. No one knows what HPV types, if any, were involved in Jade's disease. During her final months, Goody didn't focus on the details of her illness, preferring to stay positive and focus on her treatment.

In the aftermath of her death, however, the British Medical Council conducted a study titled "Coverage of Jade Goody's cervical cancer in UK newspapers: a missed opportunity for health promotion?"[5] This report analyzed 527 newspaper articles from the time of Jade's diagnosis to the time of her death. They searched for health information content and found it lacking in information on HPV vaccination. The Medical Council is a public-private partnership with industry, including GSK, the maker of Cervarix, and yet the study did not report this as a conflict of interest.[6] The study discussed the media connection between the public and government policy agendas such as the "Goody Effect," as her impact on public health policy came to be known. The study identified that the media failed to capture the opportunity to educate the public about the risks of cervical cancer and "the possibility of protecting young women against contracting the viral agent which causes cervical cancer through vaccination."[7] By 2018, however, the media in the UK reported that the "Jade Goody Effect" was gone, as smear test rates have hit a 20-year low at only 72 percent.[8]

EARLY MEDIA REPORTS A WARNING?

In the first year of the UK's program, 700,000 girls were vaccinated, and over 2,000 reactions were reported to the "Yellow Card" reporting system for adverse events.[9] According to *The Telegraph*, the reports varied from paralysis to convulsions to sight problems. Others reported nausea, muscle weakness, fever, dizziness, and numbness.[10]

Despite the enormous push to vaccinate every girl eligible in the first year of the program, there were media reports of unusual reactions to the vaccine. One case in particular was that of Carly Steele. According to the *Daily Mail*, in the summer of 2008, Steele's school participated in a clinical trial for Cervarix (the PATRICIA trial).[11] Within weeks, Carly was suffering from a number of auto-immune illnesses, which doctors found perplexing. They could not find a pathological reason and suggested that her illnesses were psychosomatic. The sudden onset of Carly's illnesses led her mother to the Internet. Piecing together the research, she realized that the timing and symptoms correlated with Carly's first injection with Cervarix. She wasn't alone. The *Daily Mail* reported on four other girls with similar symptoms at that time.[12] One girl reacted within minutes of the vaccine and soon became partially paralyzed and wheelchair-bound. Another developed seizures and is also in a wheelchair. The girls' reactions could not be proven to be associated with the vaccine, but it is clear something was causing these symptoms, which had, and in some cases continue to have, a debilitating effect on their ability to work and lead a normal life.

A Girl's Death in the UK Sparks Controversy

A few months later, and only a year into the vaccination program, there was news of the first death associated with the vaccine. Natalie Morton, a fourteen-year-old girl from Coventry, in the Midlands of England, died ninety minutes after receiving the vaccine at her school on September 28, 2009.[13] *The Telegraph* reported the following day that parents in the school were notified about Natalie's death and three others who also suffered a reaction.[14] Natalie's friends told how there was "panic in the school" when everyone heard about Natalie and the other girls. Initially the principal of the school announced that Natalie suffered "a rare, but extreme reaction to the vaccine."[15] This explanation was reversed in the days that followed, however.

According to the *Daily Mail*, this is how a schoolmate described the incident:

> About an hour after having the jab Natalie went really pale and wasn't breathing. I think it was around lunchtime.

She fainted in the corridor. I saw ambulance men pumping her chest then the teachers told us to go outside.

A lot of people were crying afterwards and we were all very worried.

We have to have three of the jabs in all and a lot of us don't want to take the rest, but they're telling us we have to because there will be side effects if we don't have them all.[16]

A day after her death, the National Health Service (NHS) temporarily recalled the batch of Cervarix used to immunize Natalie, batch number AHPVA043BB.[17] It caused panic around the UK, and parents immediately feared and questioned the vaccine side effects. Vaccination rates in Coventry City plummeted from a high of over 90 percent to 65 percent.[18]

On October 1, just three days following Natalie's death, a coroner's inquest found that the teenager had a rare malignant tumor in her heart and lungs.[19] The coroner determined that this was the cause of her sudden death and not the vaccine. A BBC article described Natalie's death as one of "natural causes."[20] Natalie's family supported this finding and disassociated themselves from the controversy. Natalie's mother publicly pledged her support for the vaccine, telling her local newspaper, the *Coventry Telegraph*, "We're confident that the vaccine is safe and parents should consider having their daughters vaccinated. It's clear from the postmortem that there was no link between the vaccine and Natalie's death."[21]

The newspaper also reported that her sister Abigail, who was eighteen at the time, took the vaccine a few months later. Abigail explained: "I know Natalie died of a tumor and not the vaccine. That's why I really want other girls and their parents to consider the vaccine to prevent cervical cancer."[22]

Over time, vaccine uptake rates recovered in Coventry City, and fears about Cervarix side effects abated. The NHS conducted an extensive opinion survey to determine the actual long-term effect on the public. The NHS was satisfied that confidence rebounded among mothers and daughters, with around 90 percent reporting being "very" or "fairly" positive about the HPV vaccine.[23]

The Medicines and Healthcare products Regulatory Agency (MHRA), the UK's equivalent of the US FDA, reviewed Natalie's case and found that "the vaccine did not play a role."[24] Natalie's case caused concern at the WHO, however, which monitors possible threats to vaccination programs worldwide through bad press and what it considers misinformation on adverse events. In fact, the WHO heralded the NHS's handling of Natalie's death as exemplary and a lesson in what to do to protect vaccines from negative publicity, such as the headline, "GIRL, 14 DIES AFTER TAKING THE CERVICAL CANCER VACCINE" as was reported by *The Telegraph*.[25] Natalie's death became "Case Study C" in a comprehensive WHO tutorial on "Managing the media following an adverse event following immunization."[26]

The NHS acted swiftly to avoid panic. It worked to get information out to the public as quickly as possible following the postmortem that Natalie's death was due to a previously undiagnosed tumor.

ADVOCACY IN THE UK

Around this time, Steve and Pauline Hinks's teenage daughter, Lucy, received three prescribed Cervarix doses. Lucy experienced only mild flu-like symptoms after the first two doses, but following her third dose, on May 4, 2011, her health began to decline precipitously. Within months, she was bedridden. In an interview with *The Guardian*, her father described her as existing in a "waking coma." Her mother described it as a "living hell."[27] Lucy slept twenty-three hours a day. She couldn't speak more than a few words at a time. She couldn't walk or support herself and had to be spoon-fed. Her first pediatric consultant wrote a note in her medical chart: "It is quite possible that this will turn out to be a reaction to the HPV vaccine." A second consultant diagnosed Lucy with chronic fatigue syndrome.

Steve Hinks wrote an article for SaneVax, where he describes how homeopathy helped Lucy recover from many of her symptoms and returned her to being a functioning teenager.[28] Lucy's journey was not easy, though. In early 2012, even though her condition was improving somewhat, Lucy's doctors recommended that she be sent to a psychiatric hospital for in-patient evaluation where she could be admitted and stay for three to six months. Reluctantly, Steve brought his daughter for an intake assessment, wishing to comply with what was recommended. The attending senior psychiatrist did not think it was an appropriate placement for Lucy so did not admit her. The Hinks family was relieved. Lucy, still only 14, was happy at home and did not want to be in a psychiatric hospital. She needed her family's support.

Later that year, as Lucy was feeling better, they decided to take a vacation to help the family recuperate. The previous year had taken its toll on everyone. Lucy's doctors and consultants agreed that she was well enough to travel for a short vacation. Her psychiatric caseworker, however, did not agree. A few hours before they planned to leave for the airport, police and social workers arrived at their home unannounced. A stressful few hours of phone calls, bureaucracy, and negotiation ensued. The family was finally allowed to leave the UK for their much-needed holiday. Steve felt that his parental rights had been infringed, and he couldn't shake the feeling that he might lose Lucy, as irrational as that seemed to him at the time.

Steve's instinct proved to be right. Upon the family's return, they faced more questions from government caseworkers. The pressure on Steve and Pauline was intense. They faced accusations that they had fabricated or induced Lucy's illness. They didn't know it at the time, although Steve suspected it, that the state was investigating them under the suspicion of Munchausen Syndrome by Proxy, a controversial diagnosis suggesting that the parents colluded with Lucy to fake her condition. The very notion of this syndrome is like nails on a chalkboard to families of children with poorly understood autoimmune illnesses. Steve was desperate to quash any notion of Munchausen's Syndrome. How could that even be considered when they were doing all they could to help Lucy recover from her illness? Eventually all the investigations were dropped, but their effect on Steve was everlasting.

It was through this process that Steve discovered that he and his wife had been under investigation for Munchausen's Syndrome by Proxy (MSBP). He felt as if they had a lucky escape that the charges were dropped. MSBP is a diagnosis against caregivers of a child that accuses them of harming or abusing the child.[29] The diagnosis can also extend to the caregiver's exaggerating or inducing mental or physical manifestations of illness in the child. The motivation for MSBP is controversial, but one alleged reason is so that the caretaker, usually the mother, can receive sympathy and attention.[30] MSBP accusations can result in the state removing a child from the caregiver's care.

There is no clear definition of what MSBP is in the scientific community. Some psychiatrists believe it is overdiagnosed or even deny it exists as a syndrome. It has even been renamed as "Factitious Disorder Imposed on Another," or FDIA.[31] Despite this, however, parents have been convicted criminally in MSBP cases in the UK and elsewhere. In the Unites States, there are approximately 1,000 reports of MSBP-related child abuse each year.[32]

Accusations are extremely difficult to disprove, since they largely depend on circumstantial evidence. Whatever the outcome may be, cases are traumatizing for parents. In the UK, doctors who have never treated the child can testify as expert witnesses, adding weight to the prosecution's case.

It is understandable why Steve felt like he could lose Lucy during the state's investigation a few months prior. The fact that he and his wife were even under suspicion terrified him. Lucy regained her health slowly and was able to return to school on a part-time basis in September 2012, more than a year after she became ill. Five years later, Lucy continues to do well and maintain an active recovery plan. September 2012 is also when the UK changed the HPV vaccine from Cervarix to Gardasil, citing the addition of the protection from warts as a reason.[33]

In the UK, the vaccine injury compensation program is often considered arbitrary.[34] Rules for application for damage include such minimum standards as proving that the vaccine caused at least 60 percent disability. The rules stipulate that you can be compensated if you are "severely disabled" following vaccination. You cannot seek compensation for babies under two years old.[35] As with all compensation programs, however, the burden of proof rests with the claimant.

Steve Hinks decided to pursue this avenue of compensation as the costs associated with Lucy's care were mounting. As Steve would find out, the application procedure is not straightforward and requires an enormous amount of paperwork. Following a written submission, the claimant receives a decision by mail. Claimants cannot take part in proceedings, as they are not public. Much to his surprise, Steve's claim on behalf of his daughter was denied. Before he appealed, he requested the full file relating to his daughter's claim from the NHS. He received boxes of files at his home. Clearly, the government had carried out an extensive investigation of his daughter's claim. He examined all the records and found several inaccurate ones. He could see that his daughter's claim failed because of incorrect medical information that certain doctors who treated his daughter had provided. He appealed but was again denied compensation.

Steve had no more options in seeking justice from the Health Service. It is technically possible to sue pharmaceutical companies in the UK, but claimants do not qualify for free legal aid, making it financially prohibitive. Doctors are reluctant to testify, and lawyers are apprehensive about taking cases. The fight for his daughter's life, including his wrangling with state bureaucracies, propelled Steve into advocacy.

Like all parents who find themselves in this position, his journey had not been by his choice. He published Lucy's story on SaneVax's website, and then parents in similar situations in the UK contacted him for help and advice. At the same time, Freda Birrell, who lives in Scotland, was making headway with Norma at SaneVax with efforts in other countries.

Steve Hinks has since become an ardent campaigner for HPV vaccine safety and eventually joined forces with Freda to set up the parent advocacy group UK Association of HPV Vaccine Injured Daughters (AHVID).[36] Together Steve and Freda have taken on the difficult role of campaigning for increased risk awareness in the UK. Freda has spoken in front of the Scottish Parliament regarding HPV vaccine safety and has repeatedly requested meetings with UK officials in London. AHVID has over 400 members, not unlike REGRET in Ireland, but both Steve and Freda think that their numbers should be in the thousands given the official numbers of serious adverse events reported to the Yellow Card system. Other groups in the UK have also started advocating for their injured daughters. "Time For Action UK" is a group set up by parents of injured girls and regularly posts updates on its lobbying efforts, FOIA requests, and research.[37]

THE YELLOW CARD REPORTING SYSTEM

The Yellow Card system was set up in the 1960s to monitor adverse events to drugs following the thalidomide scandal, when thousands of babies were born with birth defects or died.[38] While one might expect a high number of reactions when a vaccine is introduced initially, since reporting is strongly encouraged, adverse event reports following the HPV vaccine have remained higher than all other vaccines. There have been over 9,000 Yellow Card or adverse drug reports (ADRs) following the HPV vaccine since 2008.[39] The HPV vaccine made up more than 50 percent of all reports to the system from 2008 to 2012, when Cervarix was being administered (see chart below).[40] Additionally, the 2012 ADR report from the UK government states that "over 80 percent of all vaccine ADR reports in 2009 and 2010 relate to female patients as a result of the volume of HPV vaccine reports."[41]

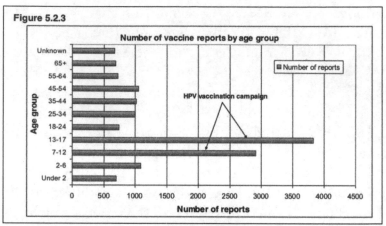

Source: MHRA UK, *Trends in UK Spontaneous Adverse Drug Reaction (ADR) Between 2008–2012.*[42]

In the four-year Cervarix review published in 2012, the MHRA dismissed all 6,403 reports as either minor or as being unrelated to the vaccine.[43] All serious reported side effects, even major neurological events like fainting and "jerking" seizures, are considered coincidental. Around 30 percent of the cases were dismissed as psychosomatic in nature:

> "Psychogenic reactions" can also manifest as loss of consciousness/altered state of consciousness, vision disturbance, injury, limb jerking (often misinterpreted/reported as a seizure/convulsion), limb numbness or tingling and difficulty in breathing.[44]

In 2017, Secretary for State and Health Nicola Blackwood was asked about the reactions in the UK to the HPV vaccine. In a written answer documented in Parliament, she stated that since 2008, there were 8,835 reported reactions to Cervarix, Gardasil, and Gardasil 9 and that over 34 percent of them were "serious" (see chart below).[45] The regulatory body, the Medicines and Healthcare products Regulatory Authority (MHRA), defines "serious reactions" as those that result in death, are life-threatening, or result in hospitalization or disability.[46]

Vaccine Brand	Total number of reports	Number of serious reports (% of total)
Cervarix	6,312	1,812 (29%)
Gardasil	1,858	767 (41%)
Gardasil 9	10	6 (60%)
HPV Brand unspecified	658	456 (69%)
Total for Human Papilloma virus vaccines	8,835*	3,038 (34%)

Source: MHRA sentinel database for adverse reactions.
Note that the total number of reports received will not be equal to the totals in the table above as some reports of suspected adverse reactions may have included more than one vaccine.

Source: see note 45.

The authors received a FOIA-requested "Case Series Drug Analysis" report for Cervarix and Gardasil through May 2018 from the MHRA.[47] The latest figures show that 9,156 adverse event reports were filed in the vaccine's first ten years, reporting 24,000 symptoms. This means that each case has on average two or three symptoms. Eight deaths were reported in total, three of them from cancer, although none is considered by the MHRA to be related to the vaccine.[48]

In its assessments, the MHRA states that there is no link to the vaccine, even though it makes no attempt to investigate any symptom class. There appear to be patterns and hundreds of similar reports, but the MHRA claims no connection. There appears to be a pervasive denial of vaccine injury in the UK, despite the relatively high rates of HPV adverse event reports. Doctors rarely speak out publicly about vaccine risks, and parents are afraid to refuse vaccines or claim harm from them. Dr. Heidi Larson associates the lack of "vaccine hesitancy" in the UK with the Wakefield scandal over the MMR and told *The Guardian*, "The backlash against the disgraced doctor Andrew Wakefield has shielded Britain from the worst of the 'antivax' trend. However, health officials have been warned to guard against emerging mistrust of the anticancer HPV jab."[49]

It is difficult to attribute any case to the vaccine, since so few are investigated. Those injured don't appear to bring cases to the UK vaccine injury compensation program. Unlike in the US, there have been no cases compensating injuries related to the HPV vaccine, and due to lack of transparency, we cannot assess why. In fact, as *Age of Autism* reported in 2017, the compensation program in the UK has largely shut down, and no monetary payments have been made following vaccine injuries in recent years.[50]

Despite some areas of high uptake, a government report published at the end of 2017 shows that vaccination coverage has declined from a high of over 90 percent who completed the three-dose series in the 2013–14 school year to around 80 percent in 2016 who completed the new 2-dose series.[51]

Current marketing of the vaccine to males in the UK targets men who have sex with men (MSM). These men are at higher risk for anal and penile cancer.[52] The government offers the vaccine at no cost to men up to the age of 45 who request it. Professor Margaret Stanley, industry spokesperson and government consultant, published an article in *Nature* in 2012 advocating the vaccine for all boys, although admitting that the men at highest risk are those who have sex with men.[53] Professor Stanley argues against targeting that population alone because of "access, equality, and ethics."[54] She also argues that it would be tricky to reach at-risk boys at the appropriate age, i.e., before sexual activity, because this approach would likely miss many boys who are not forthcoming about their sexual orientation.[55] Professor Stanley told *The Guardian* that she also would like to lower the age of vaccination to nine in the UK to remove any association with promiscuity that parents seem to have with slightly older children.[56]

In the summer of 2017, the government committee once again revisited the policy of vaccinating boys. Only four countries recommend the vaccine for boys to this point: Canada, the United States, Australia, and New Zealand. In the months running up to the deliberations, a lobbying group, *HPVAction.org*, launched a social media campaign to encourage public support for the program.[57] HPVAction.org represents 48 groups in the UK, including gay rights groups, dentists, and other special interest groups.[58] The group receives an educational grant from Merck.[59]

The Throat Cancer Foundation, a small charity in Scotland, runs *HPVAction.org*.[60] Vaccine inventor Ian Frazer, a native of Scotland, supported the Foundation as a member of their scientific advisory board, a post from which he resigned in early 2018.[61] At the time of writing, Professor Margaret Stanley is a clinical and scientific adviser, according to their website.[62]

Ultimately, when they considered the issue in 2017, the committee could not justify the cost of vaccinating boys.[63] The rationale offered was that since the rate of vaccination among girls was generally very high, it would not be cost-effective to add boys. By protecting girls, this would be enough to protect boys.[64] The Throat Cancer Foundation and *HPVAction.org* assert that this policy decision amounts to sexual discrimination, since homosexual boys would not be protected under this policy.[65]

In May 2018, according to the *Daily Mail*, the Throat Cancer Foundation filed a high court case against the NHS, citing sexual discrimination under the 2010 Equality Act.[66] The JCVI met again in June 2018 to review the case for adding boys to the vaccine program, and this time they recommended expanding the program.[67] The mathematical models had not changed, still showing no cost benefit with a high uptake among girls, but adjustments were made to the "discount rate" after the JCVI assumed that the vaccine would protect for up to 30 years.[68] It predicts that by offering boys the vaccine, the greatest effect in reducing cancers will be in unvaccinated girls and the MSM community.[69]

The UK has achieved and sustained a high vaccination rate of over 80 percent despite a growing grassroots resistance movement. The vaccination program has survived some remarkable injury stories, including the death of Natalie Morton. It has survived the changeover from Cervarix to Gardasil in 2012, despite high reaction rates with both vaccines. As lobbyists continue to push for male inclusion in the vaccination program, the UK remains a strong ally for HPV vaccine manufacturers.

28.

COLOMBIA: FAMILIES FIGHTING BACK

As an anthropologist and journalist fluent in English, Mario Lamo seemed to fall into the HPV vaccine controversy in Colombia just by doing what he is trained to do: to look for the truth and report it as he sees it. Mario conjures up an image of a journalist from another time. He is rarely without his fedora, tipped slightly forward on his head, and his satchel on his shoulder. He has a passion for photography and for his country. He affectionately refers to the Colombian girls injured in this controversy as "the girls," as if he knew each and every one.

Cervical cancer rates in Colombia have been historically high, with rates of 120 per 100,000 in the 1960s, but have reduced to 20 per 100,000 today.[1] The most prominent epidemiological expert on HPV prevalence worldwide, Dr. Nubia Muñoz—a former unit chief at the International Agency for Research on Cancer in Lyon and an emeritus professor of the National Cancer Institute of Colombia—has credited the decline in cervical cancer to improvement in socioeconomic conditions, reduced parity, and advances in cancer screening.[2]

INVESTIGATING HPV VACCINES

Mario spent almost two decades in the US and learned a great deal about vaccines while there. When Colombia announced in 2013 that it would soon offer the HPV vaccine for "free and compulsory by law of the republic," he knew there was more to the story.[3] The law introducing the vaccine, Bill #1626, contained only three lines and offered no information on the vaccine or the mechanism for opting out. The vaccine was not, in fact, compulsory, as the Colombian Constitution prohibits any medical intervention without informed consent. But cervical cancer is a reality in Colombia, affecting 5,000 women a year, almost half of whom lose their lives to the disease.[4]

By 2013, Mario had heard about side effects from this vaccine from all over the world. He suspected lobbying by pharmaceutical companies to the Colombian Congress might account for the new law, as there seemed to have been no public debate about it. It was the first vaccine "mandate" to have ever been passed by Congress. According to the *Canadian Medical Association Journal*, Colombia's medical industry is in crisis at the highest levels, meaning that perhaps Colombian officials could be quite vulnerable to lobbying or worse.[5]

Before the vaccine program rolled out, Mario wrote an article about his concerns called "Gardasil the Killer Vaccine!" which he hoped would provoke attention and warn people of what could come.[6] He had access to an online column in a major mainstream newspaper, *El Tiempo*, and it was there he published it. The article was a scathing attack on the Colombian Ministry for Health for putting the lives of 3.5 million girls in danger without good cause. He claimed that the proposed HPV vaccine program was a mass experiment on young Colombian girls without informed consent. He cited injuries and deaths in other parts of the world and said that Colombian parents must be informed.[7]

El Tiempo immediately received demands for citations and evidence to back up Mario's article from an online blogger at the propharma website "Skeptical Way of Life."[8] In response, Mario wrote a long article explaining why he opposed the vaccine program, citing the risks and providing links to supporting information.[9] The newspaper was afraid to publish his rebuttal, saying it feared they might be sued by Merck. Mario's access to his column was revoked, and his article was deleted from its website. In response, Mario then published his rebuttal piece, including all email exchanges with *El Tiempo* elsewhere online.[10]

Despite Mario's warnings, the vaccination program went ahead. A radio station asked Mario to talk about his concerns. By this time, Mario was in touch with SaneVax to find out as much as he could about the vaccine and what was happening elsewhere. He invited Norma Erickson on the radio show with him, and together they explained why they thought there was a looming tragedy about to befall some Colombian girls, based on what they were seeing around the world. While these reports in other countries were not proof that any illness was related to the vaccine, they suggested that this phenomenon of unexplained illness in teenage girls might land on Colombia's doorstep soon after the program began.

It was thus not a coincidence in Mario's mind when reports of reactions, similar to those reported around the world, began to come in from all over Colombia once the HPV vaccine program started. At first, cases seemed sporadic and isolated. Then a vaccination team came to the schools in El Carmen de Bolívar.

The Girls of El Carmen de Bolívar

With a population of 95,000, El Carmen de Bolívar is a small town in Northwest Colombia, seventy miles south of Cartagena. Mario describes it is an ethnic enclave, nestled in the hills of Bolívar and largely closed off from the outside world. It's an agricultural town, mainly exporting tobacco and avocados. The HPV vaccination teams came to the schools in July 2013, one month after Japan suspended its national program. Very little information was given to the girls and their families, and most girls complied even without obtaining parental consent. Reactions to the first dose were relatively mild and in line with reactions to other vaccines.

When the second dose was administered on March 20, 2014, however, girls began to react to the vaccine en masse, some immediately and severely. Within ten days, according to a teacher, as reported on SaneVax's website, "the situation has turned into a full-blown crisis."[11] The girls experienced convulsions, fainting, and severe headaches. In all, over 800 girls reported reactions, ranging from fainting to dizziness and paralysis. The town's mayor, a physician, told the Associated Press that hundreds received treatment in local hospitals on one particular weekend, but most recovered quickly. While he did not confirm that they suffered adverse vaccine reactions, parents were sure that this was the case.[12]

News of the girls' reactions travelled fast on social media, angering Colombia's Health Minister Alejandro Gaviria Uribe, who criticized the media for creating panic around a safe vaccine.[13] The media did not control social media, however, and stories of the girls' reactions spread. A vivid video on Facebook shows boys tending to girls violently seizing and writhing on floor mats after receiving the vaccine. It has over a half million views from around the world.[14]

The government moved to dismiss the girls' claims immediately. It declared their reactions psychosomatic in nature, even though officials never medically examined the girls. Colombian President Juan Manuel Santos hosted a press conference in September 2014 to address the public's concerns about the reactions in El Carmen de Bolívar, claiming the vaccine was safe.[15] He denied that the girls' reactions were due to the vaccine and said that many scientists had theories about what had happened in the small town, including mass hysteria. Days later, Minister Alejandro Gaviria Uribe visited the town and publicly stated that the vaccine was perfectly safe as evidenced by scientific studies and that "170 million doses have been given worldwide and nothing has happened."[16]

Mario knew he had to cover this story. Although he had tried to warn the people of Colombia, even he could not have foreseen this catastrophe. He felt drawn to El Carmen de Bolívar. It was with a heavy heart that he traveled there, imagining what he would find. Even armed with the knowledge he had, he could not take in the sheer scale of what had occurred. It wasn't long before he had met with hundreds of parents and daughters, all telling virtually the same story.

The girls got the vaccine at school, and within weeks of the second shot, their health deteriorated. Some were bedridden or having seizures, some were having menstrual problems, some were in so much pain that their parents feared they would take their own lives. It was beyond what Mario could comprehend. The government vaccinated thousands of healthy teenage girls, and, over a matter of months, hundreds fell seriously ill. Could that be just a coincidence or hysteria? Mario did what he knew how to do: He listened to the girls and their families, documenting their stories on video and in print.

Media attention began to mount, and the government recognized the need to investigate. It created a committee, mainly comprised of psychologists and social workers, to go to El Carmen de Bolívar. According to Mario, the investigators did not talk to the girls' doctors or seek medical records. If they had, they would have learned that there had been no phenomenon of mass hysteria or psychosomatic disorders before 2013. Not surprisingly, the committee decided that there was no link between the girls' illnesses and the HPV vaccine.

Despite this assurance that the girls' conditions must be psychosomatic, a number of the El Carmen de Bolívar girls did not recover. The parents founded a group called "Association for Rebuilding Hope" to raise awareness of the girls' plight so that they could get medical help. Local doctors were unable to offer any solutions and, for the most part, did not accept that the girls' symptoms were physical. Parent groups in India, Japan, Ireland, and Denmark had faced similar disbelief from doctors. Building Hope also began to look at the girls' cases from a legal perspective. The parents wanted to compel the government to help them get medical treatment.

On May 22, 2015, Colombia reported its first death after Gardasil.[17] Sixteen-year-old Karen Durán-Cantor, from a town just outside the city of Bogotá, died of complications related to autoimmune disorders, believed by her family to have been triggered by the HPV vaccine.[18] Karen received her first dose of Gardasil at the end of 2013 and her second one a few months later, in early 2014. Karen then developed rheumatoid arthritis, lost the ability to walk, lost her hair, had difficulty breathing, and was in constant pain. She died in the hospital in Bogotá, where she suffered respiratory failure.[19] Karen also prepared a video about her injury a few weeks before her death, translated by Mario Lamo.[20] In this video, she says, "this was indeed due to the HPV vaccine . . . let's say yes to life and no to the HPV vaccine. Why? Because we women are sacred and blessed. I love you very much."[21]

THE FIGHT MOVES TO THE COURTS

A case involving a girl who became crippled after receiving the vaccine was filed by her mother in 2013 and heard in the High Court of Cali.[22] The child's mother presented evidence from US labs, showing that her daughter's body had toxicity from aluminum, cadmium, silver, and lead. The court ruled in favor of the girl and required the Ministry of Health to investigate the vaccine's toxicity and side effects and to monitor future reactions. The High Court granted the child the right to the healthcare she needed. The Court also raised concerns about whether the doctors involved had obtained proper informed consent. The court recommended that vaccine program be suspended pending the outcome of further tests on the vaccine's toxicity, but this was not acted upon.[23] This was the first legal case involving the vaccine. More would follow.

Monica León del Rio, a lawyer and mother of a girl who fell ill after the vaccine, soon became a central figure in the legal battles around this issue in Colombia. She vowed to fight for her daughter Alejandra, and the other girls like her, to get them the help they so desperately needed. Monica took on many cases of suspected vaccine injury from El Carmen de Bolívar. The families of injury victims needed help to pay for mounting medical bills beyond their reach.

In November 2014, with del Rio's representation, a 15-year-old injured girl from El Carmen de Bolívar won a judgment for herself and her newborn daughter to receive all necessary healthcare to ameliorate their injuries, regardless of insurance coverage.[24] This was a landmark judgment, favoring the rights of the vaccine victim and her baby. The judge also ordered that the teenager not receive the third Gardasil dose.

A month later, a magistrate judge ruled in favor of ten victims of HPV injury, again represented by Monica León del Rio, similarly requiring the Health Ministry to coordinate treatment at the government's expense.[25] The magistrate also ordered an immunologist to examine the ten plaintiffs to explore the relationship between the vaccine, their conditions, and other possible causes of their disabilities.[26]

Shortly after this ruling, the Attorney General Alejandro Ordóñez issued an order to the National Institute of Health that children claiming HPV vaccine injury be given access to medical help to recover.[27] He also called for transparency about the technical and scientific information that led to the vaccine's approval in Colombia and all information relating to its manufacture and distribution. In other words, he was seeking a full audit on the vaccine in Colombia.[28] The outcome of this order for transparency is unclear. Attorney General Ordóñez is a controversial figure whose conservative views clashed with those of liberal Health Minister Dr. Alejandro Gaviria Uribe. According to the *Bogotá Post* in 2016, Mr. Ordóñez was removed from his post following a state council ruling that his second-term election was illegal—a ruling he respected although he did not agree with it.[29] This ended his investigation into the HPV vaccine.

THE PUBLIC RELATIONS BATTLE

During this time, a public relations war broke out as HPV vaccine defenders reacted to the reports of adverse events. The main HPV vaccine advocate, Dr. Muñoz, repeatedly denounced del Rio's legal efforts publicly, accusing her of being an antivaccine activist, which del Rio denies. Dr. Muñoz has been well respected in HPV epidemiological research for many decades. As we learned in Chapter 3, her research finds that the HPV virus is a necessary cause of cervical cancer. She has written hundreds of scientific articles, received many awards, and even been nominated for a Nobel Prize. Dr. Muñoz is also currently a member of Merck's Global HPV Advisory Board and conducts research on HPV prevalence and incidence. She did not disclose her conflict of interest, however, in an article in *El*

País in October 2014, explaining how important it is for girls to get the HPV vaccine.[30] She describes her contribution to the vaccine's development as one of epidemiological importance. She designed studies in 30 countries over 25 years, and without Dr. Muñoz's research, it is unlikely that such large investments would have been made in HPV vaccine research and development.

Dr. Muñoz denied that the vaccine could cause the effects seen in El Carmen de Bolívar; she asserts that there must have been other reasons for the girls' injuries. She reassured the public that the vaccine is safe and effective based on worldwide epidemiological studies.[31]

In January 2015, shortly after the article in *El País*, the National Institute of Health of Colombia "leaked" a final report on the events following the second dose of the Gardasil vaccine in El Carmen de Bolívar, concluding that the girls' illnesses and disabilities were "episodes of psychogenic cause."[32] This echoed a similar report from Japanese officials published the year before. The report also stated that every child received a vaccine from the same lot and batch and that the vaccines were properly handled. Despite this obvious clue, authorities did not investigate this as a possible "hot lot," or a contaminated batch, despite the sheer number of girls who reacted.

This leaked report was important. If the girls' reactions were deemed psychosomatic, they could not access medical care other than psychiatric care. Shortly after this report was made public, Director General of the National Institute of Health Fernando de La Hoz resigned. He denied that his resignation had anything to do with the growing controversy over the HPV vaccine.

In February 2015, the Center for Autoimmune Diseases at Del Rosario University in Colombia hosted a Third Colombian Symposium of Autoimmunity and invited several prominent doctors and scientists who had been involved in the HPV vaccine injury issue.[33] At the Symposium, autoimmunity expert Dr. Yehuda Shoenfeld dismissed as improbable that the symptoms the girls suffered were psychological.[34] He pointed out that girls around the world are reporting the same symptoms after Gardasil. While arguing that vaccines are "the greatest invention for medicine in the last

300 years," he stressed that medicine cannot simply ignore vaccine side effects, including weakness, fatigue, memory loss, and others.[35]

On March 16, 2016, the Health Commission of the Colombian National Academy of Medicine ad hoc Subcommittee on the HPV Vaccine released a letter addressed to Minister of Health Alejandro Gaviria Uribe, urging the ministry to change its current protocols for the HPV vaccine.[36] The letter was based on the growing national and international information linking the vaccine with the onset of autoimmune diseases.

The letter makes several points:

- the risk-benefit ratio is as yet uncertain;

- data about adverse events are limited;

- studies with sufficient sample size can be done to confirm or disconfirm safety;

- the effectiveness of the vaccine to prevent cervical cancer is uncertain, as existing data refer only to precancerous lesions, which have a high rate of spontaneous remission;

- the safety of the vaccine should be exceedingly high as the vaccine is given to healthy teenagers;

- the Hippocratic oath of "first do no harm" must pervade public health;

- experts must disclose conflicts of interest, or public confidence in all vaccines will wane; and

- the ministry must explicitly exclude from vaccination those individuals with a family history or presence of any autoimmune condition. To achieve this higher level of individual screening, the subcommittee advised that the current HPV protocol must change to exclude those most at risk for autoimmune disorders, and people must become aware of this change.

In addition, the subcommittee stated that a strong program of sexual and reproductive education, which they argue is not happening now, should accompany HPV vaccination. It insists that there must be informed consent. The Commission does not dismiss the benefits of the vaccination program but argues for the necessity of a rigorous screening program to avoid the infliction of harm.

A former investigator with the Colombian National Institute of Health studied the girls of El Carmen de Bolívar and published his research in 2016.[37] Dr. Pompilio Martinez, with the help of Mario Lamo and Rebuilding Hope, described in detail the neurological symptoms of 62 girls from the small town in his paper. He determined that the general disease pattern he observed in the girls was consistent with a demyelinating disorder, or an autoimmune neurological disease, although each case was different and deserved individual examination.[38]

THE FAMILIES TAKE ACTION

Rebuilding Hope began to get more impatient as time went on without answers or help for their daughters. In July 2016, the group's hopes were lifted when the attorney general's office called on the Constitutional Court of Colombia to enforce the suspension of the vaccine, following a ruling by the Superior Court of Cali in 2014.[39] The call from the attorney general to suspend the vaccine coincided with protests erupting all over the country and, in particular, in El Carmen de Bolívar. On July 11, 2017, parents and children took to the streets in what turned out to be a day-long standoff with officials in El Carmen de Bolívar.[40] The following day, mothers padlocked the school gates shut to further protest the vaccine being given in schools. Mario Lamo reported to Norma from Colombia and relayed what the protesters were saying. He told her that they had padlocked the doors of the schools and blocked access to classes. They wanted to be heard by the national and municipal government because the vaccine had affected hundreds of girls, and so far, no one was listening to them. They wanted an investigation.[41]

The situation resolved when officials finally agreed to meet with Monica and 60 parents from Rebuilding Hope on July 14th. The mayor of El Carmen de Bolívar, Dumek Turbay, brokered a meeting between the parents and the Minister Alejandro Gaviria Uribe in government offices in Cartagena, over seventy miles away.[42]

According to Monica León del Rio, who attended on behalf of many of the girls, the meeting lasted three hours, and the minister initially listened with empathy to the families' plight.[43] However, this sympathy was limited by Minister Gaviria's assertion that the girls in El Carmen de Bolívar may have had an underlying condition that caused their illness. Having said that, though, he would not consent to medical examinations to test his hypothesis. He would also not consent to diagnostic testing for the girls to establish the extent of neurological damage or POTS as a diagnosis.[44]

The parents stressed their concerns that their girls were experiencing a new medical condition and they needed basic treatment and a government investigation. The minister and other health officials reiterated their denial that these injuries were caused by the vaccine and repeated that the World Health Organization considers the vaccine to be safe.[45] It seemed to Monica that they refused to hear what the parents were saying. This was an impasse that seemed unresolvable. Just a few months following this meeting, the minister posted on Twitter that the vaccine was "still" safe and promoted the next generation of the vaccine, Gardasil 9.[46] In December, he retweeted an article by anthropologist Heidi Larson, of the Vaccine Confidence Project, that "The world must accept that the HPV vaccine is safe."[47]

Uptake of the vaccine in Colombia has plummeted. The Vaccine Confidence Project documented the Colombian HPV vaccine controversy in a report published in June 2017. It reported that the vaccine uptake rate is now 5 percent, a collapse from the target uptake rate of 80–90 percent.[48] The report states the reason is undoubtedly due to the publicity that the incident in El Carmen de Bolívar received.[49] In reality, the people of Colombia saw the controversy play out on social media and know that the government has refused to acknowledge the girls' injuries or the connection to the vaccine.

Rebuilding Hope continues its advocacy on behalf of the sick girls, and Monica León del Rio continues to represent them. On August 7, 2017, Monica announced a class action lawsuit on behalf of 700 sick girls from all over Colombia, some of whom are from El Carmen de Bolívar, against Merck Sharpe and Dohme for injuries from the HPV vaccine.[50] Among the claims are six on behalf of girls who died following the vaccine; Karen Durán-Cantor is one of those wrongful death plaintiffs. The aim of the lawsuit is to claim compensation for the injured girls and their families, and closure for the families of those who have died. An article featured in *Medscape* on the same day, by Carlos Guevara-Casas, quoted Dr. Lina Maria Trujillo of the National Institute of Oncology:

> . . . the lack of trust started in 2014, when a group of girls who had recently been vaccinated presented various symptoms, possibly associated with food poisoning. Although a causal link was never shown, the rumor that the vaccine had caused the symptoms spread.[51]

Just six days after the class action was filed, the attorney general ordered an investigation into the health authorities' handling of the vaccine in El Carmen de Bolívar.[52] Perhaps the implication is that the locals did not properly store the vials or follow the cold chain process. This would not explain all the other injuries in Colombia, however.

A few weeks later, another major announcement came from Colombia. Finally, the Constitutional High Court issued a ruling on a case challenging the constitutionality of the HPV vaccine mandate law, Bill #1626.[53] Monica León del Rio presented evidence from the previous favorable ruling from the 2013 High Court case in Cali. The Constitutional Court ruled that the HPV vaccine would no longer be considered mandatory in Colombia, stating that it could not rule out the vaccine as the cause of the girls' injuries.[54] It further stated that any girls presenting with symptoms after the vaccine should be given access to the appropriate medical care. The court also stipulated that informed consent must be given before administration of the vaccine, which is a huge departure from previous practices.[55]

The HPV vaccine story in Colombia continues. For now, the battleground is clear: 700 sick girls, their families, and their lawyer versus a pharmaceutical giant and the Colombian state. They join other lawsuits around the world in an effort to find answers to what happened to their children, and to seek treatment and compensation for their injuries.

29.

THE EMPEROR HAS
NO CLOTHES

Everyone in the streets and the windows said, "Oh, how fine are the Emperor's new clothes! Don't they fit him to perfection? And see his long train!" Nobody would confess that he couldn't see anything, for that would prove him either unfit for his position, or a fool. No costume the Emperor had worn before was ever such a complete success.

"But he hasn't got anything on," a little child said.

"Did you ever hear such innocent prattle?" said its father. And one person whispered to another what the child had said, "He hasn't anything on. A child says he hasn't anything on."

"But he hasn't got anything on!" the whole town cried out at last.

Hans Christian Andersen,
"The Emperor's New Clothes"[1]

If cancer has been dubbed the emperor of all maladies, then surely the HPV vaccine is the emperor of all vaccines. With cutting-edge, genetically engineered VLP technology; the promise to prevent cancer; accolades from world medical organizations; glowing endorsements from government health agencies; and soaring revenues and

---

1   Hans Christian Andersen, "The Emperor's New Clothes," http://www.andersen.sdu.dk/vaerk/hersholt/TheEmperorsNewClothes_e.html.

market penetration in more than a hundred twenty-five countries after a scant twelve years, few would cast doubt on the HPV vaccine's regal status among medicines, let alone vaccines. Yet as in the fairy tale, a child can see that the emperor has no clothes and that his regal vestments are an illusion.

In the twelve years since Gardasil gained approval, the triumphal narrative has prevailed. But the devastating narrative of harm to children worms its way into public discourse nonetheless, undermining the vaccine's international success story. We have highlighted the discrepancies and half-truths in the mainstream narrative. Just as it took time for the fairy tale crowd to catch on, so it is taking time for the world to come around to seeing the truth about the HPV vaccine.

Thus far, HPV vaccine effectiveness is showing promise in reducing the risk of cervical lesions in follow-up studies, but the vaccine is still at an experimental stage. Its effectiveness in preventing cancer remains unknown. The vaccine clinical trials were profoundly flawed for many reasons, including that no saline placebo was used as a control and that manufacturers did not adequately study the vaccines' target preteen population. Since 2006, children and young people around the world have unwittingly taken part in an uncontrolled clinical trial, without their or their parents' informed consent.

This widespread deprivation of true informed consent violates fundamental tenets of ethical medicine and human rights. It is simply unethical to put lives at risk without real informed consent, particularly when safer alternatives for cervical cancer prevention exist and the vaccine has never been proven to prevent cancer. To uphold human rights, individuals must receive full information about risks and benefits of the vaccine. It is entirely within a person's right to reject the vaccine and to defer to traditional and safe alternatives to cervical cancer prevention, such as a healthy lifestyle and Pap tests, as well as newer HPV DNA and RNA tests.

Although regulators claim the vaccine is safe, both the FDA and the WHO have received over 100,000 reports of adverse events, including deaths, from around the world. Are they all coincidences?

Although scientists now recognize that symptoms from the vaccine occur in clusters, they have not yet made this a research focus. Scientists could be doing studies that might yield a deeper understanding of long-term effects if they studied cluster symptoms now. Likewise, scientists should pay attention to the many missed safety signals in the clinical trials, which the book highlights, including effects on fertility and autoimmune conditions. As Nobel laureate Luc Montagnier reminds us in the preface, the Hippocratic Oath is "First Do No Harm."

We urgently call for more research on ways to help the children and families now suffering from HPV vaccine injury. These people have been neglected and mistreated simply because their pleas for help discredit the dominant narrative of a flawless vaccine. The medical community's impulse to disregard HPV vaccine injury or to discount it as psychogenic is deeply disheartening. Yet we are encouraged by the work of a growing number of doctors and scientists to help these victims of iatrogenic harm.

We also call for civility. We are dismayed that families who report HPV vaccine injuries are branded "antivaccine" and "antiscience" by media and government agencies alike. This marginalization and bullying destroys civil public discourse and discourages scientific inquiry, when we urgently need both. All media, including social media, should be a place where civil information sharing occurs.

As with Merck's Vioxx, the truth will come out. The HPV vaccine is on trial, both in the courts of law and public opinion. The evidence is mounting, as we've made clear. The future of the vaccine is uncertain. But in the meantime, how many children will suffer because of a pharmaceutical *nonbinding promise* that in 20 to 30 years, the vaccine will prevent some HPV-related cancers?

As the vaccine enters its second decade, it continues to be the object of high praise. But accounts of scandal, lawsuits, severe injuries, and deaths grow, challenging the prevailing narrative. This book poses many questions that regulators and manufacturers have a duty to answer. Crucial questions around the clinical trials, the ingredients in the vaccines, missed safety signals, and the potential for harm in the real world remain unanswered. It is incumbent on the scientific community to seek higher standards in clinical trial safety, especially for children. Transparency and disclosure of all clinical trial data would deter some if not all clinical trial malfeasance. This book highlights how the flawed clinical trials missed key safety signals.

Through lost lives and permanent injuries, children are resoundingly telling us that the HPV vaccine is unsafe. As in the fairy tale, adults are already starting to echo the child's truth telling. People around the world are whispering about the vaccine's risks and harms. The question is, When will the whispers turn into a roar? When will the world proclaim that the Emperor has no clothes?

ENDNOTES

NB: All endnotes accessed and links checked between June 21–August 9, 2018

CHAPTER 1

1. "2017 Lasker-DeBakey Clinical Medical Research Award, HPV Vaccines for Cancer Prevention," Albert and Mary Lasker Foundation, www.laskerfoundation .org/awards/show/hpv-vaccines-cancer-prevention/.
2. "2017 Lasker DeBakey Clinical Medical Research Award," Albert and Mary Lasker Foundation video, www.laskerfoundation.org/awards/show/hpv-vaccines -cancer-prevention/#video.
3. "Dr. Douglas R. Lowy, Acceptance Remarks, 2017 Awards Ceremony," Albert and Mary Lasker Foundation, www.laskerfoundation.org/awards/show/hpv-vaccines -cancer-prevention/#douglas-r-lowy.

CHAPTER 2

1. Frederik Joelving, "What the Gardasil Testing May Have Missed," *Slate*, December 17, 2017, https://slate.com/health-and-science/2017/12/flaws-in-the -clinical-trials-for-gardasil-made-it-harder-to-properly-assess-safety.html.
2. Ibid.
3. Danish FUTURE II recruitment brochure (2002), a copy of which is in the authors' files.
4. Signe Daugbjerg and Michael Bech, *The Vaccinated Girls* (no longer available on-line or archive), formerly at https://www.youtube.com/watch?v=GO2i-r39hok. Article in Politiken: (translation on Google) https://translate.google.com /translate?hl=en&sl=auto&tl=en&u=https%3A%2F%2Fpolitiken.dk%2Fkultur %2Fmedier%2Fart5605586%2FCavling-nomineret-film-kritiseres-for-dårligt- håndværkhttp%3A%2F%2F.
5. Danish FUTURE II recruitment brochure, note 3 above.
6. V501 Protocol/Amendment No: 015–00, at 23, https://www.scribd.com/document /367386168/V501-015-00-PRO-VD?secret_password=j4BXCUs76g4wRtDxk- 5cy.

7. Ibid.
8. Ibid., 9.

CHAPTER 3

1. J. T. Schiller and D. R. Lowy, "Developmental History of HPV Prophylactic Vaccines," in *History of Vaccine Development*, 265–284, at 266, ed. S. A. Plotkin (New York, Springer, 2011); J. T. Bryan, *et al.*, "Prevention of Cervical Cancer: Journey to Develop the First Human Papillomavirus Virus-like Particle Vaccine and the Next Generation Vaccine," *Current Opinion in Chemical Biology*, 32:34–47, at 34, 2016; H. zur Hausen, "Papillomaviruses in the Causation of Human Cancers-a Brief Historical Account," *Virology*, 384:260–65, at 260, 2009.
2. Schiller and Lowy, note 1 above, at 267.
3. "Harald zur Hausen – Biographical," The Official Website of the Nobel Prize, https://www.nobelprize.org/nobel_prizes/medicine/laureates/2008/hausen -bio.html.
4. Ibid.
5. *See* https://www.nobelprize.org/nobel_prizes/lists/year/index.html?year=2008 &images=yes.
6. Nobel Prize zur Hausen biography, note 3 above; zur Hausen, "Papillomaviruses in the Causation of Human Cancers-a Brief Historical Account," note 1 above, at 261.
7. "HeLa" is an abbreviation for Henrietta Lacks, a woman who died from cervical cancer, and the namesake of the well-known book *The Immortal Life of Henrietta Lacks* by Rebecca Skloot. The book documents Lacks's life and death as an African-American woman whose cervical cancer cells were taken from her body and marketed globally, particularly for use in research labs, without her or her family's knowledge or consent.
8. *See, e.g.*, Bryan 2016, note 1 above, at 35; E. M. Burd, "Human Papillomavirus and Cervical Cancer," *Clinical Microbiology Reviews*, 16(1):1–17, at 4, January 2003, www.ncbi.nlm.nih.gov/pmc/articles/PMC145302/pdf/0007.pdf.
9. N. Munoz, "Human Papillomavirus and Cancer: The Epidemiological Evidence," *Journal of Clinical Virology*, 19(1–2):1–5, October 2000.
10. Donald G. McNeil, "How a Vaccine Ended in Triumph," *New York Times*, August 29, 2006, www.nytimes.com/2006/08/29/health/29hpv.html.
11. Ibid.
12. Ibid.
13. Ibid.
14. C. McNeil, "Who Invented the VLP Cervical Cancer Vaccines?" *Journal of the National Cancer Institute*, 98(7):433, April 5, 2006, www.academic.oup.com /jnci/article/98/7/433/2522050.
15. S. Padmanabhan, *et al.*, "Intellectual Property, Technology Transfer and Manufacture of Low-cost HPV Vaccines in India," *Nature Biotechnology*, 28(7): 671–678, at 673, July 2010.

16. Ibid. *See also* Georgetown University, "Richard Schlegel, Biographical Information," http://explore.georgetown.edu/people/schleger/.
17. McNeil, "Who Invented the VLP Cervical Cancer Vaccines?" note 14 above.
18. Schiller and Lowy, "Developmental History of HPV Prophylactic Vaccines," note 1 above, at 270.
19. Padmanabhan, "Intellectual Property, Technology Transfer and Manufacture of Low-cost HPV Vaccines in India," note 15 above, at 673; Corydon Ireland, "A Cancer Vaccine Is Born," *Rochester Review*, Vol. 68(3), Spring 2006, www.rochester.edu/pr/Review/V68N3/feature1.html.
20. McNeil, "Who Invented the VLP Cervical Cancer Vaccines?" note 14 above.
21. "Dr. Nubia Muñoz," International Epidemiological Association: http://ieaweb.org/biographies/dr-nubia-munoz/.
22. *IARC Monographs on the Evaluation of Carcinogenic Risks to Humans*, Vol 64, Human Papillomaviruses, International Agency for Research on Cancer (IARC), at 24: http://monographs.iarc.fr/ENG/Monographs/vol64/mono64.pdf.
23. J. M. Walboomers, *et al.*, "Human papillomavirus is a necessary cause of invasive cervical cancer worldwide." *Journal of Pathology*,189(1):12–9, September 1999.
24. Ibid.
25. Ruth Beran, "Ian Frazer's Patent Problem," *Lab+Life Scientist*, July 2006, www.labonline.com.au/content/life-scientist/news/ian-frazer-s-patent-problem-1263005711.
26. *Frazer v. Schlegel*, 498 F.3d 1283 (Fed. Cir. 2007).
27. Schiller and Lowy, "Developmental History of HPV Prophylactic Vaccines," note 1 above, at 270.
28. National Archives and Records Administration, Office of Government Information Services, "In Re: Case No. 2011–0059," November 24, 2010, www.vietnamcervicalcancer.org/dmdocuments/ogis%20suba%2024%20november%202010.pdf.
29. "Top 20 Commercially Successful Inventions," National Institutes of Health (NIH), www.ott.nih.gov/top-20-commercially-successful-inventions.
30. Ibid.
31. Mark Blaxill and Dan Olmsted, "A License to Kill," *Vaccine Epidemic*, 175–205, at 184–185 (Skyhorse Pub. 2012).
32. Ibid., 185.
33. "Harald zur Hausen - Banquet Speech," Official Website of the Nobel Prize www.nobelprize.org/nobel_prizes/medicine/laureates/2008/hausen-speech_en.html .
34. "From Lab to Market: The HPV Vaccine," *NIH Record*, Vol. LIX(4), at 5, February 23, 2007, https://nihrecord.nih.gov/newsletters/2007/02_23_2007/story2.htm.
35. "HPV Vaccines for Cancer Prevention," Albert and Mary Lasker Foundation, www.laskerfoundation.org/awards/show/hpv-vaccines-cancer-prevention/.
36. For example, see discussion of various HPV vaccine studies in A. Hildesheim, *et al.*, "Efficacy of the HPV-16/18 vaccine: Final according to protocol results

from the blinded phase of the randomized Costa Rica HPV-16/18 vaccine trial," *Vaccine*, 32(39):5087–5097, at 5088, September 3, 2014, www.sciencedirect
.com/science/article/pii/S0264410X14008275?via%3Dihub.

37. Ibid.

38. Ibid.

39. Caroline Chen, "FDA Repays Industry by Rushing Risking Drugs to Market,"
Pro Publica, June 26, 2018, https://www.propublica.org/article/fda-repays-industry
-by-rushing-risky-drugs-to-market.

40. US Food and Drug Administration (FDA), PDUFA User Fee Rates Archive,
www.fda.gov/ForIndustry/UserFees/PrescriptionDrugUserFee/ucm152775
.htm.

41. G. DeLong, "Conflicts of Interest in Vaccine Safety Research," *Accountability in
Research*, 19:65–88, at 68, February 29, 2012.

42. Chen, "FDA Repays Industry by Rushing Risking Drugs to Market." note 39
above.

43. M. Angell, "Drug Companies and Doctors: A Story of Corruption," *New York
Review of Books*, January 15, 2009, www.nybooks.com/articles/2009/01/15
/drug-companies-doctorsa-story-of-corruption/.

44. L. Tomljenovic and C.A. Shaw, "Too Fast or Not Too Fast: The FDA's Approval
of Merck's HPV Vaccine Gardasil," *Journal of Law, Medicine and Ethics*, 673–681,
at 677, Fall 2012, quoting M. Angell, "Industry-Sponsored Clinical Research: A
Broken System," JAMA, 300(9):10691–1071, 2008.

45. DeLong, "Conflicts of Interest in Vaccine Safety Research," note 41 above, at 67.

46. Ibid.

47. Ibid.

48. Ibid.

CHAPTER 4

1. M. Angell, "Drug Companies and Doctors: A Story of Corruption," *New
York Review of Books*, January 15, 2009, http://www.nybooks.com/articles
/2009/01/15/drug-companies-doctorsa-story-of-corruption/.

2. "Harald zur Hausen - Banquet Speech," Official Website of the Nobel
Prize, https://www.nobelprize.org/nobel_prizes/medicine/laureates/2008
/hausen-speech_en.html.

3. "Genital HPV Infection - Fact Sheet," US Centers for Disease Control and
Prevention (CDC), www.cdc.gov/std/hpv/stdfact-hpv.htm.

4. "Human papillomavirus (HPV) and cervical cancer," World Health Organization
(WHO), http://who.int/mediacentre/factsheets/fs380/en/; A. C. de Freitas,
et al., "Susceptibility to cervical cancer: An overview," *Gynecologic Oncology*,
126:304–311, at 306, 2012.

5. B. W. Stewart and C. P. Wild, *World Cancer Report 2014*, at 468, 471 (IARC 2014),
http://publications.iarc.fr/Non-Series-Publications/World-Cancer-Reports
/World-Cancer-Report-2014.

6. *See, e.g.*, M. Komiyama and K. Hasegawa, "Comparison of Preventive Care for Cervical Cancer Between Japan and Western Countries: A Review," *Journal of Pharmaceutical Care & Health Systems*, 4(4), 2017, www.omicsonline.org/open-access/comparison-of-preventive-care-for-cervical cancer-between-japan-and-western-countries-a-review-2376-0419-1000185.pdf ; *see also Shimuraomiya Hospital*, www.hakujinkai.com/hospital_cervical.php (in Japanese); V. Kesic, "Cervical Cancer – State of Art," *HealthMED*, November 30, 2011, www.slideshare.net/ESOSLIDES/3-kesic-state-of-the-art; http://allwomen.jp/factor/hpv.html (in Japanese).

7. "Cancer Stat Facts: Cervical Cancer," National Cancer Institute (NCI), https://seer.cancer.gov/statfacts/html/cervix.html.

8. Ibid.

9. Ibid.

10. Ibid.

11. de Freitas, *et al.*, "Susceptibility to cervical cancer: An overview," note 4 above; at 305; IARC, "Cervical Cancer Incidence, Mortality and Prevalence Worldwide in 2012," http://globocan.iarc.fr/old/FactSheets/cancers/cervix-new.asp.

12. IARC Cervical Cancer Incidence, note 11 above.

13. Ibid.

14. V. Kumar, *et al.*, *Robbins Basic Pathology (8th ed.)*, at 718–21 (Elsevier Health Sciences 2007); D. W. Kufe, *et al.*, *Holland Frei Cancer Medicine (8th ed.)*, at 1299 (PMPH-U.S.A. 2009); "Inside Knowledge: Get the Facts about Gynecologic Cancer," CDC, www.cdc.gov/cancer/knowledge/provider-education/cervical/risk-factors.htm.

15. *See, e.g.*, "Inside Knowledge: Get the Facts about Gynecologic Cancer," CDC, note 14 above; "What are Risk Factors for Cervical Cancer?" American Cancer Society www.cancer.org/cancer/cervicalcancer/detailedguide/cervical-cancer-risk-factors; J. McKay, *et al.*, "Immuno-Related Polymorphisms and Cervical Cancer Risk: The IARC Multicentric Case-Control Study," *PLOS One*, 12(7): e0181285, http://journals.plos.org/plosone/article?id=10.1371/journal.pone.0177775; A. W. Batieha, *et al.*, "Serum Micronutrients and the Subsequent Risk of Cervical Cancer in a Population-based Nested Case-Control Study," *Cancer Epidemiology, Biomarkers & Prevention*, 2:335–339, July/August, 1993; R. L. Sedjo, *et al.*, "Human Papillomavirus Persistence and Nutrients Involved in the Methylation Pathway among a Cohort of Young Women," *Cancer Epidemiology, Biomarkers & Prevention*, 11:353–359, 2002; D. Huo, *et al.*, "Incidence Rates and Risks of Diethylstilbestrol-Related Clear-Cell Adenocarcinoma of the Vagina and Cervix: Update After 40-year Follow-Up," *Gynecologic Oncology*, 146:566–571, 2017. Risk factors for other HPV-associated cancers often overlap with cervical cancer risk factors. *See* https://www.cancer.org/ for more comprehensive risk factors for vaginal, vulvar, anal and other cancers.

16. *See, e.g.*, M. Plummer, *et al.*, "Smoking and Cervical Cancer: Pooled Analysis of the IARC Multi-Centric Case-Control Study," *Cancer Causes &*

Control, 14:805–814, at 812, 2003; "Global Smoking," CDC, www.cdc.gov /healthcommunication/toolstemplates/entertainmented/tips/globalsmoking. html; Larisa Brown and Michelle Nichols, "Home Fires: the World's Most Lethal Pollution," *Independent*, January 23, 2011, http://www.independent. co.uk/life-style/health-and-families/health-news/home-fires-the-worlds-most-lethal-pollution-2192000.html.

17. *See, e.g.*, J. A. den Boon, *et al.*, "Molecular Transitions from Papillomavirus Infection to Cervical Cancer and Cancer: Role of Stromal Estrogen Receptor Signaling," *Proceedings of the National Academy of Sciences of the United States of America*, 112 (25):E3255–E3264, June 8, 2015, www.pnas.org/content/112/25/ E3255; S.-H. Chung, *et al.*, "Estrogen and ERα: Culprits in Cervical Cancer?" *Trends in Endocrinology and Metabolism*, 21(8): 504–511, August, 2010; L. Fickman, "Estrogen Suspected, Examined as Cause of Cervical Cancer", University of Houston, March 1, 2018, http://www.uh.edu/nsm/news-events/stories/2018/0301-cervical-cancer.php; A. Mitra, *et. al.*, "The Vaginal Microbiota, Human Papillomavirus Infection and Cervical Intraepithelial Neoplasia: What Do We Know and Where Are We Going Next?" *Microbiome*, 4:58, 2016; Christine Kent "The Role of Glycogen in Vulvovaginal Health," *Whole Woman Blog*, February 1, 2012, https://wholewoman.com/blog/?p=1041.

18. A. Audirac-Chalifour, *et al.*, "Cervical Microbiome and Cytokine Profile at Various Stages of Cervical Cancer: A Pilot Study," *PLOS One*, 11(4): e0153274, April 26, 2016, http://journals.plos.org/plosone/article?id=10.1371/jour-nal.pone.0153274; Mitra, "The Vaginal Microbiota, Human Papillomavirus Infection and Cervical Intraepithelial Neoplasia", note 17 above; Kent "The Role of Glycogen in Vulvovaginal Health," note 17 above; J. W. Sellors and R. Sankaranarayanan, "An Introduction to the Anatomy of the Uterine Cervix," *Colposcopy and Treatment of Cervical Intraepithelial Neoplasia: a Beginners' Manual* (IARC 2003/4), https://screening.iarc.fr/colpochap.php?lang=1and https:// screening.iarc.fr/doc/Colposcopymanual.pdf.

19. Mitra, "The Vaginal Microbiota, Human Papillomavirus Infection and Cervical Intraepithelial Neoplasia," note 17 above; M. Kyrgiou, *et al.*, "Does the Vaginal Microbiota Play a Role in the Development of Cervical Cancer?" *Translational Research*, 168–182, January 2017.

20. Gardasil package insert, at 1, https://www.fda.gov/downloads/biologicsblood vaccines/vaccines/approvedproducts/ucm111263.pdf; Gardasil 9 package insert, at 1, https://www.fda.gov/downloads/BiologicsBloodVaccines/Vaccines/Approved Products/UCM426457.pdf; Cervarix package insert, at 1, https://www.fda.gov /downloads/BiologicsBloodVaccines/Vaccines/ApprovedProducts /UCM240436.pdf.

21. Gardasil package insert, note 20 above, at 7–8 (Sec. 6.1).

22. IARC Cervical Cancer Incidence, note 11 above.

23. D. M. Harper, *et al.*, "Cervical cancer incidence can increase despite HPV vaccination," *Lancet Infectious Diseases*, 10(9):594–595, September 2010.

24. T. P. Canavan and N. R. Doshi, "Cervical Cancer," *American Family Physician*, 61(5):1369–1376, March 1, 2000.

25. de Freitas, *et al.*, "Susceptibility to cervical cancer: An overview," note 4 above, at 305.

26. "Cervical Cancer is Preventable," CDC, November 2014, https://www.cdc.gov/vitalsigns/cervical-cancer/index.html.

27. "What's an HPV test?" Planned Parenthood, www.plannedparenthood.org/learn/cancer/cervical-cancer/whats-hpv-test.

28. D. M. Harper and K. B. Williams, "Prophylactic HPV Vaccines: Current Knowledge of Impact of Gynecologic Premalignancies," *Discovery Medicine*, July 3, 2010, www.discoverymedicine.com/Diane-M-Harper/2010/07/03/prophylactic-hpv-vaccines-current-knowledge-of-impact-on-gynecologic-premalignancies/; "HPV and Cancer," NCI, www.cancer.gov/about-cancer/causes-prevention/risk/infectious-agents/hpv-fact-sheet#q7; Stewart and Wild, *World Cancer Report 2014*, note 5 above, at 470.

29. Harper and Williams, "Prophylactic HPV Vaccines: Current Knowledge of Impact of Gynecologic Premalignancies," note 28 above.

30. "What are the Symptoms of HPV?" Planned Parenthood, www.plannedparenthood.org/learn/stds-hiv-safer-sex/hpv/what-are-symptoms-hpv.

31. Harper and Williams, "Prophylactic HPV Vaccines: Current Knowledge of Impact of Gynecologic Premalignancies," note 28 above.

32. Harper and Williams, "Prophylactic HPV Vaccines: Current Knowledge of Impact of Gynecologic Premalignancies," note 28 above; *see also* Harper, *et al.*, "Cervical cancer incidence can increase despite HPV vaccination," note 23 above.

33. D. M. Harper and L. R. DeMars, "HPV vaccines—A review of the First Decade," *Gynecologic Oncology*, 146(1):196–204, at 202, July 2017. A study in Manitoba, Canada highlighted these concerns. When looking at women who had and had not received HPV vaccines, researchers found that many vaccinated women were not protected against serious cervical lesions, particularly if they were older when they received the vaccines or had had abnormal cervical screening results in the past. The study's authors noted the importance of continuing cervical screening regardless of whether a woman had received an HPV vaccine or not; S. M. Mahmud, *et al.*, "Effectiveness of the Quadrivalent Human Papillomavirus Vaccine Against Cervical Dysplasia in Manitoba, Canada," *Journal of Clinical Oncology*, 22(5):438–443, February 10, 2014, http://asco-pubs.org/doi/abs/10.1200/JCO.2013.52.4645?url_ver=Z39.88-2003&rfr_id=ori%3Arid%3Acrossref.org&rfr_dat=cr_pub%3Dpubmed&.

34. C. A. Paynter, *et al.*, "Adherence to Cervical Cancer Screening Varies by Human Papillomavirus Vaccination Status in a High-Risk Population," *Preventative Medicine Reports*, 2:711–716, at 711, 2015; *see also* Harper and DeMars, "HPV vaccines—A review of the First Decade," note 33 above, at 202.

35. C. I. Fowler, *et al.*, "Trends in Cervical Cancer Screening in Title X-Funded Health Centers–United States, 2005-2015," *Morbidity and Mortality Weekly*

Report, 66(37):981–985, September 22, 2017, www.cdc.gov/mmwr/volumes/66/wr/mm6637a4.htm.

36. Harper and DeMars, "HPV vaccines—A review of the First Decade," note 33 above, at 202.

37. *See, e.g.,* S. M. Garland, *et al.,* "Impact and Effectiveness of the Quadrivalent Human Papillomavirus Vaccine: A Systematic Review of 10 Years of Real-world Experience," *Clinical Infectious Diseases,* 63(4):519–527, August 15, 2016; D. Ferris, *et al.,* "4-Valent Human Papillomavirus (4vHPV) Vaccine in Preadolescents and Adolescents After 10 Years," *Pediatrics,* 140(6):1–9, at 2–3, November 2017; M. Lehtinen, *et al.,* "Ten-Year Follow-Up of Human Papillomavirus Vaccine Efficacy Against the Most Stringent Cervical Neoplasia End-Point – Registry-Based Follow Up of Three Cohorts from Randomized Trials," *BMJ Open,* 7:e015867 (2017), http://bmjopen.bmj.com/content/bm-jopen/7/8/e015867.full.pdf; Harper and DeMars, "HPV vaccines—A review of the First Decade." (also including information about protection against persistent infection discussed below), note 33 above.

38. T. Luostarinen, *et al.,* "Vaccination protects against invasive HPV-associated cancers," *International Journal of Cancer,* 142(10):2186–2187, 2018. In a brief letter to the editor, researchers reported eight cases of cervical cancer over an eight-year period and appear to assume all cases were caused by vaccine-relevant HPV types. Absent more information about key data such as distribution of the cancer cases during the time period studied, the HPV types (if any) found in each cancer case and cervical screening, lack of screening, and any treatment of CINs in both cohorts, the pronouncement seems premature. Additionally, these women are still young, and, whether vaccinated or not, all will need to be followed for CINs as well as cancer as they enter the age ranges when cervical cancer is most often diagnosed. Recently an analysis of US data showed a drop in incidence in cervical cancer in very young women when comparing pre- and post-HPV vaccine time periods. F. Guo, et al., "Cervical Cancer Incidence in Young U.S. Females After Human Papillomavirus Vaccine Introduction," *American Journal of Preventive Medicine,* 55(2):197-204, at 202, 2018. Not only is cervical cancer quite rare in this cohort, but this study did not account for HPV vaccination status and HPV type and results may further be confounded by changes in screening protocols and behaviors. Thus the observed decrease in cervical cancer in these younger age groups cannot be definitively attributed to vaccination. In fact, the authors note the potential for an increase in cervical cancer "in the long run" because of changes to screening protocols. *Ibid.*

39. I. Frazer, "God's Gift to Women: The Human Papillomavirus Vaccine," *Immunity,* 25:179–184, August 2006; *see also* T. R. Broker, then President of the International Papillomavirus Society, speaking at a Center for American Progress Special Presentation: "Preventing HPV, Easy as 1, 2, 3 Shots? Ensuring Access to the New Anti-Cancer Vaccines," January 27, 2006, https://web.archive

.org/web/20081028100942/https://www.americanprogress.org/kf/hpv_event
_transcript.pdf.

CHAPTER 5

1. P. A. Offit, in "The Greater Good," a film by Leslie Manookian, *et al.*, 2011, http://www.greatergoodmovie.org/TGG/wp-content/uploads/2012/06 /TheGreaterGoodMovie-PressKit.pdf.

2. L. Jørgensen, *et al.*, "Index of the Human Papillomavirus (HPV) Vaccine Industry Clinical Study Programmers and Non-Industry Funded Studies: a Necessary Basis to Address Reporting Bias in a Systematic Review," *Systematic Reviews*, 7:8, January 18, 2018, https://www.ncbi.nlm.nih.gov/pmc/articles /PMC5774129/pdf/13643_2018_Article_675.pdf.

3. Ibid.; *see also* T. Jefferson and L. Jørgensen, "Redefining the 'E' in EBM," *BMJ Evidence-Based Medicine*, 23(2):46–47, April 2018, https://ebm.bmj.com/content /23/2/46.

4. M. Arbyn, *et al.*, "Prophylactic vaccination against human papillomaviruses to prevent cervical cancer and its precursors," *Cochrane Database of Systematic Reviews*, Issue 5. Art. No.: CD009069.DOI: 10.1002/14651858.CD009069. pub3, at 2 (2018), www.cochranelibrary.com.

5. D. Healy, "In the Name of the BMJ," August 7, 2018, https://davidhealy.org /in-the-name-of-the-bmj/.

6. L. Jørgensen, *et al.*, "The Cochrane HPV vaccine review was incomplete and ignored important evidence of bias," *BMJ Evidence-Based Medicine*, July 27, 2018, at 1, https://ebm.bmj.com/content/early/2018/07/27/bmjebm-2018-111012.

7. Ibid.

8. Ibid., 3.

9. N. Hawkes, "HPV vaccine safety: Cochrane launches urgent investigation into review after criticisms," *BMJ*, August 9, 2018, https://www.bmj.com/content /362/bmj.k3472.

10. Ibid.

11. 21 C.F.R. § 314.126(a).

12. 42 U.S.C. § 262(a)(2)(C)(i)(I).

13. "Vaccine Product Approval Process," FDA, www.fda.gov/BiologicsBlood Vaccines/DevelopmentApprovalProcess/BiologicsLicenseApplications BLAProcess/ucm133096.htm.

14. For example, Gardasil was tested for immunogenicity in African Green monkeys. L. Shi, *et al.*, "Gardasil®: Prophylactic Human Papillomavirus Vaccine Development—From Bench Top to Bed-side, *Clinical Pharmacology & Therapeutics*, 81(2):259–264, at 259, February 2007.

15. "Vaccine Product Approval Process," FDA, note 13 above.

16. "Step 3: Clinical Research," FDA, www.fda.gov/ForPatients/Approvals/Drugs /ucm405622.htm#Clinical_Research_Phase_Studies; "What Are the Different

Types of Clinical Research?" FDA, www.fda.gov/ForPatients/ClinicalTrials /Types/ucm20041762.htm; "Vaccine Product Approval Process," FDA, see note 13 above; V. Marshall and N. W. Baylor, "Food and Drug Administration Regulation and Evaluation of Vaccines," *Pediatrics*, 127(S1):S23-S30, May 2011, http://pediatrics.aappublications.org/content/127/Supplement_1/S23.long.

17. "Vaccines and Related Biological Products Advisory Committee," FDA, www.fda.gov/AdvisoryCommittees/CommitteesMeetingMaterials/Blood VaccinesandOtherBiologics/VaccinesandRelatedBiologicalProducts AdvisoryCommittee/default.htm.

18. M. Marquardsen, *et al.*, "Redactions in Protocols for Drug Trials: What Industry Sponsors Concealed," *JRSM*, 111(4):136–141, http://journals.sagepub.com/doi /pdf/10.1177/0141076817750554.

19. N. B. Miller, "Clinical Review of Biologics License Application for Human Papillomavirus 6, 11, 16, 18 L1 Virus Like Particle Vaccine (*S. cerevisiae*) (STN 125126 GARDASIL), manufactured by Merck, Inc.," at 44–45, June 8, 2006, archived at http://wayback.archive-it.org/7993/20161024002027/http://www .fda.gov/downloads/BiologicsBloodVaccines/Vaccines/ApprovedProducts /UCM111287.pdf.

20. Ibid., 44.

21. *See, e.g.*, ibid., 45, 50, 127, 265, 301; ClinicalTrials.gov, "Dose-Related Study of Quadrivalent Human Papillomavirus (HPV) (Types 6, 11, 16, 18) L-1 Virus-Like Particle (VLP) Vaccine (V 501–007) (Completed)," https://clinicaltrials .gov/ct2/show/results/NCT00365716?term=v501-007&rank=1; "Cervical Intraepithelial Neoplasm (CIN)-Warts Efficacy Trial in Women Gardasil (V501-013) (Completed)," ClinicalTrials.gov, https://clinicaltrials.gov/ct2/show /results/NCT00092521?term=v501-013&rank=1; "Cervical Intraepithelial Neoplasm (CIN) in Women (Gardasil)(V501-015)," ClinicalTrials.gov, https: //clinicaltrials.gov/ct2/show/results/NCT00092534?term=v501-015&rank=1; "Study of an Investigational Vaccine in Pre-Adolescents and Adolescents (Gardasil)(V501-016)," ClinicalTrials.gov, https://clinicaltrials.gov/ct2/show /results/NCT00092495?term=v501-016&rank=1; "A Study of Gardasil (V501) in Preadolescents and Adolescents (Gardasil)(V501-018), ClinicalTrials.gov, https://clinicaltrials.gov/ct2/show/results/NCT00092547?term=v501-018 &rank=1. Merck conducted two substudies under protocol 013. Protocol 011 was a study of concomitant administration of hepatitis B vaccine (HBV) comparing: (a) women receiving both HPV vaccine and HBV vaccine, (b) those who received HPV vaccine and HepB control (420 mcg aluminum adjuvant), (c) those who received HPV control (225 mcg AAHS) and HBV, and (d) those who received both HPV and HBV controls. In protocol 012, a group received monovalent HPV 16 L1 VLP (40 mcg) vaccine with 225 mcg AAHS, in addition to the standard Gardasil formulation group and the AAHS placebo group. Miller 2006 Gardasil Review, note 19 above, at 127, 137–38.

22. V501 Protocol/Amendment No: 015–00, at 30–32, https://www.scribd.com /document/367386168/V501-015-00-PRO-VD?secret_password=j4BXCUs 76g4wRtDxk5cy.
23. *See, e.g.,* R. E. Chandler, "Safety Concerns with HPV Vaccines Continue to Linger: Are Current Vaccine Pharmacovigilance Practices Sufficient?" *Drug Safety,* 40(12):1167–70, August 30, 2017, https://link.springer.com/article/10.1007 /s40264-017-0593-3; J. L. Cervantes and A. H. Doan, "Discrepancies in the Evaluation of the Safety of the Human Papillomavirus Vaccine," *Memorias do Instituto Oswaldo Cruz,* 113(8), May 28, 2018, https://www.ncbi.nlm.nih.gov /pmc/articles/PMC5967601/pdf/0074-0276-mioc-113-08-e180063.pdf.
24. Miller 2006 Gardasil Review, note 19 above, at 44–45.
25. V501 Protocol/Amendment No: 015–00, note 22 above, at 32.
26. Ibid.
27. Nuremburg Code, https://history.nih.gov/research/downloads/nuremberg.pdf.
28. Ibid.
29. Danish Cancer Society, https://www.cancer.dk/dyn/resources/File/file/0 /5170/1450196565/samtykkeerklaering-hpv-forsoeg.pdf.

CHAPTER 6

1. Transcript of FDA Center For Biologics Evaluation And Research VRBPAC Meeting, May 18, 2006, at 13–14, archived at https://wayback.archive-it.org /7993/20170404052136/https://www.fda.gov/ohrms/dockets/ac/06/tran scripts/2006-4222t1.pdf.
2. J. T. Schiller, *et al.,* "A Review of Clinical Trials of Human Papillomavirus Prophylactic Vaccines," *Vaccine,* 30(5): F123–F138, at F124, November 20, 2012, www.sciencedirect.com/science/article/pii/S0264410X12009516?via%3Dihub.
3. "Accelerated Approval," FDA, https://www.fda.gov/ForPatients/Approvals /Fast/ucm405447.htm; A. Gerhardus and O. Razum, "A long story made too short: surrogate variables and the communication of HPV vaccine trial results," *Journal of Epidemiology and Community Health,* 64(5):377–378, at 378, May 2010.
4. Gerhardus and Razum, note 3 above, at 377; *see also* "Surrogate markers may not tell the whole story," *HealthNewsReview,* www.healthnewsreview.org/toolkit /tips-for-understanding-studies/surrogate-markers-may-not-tell-the-whole-story/.
5. "Gardasil (Human Papillomavirus Vaccine) Questions and Answers-Gardasil, June 8, 2006," FDA, archived at http://wayback.archive-it.org/7993/20170722025101 /https://www.fda.gov/BiologicsBloodVaccines/Vaccines/Questionsabout Vaccines/ucm096052.htm.
6. *See* April 19, 2006 Final Briefing Document, at 16, appended to the April 19, 2006 letter from Patrick Brill-Edwards, M.D., Merck's Director of Worldwide Regulatory Affairs for Vaccines/Biologics, to Christine Walsh, R.N. of the FDA's CBER, archived at http://wayback.archive-it.org/7993/20180126170209/https: //www.fda.gov/ohrms/dockets/ac/06/briefing/2006-4222B1.pdf.

7. Ibid., 16.

8. *See, e.g., Manual for the Surveillance of Vaccine-Preventable Diseases,* "Chapter 5: Human Papillomavirus (HPV)," CDC, https://www.cdc.gov/vaccines/pubs/surv-manual/chpt05-hpv.html; "HPV and Cancer," NCI, www.cancer.gov/about-cancer/causes-prevention/risk/infectious-agents/hpv-fact-sheet#q7; *see also* J. Yingji, *et al.,* "Use of autoantibodies against tumor-associated antigens as serum biomarkers for primary screening of cervical cancer," *Oncotarget,* 8(62): 105425–105439, December 1, 2017, www.ncbi.nlm.nih.gov/pmc/articles/PMC5739648; P. E. Castle, *et al.,* "Impact of Improved Classification on the Association of Human Papillomavirus With Cervical Precancer," *American Journal of Epidemiology,* 171(2):155–163, at 161, 2009; K. Tainio, *et al.,* "Clinical course of untreated cervical intraepithelial neoplasia grade 2 under active surveillance: systematic review and meta-analysis," *BMJ Open,* 360:k499, 2018, https://www.bmj.com/content/bmj/360/bmj.k499.full.pdf.

9. *See, e.g.,* B. W. Stewart and C. P. Wild, "World Cancer Report 2014," at 472 (IARC 2014), http://publications.iarc.fr/Non-Series-Publications/World-Cancer-Reports/World-Cancer-Report-2014.

10. M. Schiffman, *et al.,* "Carcinogenic Human Papillomavirus Infection," *Nature Reviews Disease Primers,* 2:1–20, at 3–4, December 2016.

11. Ibid., 13.

12. Castle, *et al.,* "Impact of Improved Classification on the Association of Human Papillomavirus With Cervical Precancer," note 8 above, at 161.

13. Tainio, *et al.,* "Clinical course of untreated cervical intraepithelial neoplasia grade 2 under active surveillance: systematic review and meta-analysis," note 8 above.

14. "HPV and Cancer," NCI, note 8 above; Yingji, *et al.,* "Use of autoantibodies against tumor-associated antigens as serum biomarkers for primary screening of cervical cancer," note 8 above; Castle *et al.,* "Impact of Improved Classification on the Association of Human Papillomavirus With Cervical Precancer," note 8 above, at 161.

15. M. Arbyn, *et al.,* "Prophylactic Vaccination Against Human Papillomaviruses to Prevent Cervical Cancer and its Precursors," *Cochrane Database of Systematic Reviews,* Issue 5, Art. No.: CD009069, at 9, May 9, 2018, http://cochranelibrary-wiley.com/doi/10.1002/14651858.CD009069.pub3/abstract.

16. Castle, *et al.,* "Impact of Improved Classification on the Association of Human Papillomavirus With Cervical Precancer," note 8 above, at 156; *see also* "HPV & Cancer," NCI, note 8 above; *see also* Yingji, *et al.,* "Use of autoantibodies against tumor-associated antigens as serum biomarkers for primary screening of cervical cancer," note 8 above.

17. Castle, *et al.,* "Impact of Improved Classification on the Association of Human Papillomavirus With Cervical Precancer," note 8 above, at 161.

18. Rosenthal, Elisabeth, "Drug Makers' Push Leads To Cancer Vaccines' Rise," *New York Times*, August 19, 2008, https://www.nytimes.com/2008/08/20/health/policy/20vaccine.html?mcubz=0.
19. "Gardasil™ HPV Quadrivalent Vaccine May 18, 2006 VRBPAC Meeting," VRBPAC Background Document, at 2, archived at http://wayback.archive-it.org/7993/20180126170205/https://www.fda.gov/ohrms/dockets/ac/06/briefing/2006-4222B3.pdf.
20. Ibid.
21. FDA, email to authors, April 5, 2017. A copy of the FDA's April 5, 2017 correspondence with the authors is in their files.
22. "Fast Track," FDA, available at https://www.fda.gov/ForPatients/Approvals/Fast/ucm405399.htm
23. Ibid.
24. "FDA Approves Expanded Use of HPV Test," *FDA News*, March 31, 2003, archived at http://web.archive.org/web/20090120122822/https://www.fda.gov/ohrms/dockets/dockets/07p0210/07p-0210-ccp0001-01-FDA-News-vol3.pdf.
25. FDA, email to authors, April 5, 2017, note 21 above; "Fast Track," FDA, note 22 above.
26. "Fast Track," FDA, note 22 above; *see also* L. Tomljenovic and C. A. Shaw, "Too Fast or Not Too Fast: The FDA's Approval of Merck's HPV Vaccine Gardasil," *Journal of Law, Medicine & Ethics*, 673–681, at 674–75, Fall 2012.
27. *See, e.g.,* FDA, email to authors, April 5, 2017, note 21 above.
28. D. M. Harper and K. B. Williams, "Prophylactic HPV Vaccines: Current Knowledge of Impact of Gynecologic Premalignancies," *Discovery Medicine*, July 3, 2010, www.discoverymedicine.com/Diane-M-Harper/2010/07/03/prophylactic-hpv-vaccines-current-knowledge-of-impact-on-gynecologic-premalignancies/.
29. Ibid.
30. Ibid.; *see also* Tomljenovic and Shaw "Too Fast or Not Too Fast: The FDA's Approval of Merck's HPV Vaccine Gardasil," note 26 above, at 677.
31. Harper and Williams, "Prophylactic HPV Vaccines: Current Knowledge of Impact of Gynecologic Premalignancies," note 28 above.
32. "Cancer Stat Facts: Cervical Cancer," NCI, https://seer.cancer.gov/statfacts/html/cervix.html.

CHAPTER 7

1. J. F. Holland, "Ethical Issues in Randomized Clinical Trials," on file with authors.
2. "Glossary," US Department of Health and Human Services, https://www.vaccines.gov/resources/glossary/; A. Rid, *et al,* "Placebo Use in Vaccine Trials: Recommendations of a WHO Expert Panel," *Vaccine*, 32(37):4708–4712, at 4709, 4711, 2014.

3. Rid, "Placebo Use in Vaccine Trials: Recommendations of a WHO Expert Panel," note 2 above, at 4709; "Regulatory Perspective on Development of Preventive Vaccines for Global Infectious Diseases," FDA, www.fda.gov/downloads /BiologicsBloodVaccines/InternationalActivities/UCM273207.pdf; "Regulatory Perspective Development of Preventive Vaccines for Global Infectious Diseases," FDA video, http://fda.yorkcast.com/webcast/Play /b2825adab5254dc5bbc901dc5a0551541d.

4. "Expert Consultation on the Use of Placebos in Vaccine Trials," WHO, at 13, 2013, http://apps.who.int/iris/bitstream/handle/10665/94056/9789241506250 _eng.pdf?sequence=1.

5. Ibid.

6. Transcript of FDA Center For Biologics Evaluation And Research VRBPAC Meeting, May 18, 2006, at 93 (Dr. Nancy Miller), archived at https://wayback .archive-it.org/7993/20170404052136/https://www.fda.gov/ohrms/dockets /ac/06/transcripts/2006-4222t1.pdf.

7. N. B. Miller, "Clinical Review of Biologics License Application for Human Papillomavirus 6, 11, 16, 18 L1 Virus Like Particle Vaccine (S. cerevisiae) (STN 125126 GARDASIL), manufactured by Merck, Inc.," at 330, June 8, 2006, archived at http://wayback .archive-it.org/7993/20161024002027/http://www .fda.gov/downloads /BiologicsBloodVaccines/Vaccines/ApprovedProducts /UCM111287.pdf.

8. Miller, "Clinical Review of Biologics License Application for Human Papillomavirus 6, 11, 16, 18 L1 Virus Like Particle Vaccine (*S. cerevisiae*) (STN 125126 GARDASIL), manufactured by Merck, Inc.," note 7 above, at 301 (Table 210).

9. K. S. Reisinger, *et al.*, "Safety and Persistent Immunogenicity of a Quadrivalent Human Papillomavirus Types 6, 11, 16, 18 L1 Virus-Like Particle Vaccine in Preadolescents and Adolescents: A Randomized Controlled Trial," *Pediatric Infectious Disease Journal*, 26(3):201–209, at 202, March 2007.

10. Gardasil Package Insert, at 12 (Sec. 11), https://www.fda.gov/downloads/biologics bloodvacines/vaccines/approvedproducts/ucm111263.pdf.

11. "Food Additive Status List," FDA, www.fda.gov/food/ingredientspackaginglabeling/foodadditivesingredients/ucm091048.htm#ftnB.

12. *See* Chapter 21.

13. A copy of the letter from Australia's TGA to Dr. Little is in the authors' files.

14. "Product Information: Gardasil," www.seqirus.com.au/docs/392/563/Gardasil %20PI%20A160204,0.pdf.

15. Each 1-mL adult dose of Havrix contains 1440 EL.U. of viral antigen, adsorbed on 0.5 mg of aluminum as aluminum hydroxide and each 0.5-mL pediatric dose of vaccine contains 720 EL.U. of viral antigen, adsorbed onto 0.25 mg of aluminum as aluminum hydroxide. Havrix package insert at 9 (Sec. 11), www .fda.gov/downloads/BiologicsBloodVaccines/Vaccines/ApprovedProducts

4

/UCM224555.pdf. In contrast, the formulations of Havrix used in the Cervarix clinical trials were 720 EL.U. of viral antigen, adsorbed onto 0.5 mg of aluminum as aluminum hydroxide and 360 EL.U. of viral antigen, adsorbed onto 0.25 mg of aluminum as aluminum hydroxide. Cervarix package insert, at 5 (Table 1), www.fda.gov/downloads/BiologicsBloodVaccines/Vaccines/ApprovedProducts/UCM240436.pdf. *See also* N. B. Miller and J. Roberts, "Clinical Review of Biologics License Application for Human Papillomavirus 16, 18 L1 Virus Like Particle Vaccine, AS04 Adjuvant-Adsorbed (Cervarix)," at 159, October 15, 2009, https://www.fda.gov/downloads/biologicsbloodvaccines/vaccines/approvedproducts/ucm237976.pdf; C. Exley, "The Safety of Cervarix? (correspondence)," *Lancet*, 17:19–20, January 2017.

16. L. Yan, "FDA Statistical Review of Gardasil 9," at 59–60, December 10, 2014, www.fda.gov/downloads/BiologicsBloodVaccines/Vaccines/ApprovedProducts/UCM428669.pdf.

17. *See* Exley, "The Safety of Cervarix? (correspondence)," see note 15; *see also* Chapter 20.

18. C. Exley, "Aluminium-Based Adjuvants Should Not Be Used as Placebos in Clinical Trials," *Vaccine*, 29:9829, 2011.

19. *See* Chapter 20, generally.

20. 21 C.F.R. § 610.15(a).

21. A copy of the authors' correspondence with the FDA is in the authors' files.

22 L. Tomljenovic and C. A. Shaw, "Answers to Common Misconceptions Regarding the Toxicity of Aluminum Adjuvants in Vaccines," in *Vaccines & Autoimmunity*, (Y. Shoenfeld, N. Agmon-Levin & L. Tomljenovic, eds.), (Wiley Blackwell 2015) 43–55 at 43, 44.

23. *See* note 21 above.

24. Reisinger, "Safety and Persistent Immunogenicity of a Quadrivalent Human Papillomavirus Types 6, 11, 16, 18 L1 Virus-Like Particle Vaccine in Preadolescents and Adolescents: A Randomized Controlled Trial," note 9 above, at 202.

25. S. M. Garland, *et al.*, "Safety and Immunogenicity of a 9-Valent HPV Vaccine in Females 12–26 Years of Age Who Previously Received the Quadrivalent HPV Vaccine," *Vaccine*, 33(48):6855–6864, November 27, 2015.

26. Gardasil package insert, note 10 above, at 6 (Sec. 6.1,Table 5).

27. Miller, "Clinical Review of Biologics License Application for Human Papillomavirus 6, 11, 16, 18 L1 Virus Like Particle Vaccine (*S. cerevisiae*) (STN 125126 GARDASIL), manufactured by Merck, Inc.," note 7 above, at 316 (Table 229). In Protocol 018, there were five serious adverse events recorded in days 1–15 of the trial in the group of children who received Gardasil and none in the carrier solution group and overall there was a 15.5% risk difference between vaccinated and carrier solution children with the vaccinated children reporting overall more adverse events in the first 15 days of the trial. Ibid., at 316–317 (Tables 229, 230, and 231).

28. Ibid., 316 (Table 229).
29. Ibid., 377 (Table 295).
30. Ibid., 316 (Table 229).
31. Ibid., 377 (Table 295).
32. Ibid., 316 (Table 229).

Chapter 8

1. NB Miller, "Clinical Review of Biologics License Application for Human Papillomavirus 6, 11, 16, 18 L1 Virus Like Particle Vaccine (S. cerevisiae) (STN 125126 GARDASIL), manufactured by Merck, Inc.," at 301 (Table 210), June 8, 2006, archived at http://wayback.archive-it.org/7993/20161024002027 /http://www.fda.gov/downloads/BiologicsBloodVaccines/Vaccines /ApprovedProducts/UCM111287.pdf.
2. Ibid.
3. Ibid.
4. Ibid., 50 (Table 26).
5. *See, e.g.,* Ibid., 44–45, 203–205.
6. *See, e.g.,* Ibid., 301 (Table 210).
7. Ibid., 301 (Table 210).
8. Ibid., 277 (Table 188) (Protocol 016 at Month 7), 312 (Table 221) (Protocol 018 at Month 7).
9. *See, e.g.,* Ibid., 117 (Table 76), 179 (Table 122), 277 (Table 188), 312 (Table 221).
10. Ibid., 293 (indicating FDA had data).
11. Ibid., 329 (Table 245) and 393 (Table 302).
12. Ibid., 329 (Table 245).
13. Ibid., 393 (Table 302).
14. K. S. Reisinger, *et al.,* "Safety and Persistent Immunogenicity of a Quadrivalent Human Papillomavirus Types 6, 11, 16, 18 L1 Virus-Like Particle Vaccine in Preadolescents and Adolescents: A Randomized Controlled Trial," *Pediatric Infectious Disease Journal,* 26(3):201–209, March 2007; Ferris D, *et al.,* "Long-Term Study of a Quadrivalent Human Papillomavirus Vaccine," *Pediatrics,* 134(3):e657-e665, at e659 and e664, September 2014, http://pediatrics.aap-publications.org/content/pediatrics/early/2014/08/12/peds.2013-4144. full.pdf; D. Ferris, *et al.,* "4-Valent Human Papillomavirus (4vHPV) Vaccine in Preadolescents and Adolescents After 10 Years," *Pediatrics,* 140(6):1–9, at 8, November 2017, e20163947; DOI: 10.1542/peds.2016-3947, http://pediat-rics.aappublications.org/content/early/2017/11/20/peds.2016-3947.info.
15. Reisinger, *et al.,* "Safety and Persistent Immunogenicity of a Quadrivalent Human Papillomavirus Types 6, 11, 16, 18 L1 Virus-Like Particle Vaccine in Preadolescents and Adolescents: A Randomized Controlled Trial," note 14 above.

16. *See, e.g.,* Bradley Schlegel, "Merck & Co. employees honored for Gardasil creation, *The Times Herald*, April 23, 2009, http://www.timesherald.com/article/JR/20090423/NEWS01/304239982; Sino-American Pharmaceutical Professionals Assoc. – Greater Philadelphia, Dr. Eliav Barr biography, https://sapa-gp.org/sapagp/eliav-barr-md-vice-president-infectious-diseases-therapeutic-area-head-global-clinical-development-merck-co-inc/.

17. *See, e.g.,* Transcript of FDA Center For Biologics Evaluation And Research VRBPAC Meeting, May 18, 2006, at 11, 16–74, archived at https://wayback.archive-it.org/7993/20170404052136/https://www.fda.gov/ohrms/dockets/ac/06/transcripts/2006-4222t1.pdf.

18. Ferris, *et al.,* "4-Valent Human Papillomavirus (4vHPV) Vaccine in Preadolescents and Adolescents After 10 Years," note 14 above, at 8.

19. Copies of documents are maintained in the authors' files.

CHAPTER 9

1. "Gardasil™ HPV Quadrivalent Vaccine May 18, 2006 VRBPAC Meeting," VRBPAC Background Document, at 13 (Table 17, Study 013), archived at http://wayback.archive-it.org/7993/20180126170205/https://www.fda.gov/ohrms/dockets/ac/06/briefing/2006-4222B3.pdf.

2. Ibid.

3. Ibid., 14 (Table 19, Study 013).

4. Ibid.

5. "Gardasil™ HPV Quadrivalent Vaccine May 18, 2006 VRBPAC Meeting," VRBPAC Background Document, note 1 above, at 14, 15; N. B. Miller, "Clinical Review of Biologics License Application for Human Papillomavirus 6, 11, 16, 18 L1 Virus Like Particle Vaccine (S. *cerevisiae*) (STN 125126 GARDASIL), manufactured by Merck, Inc.," at 15, June 8, 2006, archived at http://wayback .archive-it.org/7993/20161024002027/http://www.fda.gov/downloads/BiologicsBlood Vaccines/Vaccines/ApprovedProducts/UCM111287.pdf.

6. N. B. Miller and J. Roberts, "Clinical Review of Biologics License Application for Human Papillomavirus 16, 18 L1 Virus Like Particle Vaccine, AS04 Adjuvant-Adsorbed (Cervarix)," at 218 (Table 136), October 15, 2009, https://www.fda.gov/downloads/biologicsbloodvaccines/vaccines/approvedproducts/ucm237976.pdf.

7. Ibid.

8. *See* "Study to Evaluate the Efficacy of the Human Papillomavirus Vaccine in Healthy Adult Women of 26 Years of Age and Older, Serious Adverse Events," https://clinicaltrials.gov/ct2/show/results/NCT00294047?sect=X30156&view=results#evnt; *see also* L. Jørgensen, *et al.,* "The Cochrane HPV vaccine review was incomplete and ignored important evidence of bias," *BMJ Evidence-Based Medicine,* July 27, 2018, https://ebm.bmj.com/content/early/2018/07/27/bmjebm-2018-111012.

9. "Committee Opinion" on Human Papillomavirus Vaccination, The American College of Obstetricians and Gynecologists (ACOG) Committee on Adolescent Health Care Immunization Expert Work Group, Number 704, June 2017, https://www.acog.org/-/media/Committee-Opinions/Committee-on-Adolescent-Health-Care/co704.pdf?dmc=1&ts=20170328T0157298695.

10. "FDA Grants Priority Review to Merck's Supplemental Biologics License Application (sBLA) for GARDASIL® 9 in Women and Men Ages 27 to 45 for the Prevention of Certain HPV-Related Cancers and Diseases," Merck, June 13, 2018, http://investors.merck.com/news/press-release-details/2018/FDA-Grants-Priority-Review-to-Mercks-Supplemental-Biologics-License-Application-sBLA-for-GARDASIL9-in-Women-and-Men-Ages-27-to-45-for-the-Prevention-of-Certain-HPV-Related-Cancers-and-Diseases/default.aspx.

CHAPTER 10

1. N. B. Miller, "Clinical Review of Biologics License Application for Human Papillomavirus 6, 11, 16, 18 L1 Virus Like Particle Vaccine (S. cerevisiae) (STN 125126 GARDASIL), manufactured by Merck, Inc.," at 195 (Table 132), June 8, 2006, archived at http://wayback.archive-it.org/7993/20161024002027/http://www.fda.gov/downloads/BiologicsBloodVaccines/Vaccines/ApprovedProducts/UCM111287.pdf.

2. Ibid., 105 (Table 73).

3. "Miscarriage: Signs, Symptoms, Treatment, and Prevention," American Pregnancy Association, http://americanpregnancy.org/pregnancy-complications/miscarriage/ (15% of women under 35 suffer miscarriage).

4. A.-M. Nybo Andersen, *et al.*, "Maternal age and fetal loss: population based register linkage study," *BMJ*, 320:1708–1712, June 24, 2000, https://www.ncbi.nlm.nih.gov/pmc/articles/PMC27416/pdf/1708.pdf.

5. Gardasil 9 package insert, at 10 (Sec. 5.1), https://www.fda.gov/downloads/BiologicsBloodVaccines/Vaccines/ApprovedProducts/UCM426457.pdf.

6. *See* Nybo Andersen, *et al.*, "Maternal age and fetal loss: population based register linkage study," for Danish background rate, note 4 above; "Miscarriage: Signs, Symptoms, Treatment, and Prevention," American Pregnancy Assoc., for US background rate, note 3 above; Miller, "Clinical Review of Biologics License Application for Human Papillomavirus 6, 11, 16, 18 L1 Virus Like Particle Vaccine (*S. cerevisiae*) (STN 125126 GARDASIL), manufactured by Merck, Inc.," note 1 above, at 14; Gardasil 9 package insert, note 5 above, at 10 (Sec. 8.1).

7. N.B. Miller and J. Roberts, "Clinical Review of Biologics License Application for Human Papillomavirus 16, 18 L1 Virus Like Particle Vaccine, AS04 Adjuvant-Adsorbed (Cervarix)," at 14, October 15, 2009, https://www.fda.gov/downloads/biologicsbloodvaccines/vaccines/approvedproducts/ucm237976.pdf.

8. Ibid.

9. S. Wacholder, *et al.*, "Risk of miscarriage with bivalent vaccine against human papillomavirus (HPV) types 16 and 18: pooled analysis of two randomised controlled trials," *BMJ Open*, March 2, 2010, at Table 3, https://www.ncbi.nlm.nih.gov/pmc/articles/PMC2831171/?report=printable.

10. Ibid.

11. L. Yan, "FDA Statistical Review of Gardasil 9," at 44 (Table 24), December 10, 2014, www.fda.gov/downloads/BiologicsBloodVaccines/Vaccines/ApprovedProducts/UCM428669.pdf.

12. Ibid.

13. Ibid., 88.

14. Ibid.

15. EMA Gardasil 9 DRAFT CHMP day 120 list of questions, at 46, https://www.scribd.com/document/367386167/Draft-Day-120-LoQ-Gardasil-9-Bortredigerad?secret_password=jl2zc1pWv03T02ddeLmi.

16. Gardasil 9 Rapporteurs' Day 150 Joint Response Assessment Report, at "Question 70" in SCRIBD Slate: https://www.scribd.com/document/367386169/Day-150-JRAR-Clinical-Bortredigerad?secret_password=xeOaPPIdg5yEMz4SK7x0.

17. EMA Gardasil 9 assessment at 113, http://www.ema.europa.eu/docs/en_GB/document_library/EPAR_-_Public_assessment_report/human/003852/WC500189113.pdf.

18. "Gardasil™ HPV Quadrivalent Vaccine May 18, 2006 VRBPAC Meeting," VRBPAC Background Document, at 24, archived at http://wayback.archive-it.org/7993/20180126170205/https://www.fda.gov/ohrms/dockets/ac/06/briefing/2006-4222B3.pdf.

19. Ibid., 25.

20. Ibid., 24 (Table 35).

21. Gardasil 9 package insert, note 5 above, at 10 (Sec. 8.1).

22. Gardasil package insert, Canada, at 60, https://www.merck.ca/static/pdf/GARDASIL-CI_E.pdf.

23. D. T. Little and H. R. Ward, "Adolescent Premature Ovarian Insufficiency Following Human Papillomavirus Vaccination: A Case Series Seen in General Practice," *Journal of Investigative Medicine High Impact Case Reports*, Oct.-Dec. 2014:1–12, https://www.ncbi.nlm.nih.gov/pmc/articles/PMC4528880/pdf/10.1177_2324709614556129.pdf.

24. Ibid.

25. Ibid.

26. D. T. Little and H. R. Ward, "Premature ovarian failure 3 years after menarche in a 16-year-old girl following human papillomavirus vaccination," *BMJ Case Reports*, September 30, 2012, https://www.ncbi.nlm.nih.gov/pmc/articles/PMC4543769/pdf/bcr-2012-006879.pdf.

27. Little and Ward, "Adolescent Premature Ovarian Insufficiency Following Human Papillomavirus Vaccination: A Case Series Seen in General Practice," note 23 above.

28. B. Komorowska, "Autoimmune Primary Ovarian Failure," *Przeglad Menopauzalny*, 15(4), February 8, 2017, https://www.ncbi.nlm.nih.gov/pmc/articles/PMC5327623/.

29. S. Colafrancesco, *et al.*, "Human papilloma virus vaccine and primary ovarian failure: another facet of the autoimmune/inflammatory syndrome induced by adjuvants," *American Journal of Reproductive Immunology*, 70(4):309–16, October 2013, https://www.ncbi.nlm.nih.gov/pubmed/23902317.

30. J. Pederson, "Primary ovarian insufficiency in adolescents: a case series," *International Journal of Pediatric Endocrinology*, 2015(1):13, March 6, 2015, https://ijpeonline.biomedcentral.com/articles/10.1186/s13633-015-0009-z.

31. "The Vaccine Adverse Event Reporting System (VAERS)," CDC Wonder, https://wonder.cdc.gov/vaers.html.

32. "New Concerns About the Human Papillomavirus Vaccine," American College of Pediatricians, January 2016, https://www.acpeds.org/the-college-speaks /position-statements/health-issues/new-concerns-about-the-human-papillomavirus -vaccine.

33. "Safety Update of HPV Vaccines," WHO, July 2017, http://www.who.int/ vaccine_safety/committee/topics/hpv/June_2017/en/.

34. G. DeLong, "A lowered probability of pregnancy in females in the USA aged 25– 29 who received a human papillomavirus vaccine injection," *Journal of Toxicology and Environmental Health Part A*, 81(14):661–674, 2018, https://www.tandfonline .com/doi/full/10.1080/15287394.2018.1477640.

35. "Statistical Bulletin: Conception in England and Wales: 2016," Office of National Statistics (ONS), https://www.ons.gov.uk/peoplepopulationandcom-munity/birthsdeathsandmarriages/conceptionandfertilityrates/bulletins/ conceptionstatistics/2016.

36. Katie Forster, "Teenage Pregnancy Rates Hit All-Time Low After Nearly Halving In Last Eight Years," *The Independent*, March 22, 2017, http://www .independent.co.uk/life-style/health-and-families/health-news/teenage-pregnancy -rates-record-low-england-wales-fall-halve-last-seven-years-a7643416.html.

37. "Statistical Bulletin: Conception in England and Wales: 2016," note 35 above.

38. Ibid.

39. "Publication Report: Teenage Pregnancy, Year of Conception Ending 31 December 2015," National Services Scotland, Information Services Division, at 4 (Chart 1), July 4, 2017, http://www.isdscotland.org/Health-Topics/Sexual-Health/Publications/2017-07-04/2017-07-04-TeenPreg-Report.pdf.

40. "Statistical Bulletin: Conception in England and Wales: 2016," note 35 above.

41. B. E. Hamilton and T. J. Mathews, "Continued Declines in Teen Births in the United States, 2015," *NCHS Data Brief*, No. 259, September 2016, https://www .cdc.gov/nchs/products/databriefs/db259.htm.

42. B. E. Hamilton, *et al.*, "Births: Provisional Data for 2016," *Vital Statistics Rapid Release*, Report No. 002, June 2017, https://www.cdc.gov/nchs/data/vsrr/report 002.pdf.

43. Susan Scutti, "U.S. teen birth rate drops to all-time low," CNN, June 30, 2017, https://www.cnn.com/2017/06/30/health/teen-birth-rate-prenatal-care-2016 /index.html.

44. Hamilton and Mathews, "Continued Declines in Teen Births in the United States, 2015," note 41 above, at 1.

CHAPTER 11

1. V501 Protocol/Amendment No: 015–00, at 7, https://www.scribd.com /document/367386168/V501-015-00-PRO-VD?secret_password=j4BXCUs76g 4wRtDxk5cy.

2. Ibid., 81–86.

3. Ibid., 86.

4. Frederik Joelving, "What the Gardasil Testing May Have Missed," *Slate*, December 17, 2017, https://slate.com/health-and-science/2017/12/flaws-in-the-clinical-trials-for-gardasil-made-it-harder-to-properly-assess-safety.html.

5. V501 Protocol/Amendment No: 015–00, note 1 above, at 104.

6. Ibid., 9, 104.

7. A. Corneli, *et al.*, "One and Done: Reasons Principal Investigators Conduct Only One FDA-Regulated Drug Trial," *Contemporary Clinical Trials Communications*, 6:31–38, 2017.

8. Joelving, "What the Gardasil Testing May Have Missed," note 4 above.

9. S. M. Garland, "Quadrivalent Vaccine against Human Papillomavirus to Prevent Anogenital Diseases," *NEJM*, 356:1928–1943, May 10, 2007, http://www .nejm.org/doi/full/10.1056/NEJMoa061760.

10. EMA scientific discussion, Gardasil, 2006, http://www.ema.europa.eu/docs /en_GB/document_library/EPAR_-_Scientific_Discussion/human/000703 /WC500021140.pdf.

11. N. B. Miller, "Clinical Review of Biologics License Application for Human Papillomavirus 6, 11, 16, 18 L1 Virus Like Particle Vaccine (*S. cerevisiae*) (STN 125126 GARDASIL), manufactured by Merck, Inc.," at 393–94 (Tables 302 & 303), June 8, 2006, archived at http://wayback.archive-it.org/7993/20161024002027 /http://www.fda.gov/downloads/BiologicsBloodVaccines/Vaccines /ApprovedProducts/UCM111287.pdf.

12. Ibid., 395–96 (Table 302).

13. Ibid., 395–96 (Table 303).

14. Ibid.

15. Ibid., 329 (Table 245).

16. Gardasil package insert, at 8 (Sec. 6.1): https://www.fda.gov/downloads/biologics bloodvaccines/vaccines/approvedproducts/ucm111263.pdf.

17. Ibid.

18. "NMCs one of EMA's major objections to approval" at 7: *EMA Assessment July 2014 Gardasil 9 "not approvable,"* www.scribd.com/document/367386167/Draft-Day-120-LoQ-Gardasil-9-Bortredigerad?secret_password=jl2zc1pWv03T02ddeLmi.

19. Gardasil 9 Rapporteurs' Day 150 Joint Response Assessment Report at "Question 68 Conclusion" in SCRIBD Slate, https://www.scribd.com/document/367386169/Day-150-JRAR-Clinical-Bortredigerad?secret_password=xeOaPPIdg5yEMz4SK7x0.
20. Ibid., "Question 61 Conclusion."
21. Ibid., "Question 68."
22. Ibid.
23. Ibid.
24. Ibid.
25. EMA final assessment report for public, no mention of NMCs: www.ema.europa.eu/docs/en_GB/document_library/EPAR_-_Public_assessment_report/human/003852/WC500189113.pdf.
26. EMA note 19 above, "Question 69."
27. Joelving, "What the Gardasil Testing May Have Missed," note 4 above.
28. EMA, note 19 above, "Question 69."
29. Ibid., "Question 67."
30. EMA final assessment report for public, note 25 above.
31. Miller, "Clinical Review of Biologics License Application for Human Papillomavirus 6, 11, 16, 18 L1 Virus Like Particle Vaccine (*S. cerevisiae*) (STN 125126 GARDASIL), manufactured by Merck, Inc.," note 11 above, at 379 (Table 297).
32. Ibid.
33. S. Yang, *et al.*, "Gardasil 9 Statistical Review," at 40 (Sec. 6.1.12.3), https://www.fda.gov/downloads/BiologicsBloodVaccines/Vaccines/ApprovedProducts/UCM428669.pdf.
34. K. D. Kochanek, *et al.*, "Deaths: Final Data 2002," *National Vital Statistics Report*, 53(5):1–116, at 24, October 12, 2004 (Table 5), https://www.cdc.gov/nchs/data/nvsr/nvsr53/nvsr53_05.pdf.
35. Miller, "Clinical Review of Biologics License Application for Human Papillomavirus 6, 11, 16, 18 L1 Virus Like Particle Vaccine (*S. cerevisiae*) (STN 125126 GARDASIL), manufactured by Merck, Inc.," note 11 above, at 379 (Table 297).
36. Ibid.
37. Miller, "Clinical Review of Biologics License Application for Human Papillomavirus 6, 11, 16, 18 L1 Virus Like Particle Vaccine (*S. cerevisiae*) (STN 125126/419 GARDASIL) to extend indication for prevention of vaginal and vulva cancers..." at 77–78 (Table 43), September 11, 2008: https://www.fda.gov/downloads/Biologicsbloodvaccines/vaccines/approvedproducts/UCM111274.pdf
38. Kochanek, *et al.*, "Deaths: Final Data 2002," note 34 above.
39. Miller, "Clinical Review of Biologics License Application for Human Papillomavirus 6, 11, 16, 18 L1 Virus Like Particle Vaccine (*S. cerevisiae*) (STN

125126 GARDASIL), manufactured by Merck, Inc.," note 11 above, at 379 (Table 297).

40. "Cancer Stat Facts: Cervical Cancer," NCI, https://seer.cancer.gov/statfacts /html/cervix.html.
41. J. N. Roberts, "Clinical Review of Biologics License Application Supplement STN# 125126/773 – mid-adult women indication for GARDASIL" at 34 (Sec. 8.1.8.6.5), archived at: http://wayback.archive-it.org/7993/20170722145326 /https://www.fda.gov/downloads/BiologicsBloodVaccines/Vaccines/Approved Products/UCM251763.pdf.
42. Ibid., 18.
43. "Statistical Review and Evaluation," (Protocol 020), FDA, at 5: https://www.fda .gov/downloads/BiologicsBloodVaccines/Vaccines/ApprovedProducts /UCM190978.pdf.
44. Ibid.
45. Gardasil package insert, at 7 (Sec. 6.1), https://www.fda.gov/downloads/biologics bloodvaccines/vaccines/approvedproducts/ucm111263.pdf
46. Ibid. and Miller, "Clinical Review of Biologics License Application for Human Papillomavirus 6, 11, 16, 18 L1 Virus Like Particle Vaccine (*S. cerevisiae*) (STN 125126 GARDASIL), manufactured by Merck, Inc.," note 11 above, at 379 (Table 297).
47. Gardasil 9 Package Insert, at 8 (Sec. 6.1): https://www.fda.gov/downloads/ BiologicsBloodVaccines/Vaccines/ApprovedProducts/UCM426457.pdf.

CHAPTER 12

1. S. Gupta, *et al.*, "Is human papillomavirus vaccination likely to be a useful strategy in India?" *South Asian Journal of Cancer,* 2(4):193–97, at 194, October-December 2014, http://www.ncbi.nlm.nih.gov/pmc/articles/PMC3889025/.
2. S. LaMontagne, *et al.*, "Human papillomavirus vaccine delivery strategies that achieved high coverage in low- and middle-income countries," Article ID: BLT.11.089862, September 1, 2011, http://www.who.int/bulletin/online_first /11-089862.pdf.
3. "72nd Report on the *Alleged Irregularities in the Conduct of Studies Using Human Papilloma Virus (HPV) Vaccine by Programme for Appropriate Technology in Health (PATH) in India,*" at paragraph 1.11, August 2013, http://164.100.47.5/new-committee/reports/EnglishCommittees/Committee%20on%20Health%20 and%20Family%20Welfare/72.pdf.
4. Ibid., generally.
5. Ibid., para 1.12 and 3.4.
6. Ibid., para 2.1.
7. Ibid., para 1.1.
8. Ibid., para 2.5.
9. Ibid.

10. Ibid., para 3.18 and 6.10.

11. Ibid., para 6.11.

12. Ibid., para 6.16.

13. Anand Rai, *et al.*, "*Fact Finding into HPV Vaccine Trial in Indore, M.P. India*," at 27–30, June 25, 2014. Submitted before the Hon'ble Supreme Court of India via an affidavit as an addendum in combined W.P. (C) No. 33/2012, 91/2004 and 79/2012, http://sanevax.org/wp-content/uploads/2014/07/Additional-Affidavit-on-V-503.doc.

14. Ibid.

15. Ibid.

16. Ibid.

17. 72nd Report, note 3 above, para 6.19.

18. Ibid.

19. Ibid., para 6.26.

20. Ibid., para 6.37.

21. Ibid., para 7.12, 7.13.

22. Ibid., para 7.13.

23. "*Supreme Court admits writ petition against licensing and trials with 'cervical cancer' vaccine implicating the Drugs Controller of India, PATH, ICMR and others ordering Government of India to immediately respond,*" Human Rights Law Network, January 7, 2013, http://www.hrln.org/hrln/peoples-health-rights/pils-a-cases /1171-supreme-court-admits-writ-petition-against-licensing-and-trials-with-cervical -cancer-vaccines-implicating-the-drugs-controller-of-india-path-icmr-and-others- ordering-government-of-india-to-; complaint available at http://www.hrln.org /hrln/images/stories/pdf/HRLN-HPV-SYNOP.pdf.

24. Christina England, "Serious Allegations Against HPV Vaccine Trials Affecting Thousands of Girls Accepted by Supreme Court of India," *Vactruth.com*, January 8, 2013, https://vactruth.com/2013/01/08/vaccine-trials-supreme-court/.

25. Ibid.

26. I. Mattheij, *et al.*, "Do cervical cancer data justify HPV vaccination in India? Epidemiological data sources and comprehensiveness," *JRSM*, 105: 250–262, 2012, http://jrs.sagepub.com/content/105/6/250.full. Royal Society of Medicine, 2012, "Controversial vaccine trial should never have been run in India, researchers say," press release at https://www.rsm.ac.uk/about-us /media-information/2012-media-releases/controversial-vaccine-trial-should- never-have-been-run-in-india,-researchers-say.aspx.

27. Royal Society of Medicine, "Controversial vaccine trial should never have been run in India, researchers say," note 26 above.

28. Gupta, "Is human papillomavirus vaccination likely to be a useful strategy in India?" note 1 above.

29. Royal Society of Medicine, "Controversial vaccine trial should never have been run in India, researchers say," note 26 above.

30. Mattheij, "Do cervical cancer data justify HPV vaccination in India? Epidemiological data sources and comprehensiveness," note 26 above.

31. Ibid. Royal Society of Medicine, "Controversial vaccine trial should never have been run in India, researchers say." note 26 above.

32. Gupta, "Is human papillomavirus vaccination likely to be a useful strategy in India?" note 1 above.

33. Ibid.

34. Ibid.

35. Ibid.

36. Ibid.

37. Ibid.

38. Ibid., 196.

39. P. Chatterjee, "India tightens regulation of clinical trials to safeguard participants," *BMJ*, 346:f1275, 2013, http://www.bmj.com/content/346/bmj.f1275 .long.

40. Pooja Agarwal, "Indian Supreme Court Demands Regulation of Clinical Trials," *Regulatory Review*, Oct. 23, 2013, https://www.theregreview.org /2013/10/24/24-agarwal-indian-trials/.

41. DGCI issues draft guidelines on audio-visual recording of informed consent process in clinical trial, Pharmabiz.com, January 15, 2014, http://www.pharm-abiz.com/NewsDetails.aspx?aid=79794&sid=1.

42. Chirag Shah and Param Dave, "Regulatory Approval in India: An Updated Review," *Applied Clinical Trials*, May 4, 2016, http://www.appliedclinicaltrial sonline.com/regulatory-approval-india-updated-review.

43. M. Feinberg, "HPV vaccine suspension in India," *Lancet*, 376:1644–65, Nov. 13, 2010, http://www.thelancet.com/journals/lancet/article/PIIS0140-6736(10) 62094-6/fulltext?elsca1=TL-121110&elsca2=email&elsca3=segment.

44. Ibid.

45. PATH, "Statement from PATH: cervical cancer demonstration project in India," updated Sept. 3, 2013, https://path.org/media-center/statement-from -path-cervical-cancer-demonstration-project-in-india/

46. Ibid.

47. Ibid.

48. Ibid.

49. GAVI, "GAVI's historical relationship with the Indian government with regard to vaccine policy in India," http://www.gavi.org/library/news/press-releases /2016/historic-partnership-between-gavi-and-india-to-save-millions-of-lives/; Gavi Board Members: https://www.gavi.org/about/governance/gavi-board /members/#.

50. Nida Najar, "India's Ban on Foreign Money for Health Group Hits Gates Foundation," *New York Times*, April 20, 2017, https://www.nytimes.com /2017/04/20/world/asia/india-health-nonprofit-gates-foundation.html?_r=0.

51. *See* Tabassum Barnagarwala, "Why the Vaccine against Cervical Cancer Is Not Such a Simple Shot," *Indian Express*, January 10, 2018 http://indianexpress .com/article/explained/why-the-vaccine-against-cervical-cancer-is-not-such-a-simple-shot-4980018/.

CHAPTER 13

1. Merck 2017 Annual Report 10-K at 40, http://d18rn0p25nwr6d.cloudfront .net/CIK-0000310158/357ac382-9a56-4879-bce6-6a4b7fb87e58.pdf.
2. GSK 2017 annual report, at 47, https://www.gsk.com/media/4629/fy-2017-results -announcement.pdf.
3. WHO, "Safety Update of HPV Vaccines," July 14, 2017, http://www.who.int/ vaccine_safety/committee/topics/hpv/June_2017/en/.
4. Merck 2017 10-K, note 1 above, at 20.
5. GSK 2017 annual report, note 2 above, at 9.
6. Merck is listed 72nd based on the Fortune 500 ranking system. http://www .rankingthebrands.com/The-Brand-Rankings.aspx?rankingID=131&.
7. "Merck Sees Slightly Higher 2007 Earnings," *New York Times*, December 7, 2006, https://www.nytimes.com/2006/12/07/business/07drug.html
8. "Congress Questions Vioxx, FDA," *PBS NewsHour*, November 18, 2004, http: //archive.is/M6f1e.
9. P. Gøeetzsche, *Deadly Medicines and Organised Crime: How Big Pharma Has Corrupted Healthcare* (CRC Press; 1st ed., August 30, 2013), at 161–62.
10. Ibid., 155.
11. Ibid.
12. Ibid., 156.
13. Ibid., 157.
14. Ibid.
15. Alex Berenson, "Evidence in Vioxx Suits Shows Intervention by Merck Officials," *New York Times*, April 24, 2005, https://www.nytimes.com/2005/04/24/business /evidence-in-vioxx-suits-shows-intervention-by-merck-officials.html.
16. Ibid.
17. Gøtzsche, *Deadly Medicines and Organised Crime*, note 9 above, at 158.
18. Jim Edwards, "Merck Created Hit List to 'Destroy,' '"Neutralize' or 'Discredit' Dissenting Doctors," *CBS Moneywatch*, May 6, 2009, https://www.cbsnews.com /news/merck-created-hit-list-to-destroy-neutralize-or-discredit-dissenting -doctors/.
19. Gøtzsche, *Deadly Medicines and Organised Crime*, note 9 above, at 158.
20. Ibid.,158–59.
21. J. Lenzer, "FDA is Incapable of Protecting Us Against Another Vioxx," *BMJ*, 329(7477):1253, November 27, 2004, https://www.ncbi.nlm.nih.gov/pmc /articles/PMC534432/pdf/bmj32901253.pdf.
22. Ibid.

23. H. M. Krumholz, *et al.*, "What Have We Learnt From Vioxx?" *BMJ*, 334(7585): 120–123, at 120, January 29, 2007.

24. Ibid., 162.

25. Lenzer, note 21 above, 1253.

26. Ibid.

27. FDA Science and Mission at Risk: Report of the Subcommittee on Science and Technology, November 2007, archived at http://wayback.archive-it.org /7993/20180126164015/https://www.fda.gov/ohrms/dockets/ac/07/briefing /2007-4329b_02_01_FDA%20Report%20on%20Science%20and%20 Technology.pdf.

28. Alex Berenson, "Merck Agrees to Settle Vioxx Suits for $4.85 Billion," *New York Times*, November 9, 2007, http://www.nytimes.com/2007/11/09/business /09merck.html.

29. Ibid.

30. Department of Justice, Office of Public Affairs, 2012. "U.S. Pharmaceutical Company Merck Sharp & Dohme Sentenced in Connection with Unlawful Promotion of Vioxx," April 19, 2012, https://www.justice.gov/opa/pr/us-phar-maceutical-company-merck-sharp-dohme-sentenced-connection-unlawful-pro-motion-vioxx.

31. Ibid.

32. Ibid.

33. Gøtzsche, *Deadly Medicines and Organised Crime*, note 9 above, at 122.

34. Merck's senior leadership in its executive committee includes several individuals who have been with the corporation for more than a decade, including Kenneth C. Frazier, current Chairman of the Board and Chief Executive Officer who formerly served as general counsel, Sanat Chattopadhyay, Miriam M. Graddick-Weir, Roger M. Perlmutter, and Adam H. Schechter.

35. Carl Elliott, *White Coat, Black Hat: Adventures on the Dark Side of Medicine*, (Boston: Beacon Press, 2010), Chapter 5, n. 25.

36. Ibid., Ch. 5.

37. Ibid., Ch. 3.

38. "Direct to Consumer Advertising under Fire,"*Bulletin of the World Health Organization*, vol. 87, 2009, 565–644, http://www.who.int/bulletin/volumes /87/8/09-040809/en/.

39. American Medical Association, 2015. "AMA Calls for Ban on Direct to Consumer Advertising of Prescription Drugs and Medical Devices," http:// www.ama-assn.org/ama/pub/news/news/2015/2015-11-17-ban-consumer -prescription-drug-advertising.page.

40. Ibid.

41. Judith Siers-Poisson, "Research, Develop, and Sell, Sell, Sell: Part Two in a Series on the Politics and PR of Cervical Cancer," *Alternet.org*, July 16, 2007, http:// www.alternet.org/story/56677/research,_develop,_and_sell,_sell,_sell%3A _part_two_in_a_series_on_the_politics_and_pr_of_cervical_cancer.

42. Ibid.
43. CDC Vaccine Price List, https://www.cdc.gov/vaccines/programs/vfc/awardees/vaccine-management/price-list/index.html.
44. Ibid.
45. Carolina Fernandez Branson, "I Want to be One Less: The Rhetoric of Choice in Gardasil Ads," *The Communication Review*, 15:144–158, 2012.
46. Elisabeth Rosenthal, "Drug Makers' Push Leads to Cancer Vaccines' Rise," *New York Times*, August 19, 2008, http://www.nytimes.com/2008/08/20/health/policy/20vaccine.html?pagewanted=all.
47. S. Grantham, *et al.*, "Merck's One Less Campaign: Using RiskMessage Frames to Promote the Use of Gardasil in HPV Prevention," *Communication Research Reports*, 28(4):318–326, 2011.
48. Ibid.
49. "Adequate Provision," FDA, Drug Advertising Glossary, http://www.fda.gov/Drugs/ResourcesForYou/Consumers/PrescriptionDrugAdvertising/ucm072025.htm#brief_summary.
50. Rosenthal, "Drug Makers' Push Leads to Cancer Vaccines' Rise," note 46 above.
51. Edelman website, https://www.edelman.com/.
52. Beth Herskovits, "Brand of the Year," *PharmExec.com*, February 1, 2007, http://www.pharmexec.com/brand-year-0.
53. CDC, "Vaccines Included in the VFC Program," Resolution No. 6/06-1, effective June 29, 2006, https://www.cdc.gov/vaccines/programs/vfc/downloads/resolutions/0606-vaccines.pdf.
54. House of Representatives Committee on Government Reform Majority Staff Report, "Conflicts of Interest in Vaccine Policy Making," June 15, 2000, https://www.gpo.gov/fdsys/pkg/CHRG-106hhrg73042/html/CHRG-106hhrg73042.htm.
55. M. Holland and R. Krakow, "The Right to Legal Redress," chapter 5 in *Vaccine Epidemic* (Habakus and Holland, Eds.) (Pub. 2012).
56. N. F. Engstrom, "A Dose of Reality for Specialized Courts: Lessons from the VICP," 163 *University of Pennsylvania Law Review*, 1631, 1673 (2014).
57. Herskovits, "Brand of the Year," note 52 above.
58. Deborah Dick-Rath, "DDR on DTC: Merck's Gardasil,'" *Medical Marketing and Media*, March 15, 2009, http://www.mmm-online.com/pharmaceutical/ddr-on-dtc-mercks-gardasil/article/129890/.
59. S. M. Rothman and D. Rothman, "Marketing HPV Vaccine: Implications for Adolescent Health and Medical Professionalism," *JAMA*, 302(7):781–786, at 783, 2009, http://jama.jamanetwork.com/article.aspx?articleid=184429.
60. Ibid.
61. American Cancer Society, "FDA Approves Gardasil 9 HPV Vaccine," January 8, 2015, https://www.cancer.org/latest-news/fda-approves-gardasil-9-hpv-vaccine.html ("Gardasil 9 will protect against 90% of cervical cancers").

62. D. M. Harper, telephone interview with authors, April 9, 2015.

63. D. M. Harper, "Prophylactic HPV Vaccines: Current Knowledge of Impact on Gynecologic Premalignancies," *DiscoveryMedicine.com*, July 3, 2010, http://www.discoverymedicine.com/Diane-M-Harper/2010/07/03/prophylactic-hpv-vaccines-current-knowledge-of-impact-on-gynecologic-premalignancies/.

64. "Be One Less" slogan on Gardasil 9 website: https://www.gardasil9.com/about-gardasil9/what-is-gardasil9/.

65. D. M. Harper, *et al.*, "Cervical cancer incidence can increase despite HPV vaccination," *Lancet Infectious Disease*, 10(9):594–595, September 2010.

66. Melissa Haussman, *Reproductive Rights and the State* (Santa Barbara, CA: Praeger, 2013), at 145.

67. Gardasil package insert, at 13 (Sec.13.1): "GARDASIL has not been evaluated for the potential to cause carcinogenicity or genotoxicity." http://www.fda.gov/downloads/BiologicsBloodVaccines/Vaccines/ApprovedProducts/UCM111263.pdf.

68. "FDA approves HPV vaccine for males ages 16–26," *AAP News*, December 16, 2015, http://www.aappublications.org/news/2015/12/16/HPV121615.

69. Information about Gardasil 9, https://www.gardasil9.com/hpv-facts/related-cancer-diseases/.

70. Charlie Cooper and Gloria Nakajubi, "Professor Harald zur Hausen: Nobel scientist calls for HPV vaccination for boys," *Independent*, July 12, 2015, https://www.independent.co.uk/life-style/health-and-families/health-news/professor-harald-zur-hausen-nobel-scientist-calls-for-hpv-vaccination-for-boys-10382796.html.

71. Australia announced that Gardasil 9 will be in the school-based National HPV Vaccination Program from 2018, http://www.hpvvaccine.org.au/about-the-vaccine/vaccine-background.aspx. European Centre for Disease Prevention and Control, vaccine schedule page, http://vaccine-schedule.ecdc.europa.eu/Pages/Scheduler.aspx.

72. Vaccine European New Integrated Collaboration Effort (VENICE), Report on the health technology assessments on human papillomavirus and rotavirus vaccinations in Europe, September 2011, at 24, http://venice.cineca.org/Venice2_HTA_HPV_rota_Report_v9.pdf .

73. "Italy adopts gender-neutral HPV vaccination programme, citing study by health economics expert from Kingston Business School," Jan. 28, 2017, http://www.kingston.ac.uk/news/article/1785/28-jan-2017-italy-adopts-genderneutral-hpv-vaccination-programme-citing-study-by-health-economics-expert-from-kingston-business/.

74. Kimberly Leonard, "HPV Vaccine in Men Would Save Costs of Treating Throat Cancer," *U.S. News & World Report*, April 13, 2015, https://www.usnews.com/news/articles/2015/04/13/hpv-vaccine-in-men-would-save-costs-of-treating-throat-cancer.

75. "Throat cancer," Mayo Clinic, https://www.mayoclinic.org/diseases-conditions /throat-cancer/symptoms-causes/syc-20366462.

76. "Anal Cancer: Statistics," *Cancer.net*, https://www.cancer.net/cancer-types /anal-cancer/statistics.

77. FUTURE II Study Group, "Quadrivalent Vaccine against Human Papillomavirus to Prevent High-Grade Cervical Lesions," *NEJM*, May 10, 2007, https://www .nejm.org/doi/full/10.1056/NEJMoa061741. *See also* Jeanne Lenzer, "Should Boys Be Given the HPV Vaccine? The Science Is Weaker than the Marketing," November 14, 2011, http://blogs.discovermagazine.com/crux/2011/11/14 /should-boys-be-given-the-hpv-vaccine-the-science-is-weaker-than-the-marketing /#.WzaYXaknaqA.

78. Ibid.

79. Rosenthal, "Drug Makers' Push Leads to Cancer Vaccines' Rise," note 46 above.

80. HPV vaccine commercial Merck, https://www.youtube.com/watch?v=sLB0M aY7luE.

CHAPTER 14

1. Ellen Goodman, "A dose of reality on HPV vaccine," *Boston Globe*, March 2, 2007, http://archive.boston.com/news/globe/editorial_opinion/oped/articles/2007 /03/02/a_dose_of_reality_on_hpv_vaccine/.

2. R. Seither, *et al.*, "Vaccination Coverage Among Children in Kindergarten– United States, 2014–15 School Year," *Morbidity and Mortality Weekly Report*, 64(33); 897–904, August 28, 2015, http://www.cdc.gov/mmwr/preview /mmwrhtml/mm6433a2.htm.

3. "How much does the HPV vaccine cost?" American Cancer Society, https: //www.cancer.org/cancer/cancer-causes.html; https://www.cdc.gov/vaccines /programs/vfc/awardees/vaccine-management/price-list/.

4. "About ACIP Members," CDC, https://www.cdc.gov/vaccines/acip/about.html.

5. CDC, Record of the Meeting of the Advisory Committee on Immunization Practices, February 21–22, 2006, at 6, https://www.cdc.gov/vaccines/acip /meetings/downloads/min-archive/min-2006-02-508.pdf.

6. Ibid., 16.

7. Ibid., 32.

8. Ibid., 33.

9. CDC, Record of Proceedings Advisory Committee on Immunization Practices, June 29–30, 2006, at 19, 22, https://www.cdc.gov/vaccines/acip/meetings /downloads/min-archive/min-2006-06-508.pdf.

10. Ibid., 19.

11. Ibid., 20–21.

12. CDC, "FDA Licensure of Bivalent Human Papillomavirus Vaccine (HPV2, Cervarix) for Use in Females and Updated HPV Vaccination Recommendations

from the Advisory Committee on Immunization Practices," *Morbidity and Mortality Weekly Report*, 59(20):626–629, at 626, May 28, 2010, https://www.cdc.gov/mmwr/pdf/wk/mm5920.pdf ("In anticipation of FDA licensure of HPV2, ACIP reviewed data on the immunogenicity, efficacy, and safety of HPV2, as well as information on HPV4. At its October 21, 2009, meeting, ACIP approved updated recommendations for use of HPV vaccines in females.").

13. CDC, Summary Report of Advisory Committee on Immunization Practices Meeting, October 25–26, 2011, at 42, 50, https://www.cdc.gov/vaccines/acip/meetings/downloads/min-archive/min-oct11.pdf.

14. CDC, Summary Report of Advisory Committee on Immunization Practices Meeting, February 26, 2015, pages 54–56, https://www.cdc.gov/vaccines/acip/meetings/downloads/min-archive/min-2015-02.pdf.

15. HHS, Healthy People.gov, IID.11.4, https://www.healthypeople.gov/2020/topics-objectives/topic/immunization-and-infectious-diseases/objectives.

16. Ibid.

17. Ibid.

18. CDC, Summary Report of Advisory Committee on Immunization Practices Meeting, October 23–24, 2013, at 115, https://www.cdc.gov/vaccines/acip/meetings/downloads/min-archive/min-oct13.pdf.

19. Ibid., 113.

20. Ibid., 115.

21. Ibid., 119.

22. "CDC doctor opposes law for vaccine," *Washington Times*, Feb. 26, 2007, https://www.washingtontimes.com/news/2007/feb/26/20070226-115014-2031r/.

23. E. F. Fowler and S. E. Gollust, "The Content and Effect of Politicized Health Controversies," *ANNALS AAPSS*, 658(1):155–171, at 160, March 2015.

24. Ibid.

25. Adam Martin, "Vaccine Maker Gave Rick Perry $30,00 Plus a Whole Lot More," *The Wire*, Sept. 14, 2011 http://www.thewire.com/politics/2011/09/vaccine-maker-gave-rick-perry-30000-plus-whole-lot-more/42463/.

26. Texas Legislature Online Actions, http://www.legis.state.tx.us/BillLookup/Actions.aspx?LegSess=80R&Bill=HB1098 .

27. Andrew Pollack and Stephanie Saul, "Merck to Halt Lobbying for Vaccine for Girls," *New York Times*, Feb. 21, 2007, http://www.nytimes.com/2007/02/21/business/21merck.html?_r=0.

28. Ibid.

29. In Protocol 016, 506 girls ages 10–15 received a full dose of Gardasil. Some additional girls in this cohort were included in an end-expiry dosing study but did not receive vaccines with the 20/40/40/20 VLP ration (all received lower). In Protocol 018, 364 9–12 year-old girls received a vaccine and 199 9–12 year-old girls received a carrier solution control. *See* N. B. Miller, "Clinical Review of Biologics License Application for Human Papillomavirus

6, 11, 16, 18 L1 Virus Like Particle Vaccine (*S. cerevisiae*) (STN 125126 GARDASIL), manufactured by Merck, Inc.," at 274 (Table 184), 275 (Table 186), 301 (Table 210), 311 (Table 220), June 8, 2006, archived at http://wayback .archive-it.org/7993/20161024002027/http://www.fda.gov/downloads/ BiologicsBloodVaccines/Vaccines/ApprovedProducts/UCM111287.pdf.

30. R. A. Whidden and T. Tuscherer, "Good Parents Vaccinate: An Analysis of Merck's Gardasil Campaign," *Conference Proceedings–National Communication Association/American Forensic Association (Alta Conference on Argumentation)*, 761–767 at 760, 2007.

31. "Flogging Gardasil," *Nature Biotechnology*, 25(3):261 (2007).

32. G. McGee and S. Johnson, "Has the Spread of HPV Vaccine Marketing Conveyed Immunity to Common Sense?" *American Journal of Bioethics*, 7(7):1–2, 2007.

33. National Conference of State Legislators, http://leg1.state.va.us/cgi-bin/ legp504.exe?ses=071&typ=bil&val=sb1230.

34. Elisabeth Rosenthal, "Drug Makers' Push Leads to Cancer Vaccines' Rise," *New York Times*, August 19, 2008, http://www.nytimes.com/2008/08/20 /health/policy/20vaccine.html?pagewanted=all.

35. National Conference of State Legislators, http://www.ncsl.org/research/ health/hpv-vaccine-state-legislation-and-statutes.aspx.

36. Malika Redmond, "A *Critical Discourse Analysis* of the Marketing of Merck & Co.'s Human Papillomavirus Gardasil," Thesis, Georgia State University, at 22, December 5, 2011, https://scholarworks.gsu.edu/cgi/viewcontent.cgi? article=1028&context=wsi_theses.

37. Rhode Island Department of Public Health School Immunization Requirements, http://www.health.ri.gov/immunization/for/schools/index.php.

38. Ibid.

39. National Conference of State Legislators, "HPV Vaccine: State Legislation and Statutes: School Requirements," http://www.ncsl.org/research/health /hpv-vaccine-state-legislation-and-statutes.aspx.

40. Felice Freyer, "Parents protest R.I. mandating HPV vaccine for teens," *Boston Globe*, Sept. 8, 2015, https://www.bostonglobe.com/metro/2015/09/07/rhode-island-mandate-for-hpv-vaccine-sparks-protests-and-interest-from-massachusetts -officials/ZKmTZNPVTVKibPgqsUAgYK/story.html.

41. Rhode Island Department of Public Health School Immunization Requirements, http://www.health.ri.gov/immunization/for/schools/index.php.

42. John Howell, "Vaccination Exemption Stays for Now," *Johnston Sunrise*, August 5, 2015, http://johnstonsunrise.net/stories/vaccination%20exemption%20 stays%20for%20now,104571.

43. CDC, "National, Regional, State, and Selected Local Area Vaccination Coverage Among Adolescents Aged 13–17 Years – United States, 2016," *Morbidity and Mortality Weekly Report*, 66(33):874–882, at 876, August 25, 2017, https://www .cdc.gov/mmwr/volumes/66/wr/mm6633a2.htm.

44. Ibid.
45. CDC, 2015. "Many adolescents still not getting HPV vaccine." https://www .cdc.gov/media/releases/2015/p0730-hpv.html.
46. CDC, Teen Vaccination Coverage, 2014 National Immunization Survey–Teen, https://www.cdc.gov/vaccines/imz-managers/coverage/nis/child/2014 -released-child-teen.html
47. "Organizations and professional societies focusing on vaccines/VPDs," Immunization Action Coalition http://www.immunize.org/resources/part_us .asp.
48. American Cancer Society, 2016. "NCI-designated Cancer Centers Urge HPV Vaccination for the Prevention of Cancer," https://www.mdanderson.org /content/dam/mdanderson/documents/prevention-and-screening/NCI _HPV_Consensus_Statement_012716.pdf.
49. Tisch Cancer Institute, 2017. "The Tisch Cancer Institute at Mount Sinai Joins Nation's Cancer Centers in Endorsement of HPV Vaccination for Cancer Prevention." http://www.mountsinai.org/about-us/newsroom/press-releases/the -tisch-cancer-institute-at-mount-sinai-joins-nations-cancer-centers-in-endorsement -of-hpv-vaccination-for-cancer-prevention.
50. *See* Chapter 4.
51. American Cancer Society, 2016. "NCI-designated Cancer Centers Urge HPV Vaccination for the Prevention of Cancer," see note 48 above.
52. Ibid.
53. "CA Law on Minor Consent for STD Prevention Services FAQ," California Immunization Coalition, Jan. 2013, http://www.immunizeca.org/wp-content /uploads/2011/06/AB_499_FAQ.pdf.
54. *See, e.g.,* NVIC 2011. "NVIC Calls New CA Vaccine Law a 'Violation of Parental Informed Consent Rights and Federal Law.'" http://www.nvic.org/pressrelease /PR-CA-AB499-Signed.aspx.
55. Ibid.
56. 42 U.S.C. § 300aa-26, https://www.gpo.gov/fdsys/pkg/USCODE-2010-title42/ pdf/USCODE-2010-title42-chap6A-subchapXIX-part2-subpartc-sec300aa-26.pdf.
57. CDC instructions for VIS for minors: https://www.cdc.gov/vaccines/hcp/vis/ about/vis-faqs.html.
58. N.C. Gen. Stat. § 90–21.5, "Minor's consent sufficient for certain medical health services," https://www.ncleg.net/EnactedLegislation/Statutes/PDF/BySection /Chapter_90/GS_90-21.5.pdf.
59. Alan Phillips,, "Stealth Vaccine Laws Allow Children to Consent to Vaccines," March 22, 2012, *GreenMedinfo*, http://www.greenmedinfo.com/blog/stealth -vaccine-laws-allow-children-consent-vaccines.
60. NY regulation adding preventative services to existing bill: https://regs.health. ny.gov/sites/default/files/pdf/recently_adopted_regulations/Expansion%20 of%20Minor%20Consent%20for%20HIV%20Treatment%20%20Access%20 and%20Prevention.pdf.

61. Planned Parenthood supports HPV regulation for minors: https://www
.plannedparenthood.org/planned-parenthood-new-york-city/our-issues
/ppnycs-legislative-and-policy-agenda.

62. "Indoor Tanning Restrictions for Minors-a state-by-state comparison," National
Conference of State Legislators, July 1, 2015, http://www.ncsl.org/research
/health/indoor-tanning-restrictions.aspx.

63. "Criteria for Vaccination Requirements for U.S. Immigration Purposes," HHS,
Federal Register, vol. 74, no. 218, Nov. 13, 2009, https://www.gpo.gov/fdsys
/pkg/FR-2009-11-13/pdf/E9-27317.pdf.

64. K. J. Hachey, *et al.*, "Requiring Human Papillomavirus Vaccine for Immigrant
Women," *Obstetrics & Gynecology*, 114(5):1135–1139, November 2009.

65. National Coalition for Immigrant Women's Rights, 2008. "Statement on HPV
Vaccination." Archived at https://web.archive.org/web/20150910145525/https:
//napawf.org/wp-content/uploads/2009/working/pdfs/NCIWR%20
HPV%20Vaccine%20FINAL-9.29.08.pdf.

66. Ibid.

67. "Criteria for Vaccination Requirements for U.S. Immigration Purposes," HHS,
Federal Register, vol. 74, no. 218, Nov. 13, 2009, https://www.gpo.gov/fdsys/pkg
/FR-2009-11-13/pdf/E9-27317.pdf.

68. Ibid.

69. Ibid.

70. R. Adm. Paul J. Higgins, Director of Health & Safety, Coast Guard,
"*Gardasil–Human Papillomavirus (HPV) Vaccine*," March 7, 2007, https:
//www.health.mil/Reference-Center/Policies/2007/03/28/ALCOAST-Gardasil
-Human-Papillomavirus-Vaccine.

71. Dr. Limone Collins, "*Information Paper, HPV and HPV Vaccines*," Milvax–VHCN,
May 12, 2014, https://www.vaccines.mil/documents/1712_MIP-HPV.pdf.

72. H. Maktabi, "Quadrivalent Human Papillomavirus Vaccine Initiation,
Coverage, and Compliance Among U.S. Active Component Service Women
2006–2011," *MSMR*, 19(5), May 2012.

73. "Most States offer HPV vaccinations to girls in juvenile justice system,"
Science Daily, April 28, 2010, https://www.sciencedaily.com/releases/2010/04
/100428110812.htm; C. E. Henderson, *et al.*, "HPV Vaccination Practices
Among Juvenile Justice Facilities in the United States," *Journal of Adolescent
Health*, 46(5):495, 2010.

74. "Most States offer HPV vaccinations to girls in juvenile justice system," *Science
Daily*, note 73 above.

75. "SaneVax Discovers Vulnerable Girls in United States Targeted for HPV
Vaccination," SaneVax, Oct. 7, 2010, https://www.prlog.org/10982888
-sanevax-discovers-vulnerable-girls-in-united-states-targeted-for-hpv-vaccination
.html.

76. Ibid.

CHAPTER 15

1. Tracy Andrews Wolf, "Gardasil changed our dreams to nightmares," May 24, 2013, http://sanevax.org/gardasil-changed-our-dreams-to-nightmares/.

2. Ibid.

3. Ibid.

4. Ibid.

5. Ibid.

6. Ibid; *see also* Tracy Andrews-Wolf, "A Day in the Life of Alexis Wolf: Six Years After Gardasil," Aug. 11, 2013, http://www.hormonesmatter.com/life-of-alexis-wolf-post-gardasil/; Kelly Brogan, "A Ruined Life from Gardasil," Aug. 14, 2012, http://www.hormonesmatter.com/ruined-life-gardasil/.

7. B. A. Slade, *et al.*, "Postlicensure Safety Surveillance for Quadrivalent Human Papillomavirus Recombinant Vaccine," JAMA, 302(7):750–757 (2009).

8. "Human Papillomavirus (HPV) Quadrivalent & Bivalent Vaccines, Global Parental Concerns Regarding Safety and Efficacy of Gardasil and Cervarix," FDA Webinar, March 12, 2010, available at http://www.wanttoknow.nl/wp-content/media/28237701-03-06-10-FDA-Presentation-Final.pdf. *See also* Christina England, "FDA Requests Meeting with Activists Exposing Gardasil Adverse Reactions," *Vactruth*, March 8, 2010; J. B. Handley, "The Truth about Gardasil? It's Destroying our Girls," *Age of Autism*, March 24, 2010, http://www.ageofautism.com/2010/03/the-truth-about-gardasil-its-destroying-our-girls.html.

9. FDA Webinar, note 8 above.

10. Ibid., slide 54.

11. Ibid., slide 2.

12. Ibid., slide 6.

13. Ibid., slides 20–30.

14. Ibid., slides 32–40.

15. Ibid., slides 52–54.

16. "*How Cecile Richards, Douglas R. Lowy and John T. Schiller Advanced Women's Health,*" The Leonard Lopate Show, Sept. 14, 2017, at minute 30, http://www.wnyc.org/story/cecile-richards-douglas-r-lowy-and-john-t-schiller-creating-hpv-vaccine/.

17. Countries and dose statistics in S. M. Garland, *et al.*, "Impact and Effectiveness of the Quadrivalent Human Papillomavirus Vaccine: A Systematic Review of 10 Years of Real-world Experience," *Clinical Infectious Diseases*, 63(4):519–527, at 519–20, August 15, 2016; WHO, http://www.who.int/vaccine_safety/committee/topics/hpv/June_2017/en/.

18. "HPV Vaccine is Safe–(Gardasil)," CDC, https://www.cdc.gov/vaccinesafety/pdf/data-summary-hpv-gardasil-vaccine-is-safe.pdf.

19. Ibid.

20. Ibid.

21. Ibid.

22. WHO Global Advisory Committee on Vaccine Safety Statement on HPV Vaccine, Dec. 17, 2015, http://www.who.int/vaccine_safety/committee/GACVS_HPV_statement_17Dec2015.pdf?ua=1.
23. Ibid., 1.
24. Ibid.
25. Ibid., 3.
26. Ibid.
27. WHO Human papillomavirus vaccines: WHO position paper, May 2017, http://www.who.int/immunization/policy/position_papers/hpv/en/.
28. Ibid., 260.
29. Ibid., 261.
30. Ibid., 261–62.
31. Ibid., 265.
32. For example, see the endorsement of national cancer centers, discussed in "Controlling the Message" (Chapter 17). Note the endorsement of the American Academy of Pediatrics and the American Academy of Family Physicians on the CDC HPV information bulletin noted above.
33. Gardasil package insert, at 11 (Sec. 8.1): ". . . GARDASIL should be used during pregnancy only if clearly needed," https://www.fda.gov/downloads/biologicsbloodvaccines/vaccines/approvedproducts/ucm111263.pdf.
34. The authors' correspondence with the FDA is in their files.
35. "Systematic Review of 58 Publications of Real-World Use of Gardasil Presented at Eurogin Congress," Merck, June 16, 2016, http://investors.merck.com/news/press-release-details/2016/Systematic-Review-of-58-Publications-of-Real-World-Use-of-GARDASIL-Presented-at-EUROGIN-Congress/default.aspx.
36. S.M. Garland et al, "Impact and Effectiveness," see note 17 above.
37. Ibid., 520.
38. Ibid., 526.
39. Ibid.
40. Ibid.
41. Ibid., at 527.
42. D. M. Harper and L. R. DeMars, "HPV vaccines—A review of the first decade," *Gynecology & Oncology*, 146(1):196–204. July 2017.
43. Ibid., 8.
44. Y. Shoenfeld, *et al.*, *"Introduction,"* 1–7, *Vaccines & Autoimmunity*, at 1 (Y. Shoenfeld, N. Agmon-Levin & L. Tomljenovic, eds.) (Wiley Blackwell 2015).
45. L. Tomljenovic and C.A. Shaw, "Adverse Reactions to Human Papillomavirus Vaccines," Chapter 17, 163-174, *Vaccines & Autoimmunity* Y Shoenfeld, N Agmon-Levin & L Tomljenovic, (Hoboken, NJ: Wiley Blackwell, 2015).
46. Ibid., 164 (Table 17.1).
47. Ibid., 167.

48. Ibid., 164.

49. Ibid., 168–69.

50. Ibid., 171.

51. Ibid., 171, 172.

52. Ibid., 171.

53. 21 C.F.R. § 201.57, Labeling Requirement for Prescription Drugs and/or Insulin, https://www.accessdata.fda.gov/scripts/cdrh/cfdocs/cfCFR/CFRSearch .cfm?fr=201.57.

54. 42 U.S.C. § 300aa-26, https://www.gpo.gov/fdsys/pkg/USCODE-2010-title42 /pdf/USCODE-2010-title42-chap6A-subchapXIX-part2-subpartc-sec300aa-26 .pdf.

55. Gardasil package insert, note 33 above, at 13 (Sec. 13.1).

56. Cervarix package insert at 12 (Sec. 13.1), https://www.fda.gov/downloads /BiologicsBloodVaccines/Vaccines/ApprovedProducts/UCM240436.pdf.

57. Gardasil package insert, note 33 above, at 8 (Sec. 6.2).

58. Cervarix package insert, note 58 above, at 9 (Sec. 6.2).

59. United States Department of Health and Human Services (DHHS), Public Health Service (PHS), Centers for Disease Control (CDC) / Food and Drug Administration (FDA), Vaccine Adverse Event Reporting System (VAERS) 1990–last month, CDC WONDER Online Database, https://wonder.cdc.gov /vaers.html.

60. Ibid.

61. Ibid.

62. Interviews with Emma and Deborah, March 31, 2017.

63. E. Laskowski, "What's a normal resting heart rate?" Mayo Clinic, https: //www.mayoclinic.org/healthylifestyle/fitness/expert-answers/heart-rate/ faq-20057979.

64. S. H. Lee, Expert Report in *Gomez v. HHS*, Sept. 25, 2015 at 2, available at http: //sanevax.org/wp-content/uploads/2015/11/Gomez-v-USDOH-expert-report .pdf.

65. Ibid., 5.

66. Ibid., 8.

67. *Gomez v. HHS*, Order Denying Petitioners' Motion for Discovery on a Non-Party Vaccine Manufacturer, December 15, 2015, https://ecf.cofc.uscourts.gov /cgi-bin/show_public_doc?2015vv0160-29-0.

68. *Gomez v HHS*, Decision Awarding Damages, September 21, 2016, https://ecf .cofc.uscourts.gov/cgi-bin/show_public_doc?2015vv0160-54-0.

69. Ibid., 4.

70. Norma Erickson, "Vaccine Injury Compensation Program: Fatality after Gardasil," *SaneVax*, November 11, 2015, http://sanevax.org/vaccine-injury-compensation-program-fatality-after-gardasil/; *see also* E. Wehbe, "A Catastrophic Failure," *American Journal of Medicine*, 124(3):e7-e9, 2011. Dr.

Wehbe writes in a letter to the editor the case study of a deceased 17-year old woman who passed away. She was diagnosed with myocarditis, and he reported that her myocarditis occurred after receiving an HPV vaccine though he was unaware of any association between myocarditis and HPV vaccines.

71. Interview with Tracie Moorman, March 9, 2018.
72. Interview with Kathleen Berrett, June 29, 2018.

CHAPTER 16

1. James Colgrove, *State of Immunity*, at 188–193 (Univ. of California Press 2006); see also *Davis v. Wyeth*, 399 F.2d 121 (9th Cir. 1968); *Reyes v. Wyeth*, 498 F.2d 1264 (5th Cir. 1974).
2. N. F. Engstrom, "A Dose of Reality for Specialized Courts: Lessons from the VICP," 163 *University of Pennsylvania Law Review*, 1631, 2015.
3. Dr. Jonas Salk, the developer of the first polio vaccine, opposed blanket liability protection and stated in Congressional hearings in 1984 that "removal of the incentive for manufacturers and the scientific community to improve existing vaccines" was a serious concern. Jonas Salk, MD, Statement on National Childhood Vaccine Injury Compensation Act (May 3, 1984) (at page 166 [Bates-stamped page 171]). A copy of this document is in the authors' files.
4. Advisory Commission on Childhood Vaccines (ACCV) and National Vaccine Advisory Committee (NVAC) Subcommittees on Vaccine Safety, May 31, 1995, at 75.
5. The 1983 vaccine schedule can be found at https://www.cdc.gov/vaccines /schedules/images/schedule1983s.jpg; the current schedule is at https://www .cdc.gov/vaccines/schedules/hcp/imz/child-adolescent.html.
6. The Vaccine Reaction, December 8, 2015, http://www.thevaccinereaction. org/2015/12/u-s-vaccine-market-forecast-at-17-4-billion-by-2018/.
7. "Medicines in Development, Update 2017: Vaccines," Pharmaceutical Research and Manufacturers of America, *Phrma.org*, http://phrma-docs.phrma.org/file s/dmfile/MID_Vaccines_2017.PDF.
8. National Childhood Vaccine Injury Act of 1986, 42 U.S.C. §§ 300aa-1 to 34 (2016).
9. H.R. Rep. No. 99–908, at 3 (1986) reprinted in 1986 U.S.C.C.A.N. 6344, 6344.
10. 42 U.S.C. § 300aa-11.
11. Sections VIII-XVI have been added to the Table of Injuries since 1986, relating to new vaccines added to the Table. Vaccine Injury Table: https://www.hrsa .gov/sites/default/files/vaccinecompensation/vaccineinjurytable.pdf.
12. Engstrom, "A Dose of Reality for Specialized Courts: Lessons from the VICP," note 2 above, at 1703, n.328.
13. "Human papillomavirus vaccines: WHO position paper," WHO, May 2017, at 251, http://www.who.int/immunization/policy/position_papers/hpv/en/. It goes on to say that the "reasons are unclear" why the HPV vaccine induces such a

strong antibody response but suggests that this is "possibly by the use of adjuvants in the existing vaccines."

14. J. Sack, "'One Less' Avenue of Recovery?: The Treatment of Gardasil Under the National Vaccine Injury Compensation Program," 19 *Federal Circuit Bar Journal*, 663 (2010), 684–86.

15. *Althen v. HHS*, 418 F.3d 1274 (Fed. Cir. 2005).

16. "Vaccine Injury Compensation: Most Claims Took Years and Many Were Settled through Negotiation," US Government Accountability Office, Nov. 21, 2014, https://www.gao.gov/products/GAO-15-142.

17. "Special Masters – Biographies," US Court of Federal Claims, http://www.us-cfc.uscourts.gov/special-masters-biographies.

18. Under 42 U.S.C. § 300aa-12(c)(4), Special Masters serve 4-year terms. Under 28 U.S.C. . § 172(a), judges at the Court of Federal Claims serve 15-year terms.

19. Information on the total number of HPV vaccine injury claims comes from scholarship of Wayne Rohde, author of *Vaccine Court: The Dark Truth of America's Vaccine Injury Compensation Program* (New York: Skyhorse Publishing, 2014).

20. "Examining the FDA's HPV Vaccine Records," Judicial Watch, June 30, 2008, https://www.judicialwatch.org/documents/2008/JWReportFDAhpv VaccineRecords.pdf.

21. Peter Lind, "U.S. court pays $6 million to Gardasil victims," *Washington Times*, December 31, 2014, quoting Judicial Watch President Tom Fitton, https://www .washingtontimes.com/news/2014/dec/31/us-court-pays-6-million -gardasil-victims/.

22. *Tarsell v HHS*, Special Master Moran, Decision Denying Compensation, Feb. 16, 2016, https://scholar.google.com/scholar_case?case=1650304742716798 3466&q=tarsell+v+secretary+of+health+and+human+services&hl=en&as _sdt=6,33.

23. Ibid.

24. *Tarsell v. HHS*, 2017 WL 3837363 (Fed. Cl. June 30, 2017).

25. Ibid.

26. Ibid., 22.

27. *Tarsell v HHS* Decision Denying Compensation, see note 22 above.

28. *Tarsell v. HHS*, Court of Federal Claims decision, see note 24 above.

29. *Tarsell v. HHS*, Decision Denying Compensation, see note 22 above.

30. Tarah Gramza, interview, April 13, 2016, court documents in *Gramza v. HHS*, and interviews June 6–7, 2017.

31. C. Perricone, *et al.*, "Immune Thrombocytopenic Purpura: Between Infections and Vaccinations," in *Vaccines & Autoimmunity*, chapter 28, see note 44. 271–282, eds, Y. Shoenfeld, N. Agmon-Levin & L. Tomljenovic, eds.) (Hoboken, NJ: Wiley Blackwell, 2015).

32. *See, e.g.*, ibid.; M. Blank and P. Cruz-Tapias, "Antiphospholipid Syndrome and Vaccines" in *Vaccines & Autoimmunity* chapter 15, 141–147, eds. Y. Shoenfeld, N. Agmon-Levin & L. Tomljenovic, (Hoboken, NJ: Wiley Blackwell, 2015).

33. M. Bizjak, *et al.*, "Vaccinations and Secondary immune Thrombocytopenia with Antiphospholipid antibodies by Human Papillomavirus Vaccine," *Seminars in Hematology*, 53(S1):S48-S50, April 2016.
34. *Gramza v. HHS*, Exhibit 66, Rebuttal Expert Report of Dr. Yehuda Shoenfeld, February 1, 2016, at 4.
35. Tarah and Patrick Gramza, "Gramza Vaccine Court Story," http://canaryparty .org/wp-content/uploads/2016/12/Gramza-Vaccine-Court-Story.pdf.
36. *Gramza v. HHS*, 2018 WL 1581674 (Fed. Cl. Feb. 5, 2018), Decision Denying Entitlement.
37. *American Home Products Corp. v. Ferrari*, 668 S.E.2d 236 (Ga. 2008).
38. *Bruesewitz v. Wyeth Inc.*, 561 F.3d 233 (3d Cir. 2009).
39. Ibid. Justice Kagan recused herself because she had been involved in the case as Solicitor General before being appointed to the Supreme Court.
40. *N.W. v. Sanofi Pasteur*, European Court of Justice, June 21, 2017, https://eur-lex .europa.eu/legal-content/EN/TXT/?uri=CELEX%3A62015CJ0621.
41. *Robi v. Merck*, Superior Court of California, Los Angeles Central District, Case No. BC628589, complaint filed July 27, 2016. A copy of this complaint is in the authors' files.
42. *Robi v. HHS*, U.S. Court of Federal Claims, April 15, 2015, Unpublished Decision Denying Compensation, https://ecf.cofc.uscourts.gov/cgi-bin/show _public_doc?2013vv0734-35-0.
43. *Robi v. Merck* complaint, note 41 above, at ¶ 14; *see also* ¶ 28.
44. *See, e.g.*, ibid., *at* ¶¶ 36–38.
45. Ibid., ¶ 35.
46. Ibid., ¶¶ 38–42.

CHAPTER 17

1. Kelly Brownell and Kenneth Warner, "The Perils of Ignoring History: Big Tobacco Played Dirty and Millions Died. How Similar is Big Food?" *The Milbank Quarterly*, 87(1): 259–294, at 287, 2009.
2. Ibid., 270–71.
3. Ibid., 265.
4. Ibid., 264–65.
5. David Bruser and Jesse McLean, "HPV vaccine Gardasil has a dark side, Star investigation finds," *Toronto Star*, Feb. 5, 2015, archived at https://web.archive.org/ web/20150205215614/http://www.thestar.com/news/canada/2015/02/05 /hpv-vaccine-gardasil-has-a-dark-side-star-investigation-finds.html (retracted from newspaper's website).
6. Ibid.
7. Ibid.
8. Juliet Guichon and Rupert Kaul, "Science shows HPV vaccine has no dark side," *Toronto Star*, February 11, 2015, http://www.thestar.com/opinion /commentary/2015/02/11/science-shows-hpv-vaccine-has-no-dark-side.html.

9. Ibid.

10. Ibid.

11. Kevin Donovan, "*Toronto Star*'s Head of Investigations Stands by HPV Story," *Canadaland*, February 12, 2015, http://canadalandshow.com/article/toronto -stars-head-investigations-stands-hpv-story.

12. Ibid.

13. "A Note from the Publisher," *Toronto Star*, Feb. 20, 2015, http://www.thestar .com/news/2015/02/20/a-note-from-the-publisher.html.

14. Sarah Kaplan, "Botched expose of HPV vaccine's 'dark side' reveals dark side of news business," *Washington Post*, February 25, 2015, www.washingtonpost.com /news/morning-mix/wp/2015/02/25/botched-newspaper-expose-of-hpv -vaccines-dark-side-reveals-dark-side-of-news-business/.

15. Ibid.

16. "Katie (talk show)," Wikipedia, https://en.wikipedia.org/wiki/Katie_(talk _show).

17. John Stone, "The Couric Incident: HPV Vaccines and Mass Bullying," *SaneVax, Inc.*, May 24, 2015, http://sanevax.org/the-couric-incident-hpv-vaccines-mass -bullying/.

18. Ibid.

19. Alexandra Sifferlin, "Is Katie Couric the Next Jenny McCarthy? A former Playboy Bunny spreading misinformation is bad enough," *Time*, December 4, 2013, http://ideas.time.com/2013/12/04/is-katie-couric-the-next-jenny-mccarthy /?iid=tsmodule.

20. Michael Hiltzik, "Katie Couric puts the anti-vaccination movement into the mainstream," *Los Angeles Times*, December 4, 2013, http://articles.latimes .com/2013/dec/04/business/la-fi-mh-katie-couric-20131204.

21. Katie Couric, "Furthering the HPV Vaccine Conversation," *Huffington Post*, December 10, 2015, http://www.huffingtonpost.com/katie-couric/vaccine-hpv -furthering-conversation_b_4418568.html.

22. Brian Shilhavy, "Mainstream Media Attacks Katie Couric for Publishing Truth on Gardasil Vaccine," *Health Impact News*, December 5, 2013, https://health impactnews.com/2013/mainstream-media-attacks-katie-couric-for-publishing -truth-on-gardasil-vaccine/.

23. "Katie (talk show)," Wikipedia, note 16 above.

24. R. Inbar *et al.*, "Behavioral abnormalities in young female mice following administration of aluminum adjuvants and the human papillomavirus (HPV) vaccine Gardasil," *Vaccine Papers*, http://vaccinepapers.org/wp-content /uploads/Behavioral-abnormalities-al-adjuvant-gardasil.pdf (original study from *Vaccine*).

25. Ibid.

26. Ibid.

27. R. Inbar, *et al.*, "WITHDRAWN: Behavioral abnormalities in young female mice following administration of aluminum adjuvants and the human

papillomavirus (HPV) vaccine Gardasil," *Vaccine*, S0264-410X(16)00016–5, January 9, 2016, https://www.ncbi.nlm.nih.gov/pubmed/26778424.

28. T. Blackwell., "Journal permanently spikes Canadian study critical of HPV vaccine," *National Post*, March 8, 2016, http://news.nationalpost.com/news /canada/journal-permanently-spikes-canadian-study-critical-of-hpv-vaccine.

29. "Study Linking Gardasil to Behavioral Abnormalities Pulled from Vaccine Journal," *Vaccine Reaction*, March 12, 2016, http://www.thevaccinereaction.org /2016/03/study-linking-gardasil-to-behavioral-abnormalities-pulled-from -vaccine-journal/.

30. Nellis B. Mayo, "Clinic Discovers African-Americans Respond Better to Rubella Vaccine," *Mayo Clinic*, February 26, 2014, http://newsnetwork.mayoclinic.org /discussion/mayo-clinic-discovers-african-americans-respond-better-to-rubella -vaccine/.

31. R. Inbar, *et al.*, "Behavioral abnormalities in young female mice following administration of aluminum adjuvants and the human papillomavirus (HPV) vaccine Gardasil," *Immunologic Research*, 65(1):136–149, February 2017.

32. S. H. Lee, "Allegations of Scientific Misconduct by GACVS/WHO/CDC Representatives *et al*, An open-letter of complaint to the Director-General of the World Health Organization, Dr. Margaret Chan," January14, 2016, http://sanevax .org/hpv-vaccine-safety-an-illusion-maintained-by-suppression-of-science/.

33. Ibid., 15.

34. Ibid., 12, citing Dr. Helen Petousis-Harris's email.

35. Ibid. at 15.

36. European Medicines Agency, 2016. "Assessment Report, HPV vaccines," at 32 (at 2.2.4.5) http://www.ema.europa.eu/docs/en_GB/document_library/Referrals _document/HPV_vaccines_20/Opinion_provided_by_Committee_for _Medicinal_Products_for_Human_Use/WC500197129.pdf.

37. European Medicines Agency, 2016. "Assessment Report, HPV vaccines," note 36 above, at 35.

38. Nordic Cochrane Centre, 2016. "Complaint to the EMA Over Maladministration at the EMA." https://nordic.cochrane.org/sites/nordic.cochrane.org/files/public /uploads/ResearchHighlights/Complaint-to-EMA-over-EMA.pdf.

39. Ibid., 2.

40. Ibid., 3.

41. Ibid., 1.

42. Ibid., 5.

43. Ibid., 7.

44. Ibid., 11–12.

45. Ibid., 12.

46. Ibid.

47. Ibid.,16.

48. EMA Letter to Nordic Cochrane Centre, Denmark, July 1, 2016, http://www .ema.europa.eu/docs/en_GB/document_library/Other/2016/07/ WC500210543.pdf.

49. Nordic Cochrane Centre complaint to the European Ombudsman over maladministration at the EMA in relation to the safety of the HPV vaccines, October 10, 2016, http://nordic.cochrane.org/sites/nordic.cochrane.org/files/public/ uploads/complaint-to-ombudsman-over-ema_101016.pdf.

50. Reply from the European Ombudsman to Nordic Cochrane Centre June 26, 2017, http://nordic.cochrane.org/sites/nordic.cochrane.org/files/public/uploads /26_june_2017_letter_from_ombudsman_to_nordic_cochrane_centre.pdf.

51. Nordic Cochrane Centre's assessment of the Ombudsman's decision, November 2, 2017, http://nordic.cochrane.org/sites/nordic.cochrane.org/files/public /uploads/nordic_cochrane_views_on_the_ombudsmans_decision_2_nov _2017.pdf.

52. H. Larson, "The World Must Accept that the HPV vaccines is safe," *Nature* 528:9, December 3, 2015, https://www.nature.com/news/the-world-must-accept -that-the-hpv-vaccine-is-safe-1.18918.

CHAPTER 18

1. Australia has lower cervical cancer rates than the US prior to introduction of the vaccine. Australian National Cervical Screening Program, Screening to Prevent Cervical Cancer: Guidelines for the Management of Asymptomatic Women with Screen Detected Abnormalities (2005), https://healthygc.com.au /MedicareLocal/media/Site-Pages-Content/Cancer%20Screening /Screening_to_prevent_cervical_cancer_guidelines.pdf.

2. Ruth Beran, "Ian Frazer's Patent Problem," *Lab & Life Scientist*, http: //www.labonline.com.au/content/life-scientist/news/ian-frazer-s -patent-problem-1263005711.

3. "Cancer in Aboriginal and Torres Strait Islander peoples of Australia: an Overview," Australian Institute of Health and Welfare, (Canberra, 2013) https://healthinfonet.ecu.edu.au/key-resources/publications/?id=26088& title=Cancer+in+Aboriginal+and+Torres+Strait+Islander+peoples+of+Australia %3A+an+overview

4. Jessica van Vonderen, "Cervical Cancer Screening Rates among Indigenous Women Show No Improvement: Study,"*ABC*, April 21, 2016, http://www.abc.net .au/news/2016-04-12/cervical-cancer-screening-rates-among-indigenous -women-low/7320974.

5. Matthew Stevens, "Howard Rescues Gardasil from Abbot Poison Pill," *The Australian*, November 10, 2006, https://www.theaustralian.com.au/archive /business/howard-rescues-gardasil-from-abbott-poison-pill/news-story /02ca88665d4ce0d7271a5f21545c53f9.

6. Ibid.
7. Leigh Dayton, "Cancer vaccine a gift to women," *The Australian*, June 11, 2012, http://www.theaustralian.com.au/archive/in-depth/q-ian-frazer/news-story/326e28927d3b68e86c119322f7eb9149.
8. Ibid.
9. Ibid.
10. "Abbott rules out cancer vaccine for his daughters," *news.com.au*, http://www.news.com.au/national/abbott-rules-out-cancer-vaccine-for-his-daughters/news-story/1a2eadd3004542ffb5ce1973de5d426a.
11. Ibid.
12. Marion Haas. "Government Response to PBAC Recommedations. Centre for Health, Economics Research and Evaluation. 2007. https://web.archive.org/web/20160426224413/http://hpm.org/en/Surveys/CHERE_-_Australia/09/Government_response_to_PBAC_recommendations.html.
13. *See* "Screening as well as vaccination is essential in the fight against cervical cancer," WHO, http://www.who.int/reproductivehealth/topics/cancers/fight-cervical-cancer/en/.
14. "HPV Vaccination Coverage 2007–2011," National HPV Vaccination Program Register, http://www.hpvregister.org.au/research/coverage-data/hpv-vaccination-coverage-2007-11.
15. Anahad O'Connor, "HPV Vaccine Showing Successes in Australia," *New York Times*, April 18, 2013, https://well.blogs.nytimes.com/2013/04/18/hpv-vaccine-showing-successes-in-australia/?mcubz=0.
16. "How dizzy school girls wiped $1bn off CSL," *Crikey.com.au*, May 25, 2007, https://www.crikey.com.au/2007/05/25/how-dizzy-school-girls-wiped-1bn-off-csl/.
17. Gavin Fang, "Abbot Plays Down Gardasil Side Effects," *The World Today*, May 22, 2007, http://www.abc.net.au/worldtoday/content/2007/s1929912.htm.
18. Ibid.
19. Reko Renni, "Vaccine is safe, says creator," *theage.com.au*, May 22, 2017, http://www.theage.com.au/articles/2007/05/22/1179601376505.html?from=top5.
20. "CSL to Reap Big Royalties on Vaccine," *Sydney Morning Herald*, October 8, 2005 http://www.smh.com.au/news/business/csl-to-reap-big-royalties-on-vaccine/2005/10/07/1128562999590.html.
21. Tim Binsted, "CSL's 100 year rise to the top had sickness and health, hardship and wealth," *Financial Review*, April 23, 2016, http://www.afr.com/business/health/biotechnology/csls-100-year-rise-to-the-top-had-sickness-and-health-hardship-and-wealth-20160421-gobscn.
22. IVIG products are a key growth driver at CSL. CSL Ltd., ASX Full-Year Information 30 June 2017, at 2, http://member.afraccess.com/media?id=CMN://3A475252&filename=20170816/CSL_01884073.pdf.
23. DAEN reporting system, http://apps.tga.gov.au/PROD/DAEN/daen-report.aspx.

The HPV Vaccine on Trial *403*

24. Ibid., search term "Gardasil."

25. No reported deaths have been associated with the vaccine in Australia. Australian Government Department of Health, 2015. "Gardasil (quadrivalent human papillomavirus vaccine) update 2." https://www.tga.gov.au/alert /gardasil-quadrivalent-human-papillomavirus-vaccine-update-2.

26. Most expenses incurred by TGA covered by fees charged to industry. "Funding Capital Expenditure and Anticipated Revenue," TGA, https://www.tga.gov .au/book-page/funding-capital-expenditure-and-anticipated-revenue.

27. "Enhanced school-based surveillance of acute adverse events following immunisation with human papillomavirus vaccine in males and females," TGA, 2013 (May 2015), https://www.tga.gov.au/sites/default/files/medicine-review -school-based-surveillance-immunisation-with-human-papillomavirus-vaccine .pdf.

28. Ibid., 8 (2013: 748 AEFIs reported to DAEN).

29. Ibid.

30. Australian Government Department of Health, 2015. "Gardasil (quadrivalent human papillomavirus vaccine) update 2." https://www.tga.gov.au/alert /gardasil-quadrivalent-human-papillomavirus-vaccine-update-2.

31. Ibid.

32. Ibid.

33. Ibid.

34. D. T. Little and H. R. Ward, "Adolescent Premature Ovarian Insufficiency Following Human Papillomavirus Vaccination: A Case Series Seen in General Practice," *Journal of Investigative Medicine High Impact Case Reports*, Oct.-Dec. 2014:1–12, https://www.ncbi.nlm.nih.gov/pmc/articles/PMC4528880/pdf /10.1177_2324709614556129.pdf; D. T. Little and H. R. Ward, "Premature ovarian failure 3 years after menarche in a 16-year-old girl following human papillomavirus vaccination" *BMJ Case Reports*, September 30, 2012, https: //www.ncbi.nlm.nih.gov/pmc/articles/PMC4543769/pdf/bcr-2012-006879 .pdf.

35. Stephen Tunley, "Herd protection from the female HPV vaccination programme," *The Lancet*, 16(12):1333–1334, December 2016, http://www.thelancet.com/journals/laninf/article/PIIS1473-3099(16)30468–6/fulltext.

36. "Ian Frazer," contributor profile, *The Conversation*, https://theconversation .com/profiles/ian-frazer-10030.

37. "Contributing institutions," *The Conversation*: https://theconversation.com /institutions.

38. J. Wilyman, "A critical analysis of the Australian government's rationale for its vaccination policy," University of Wollongong, 2015, https://alor.org /Library/Wilyman%20J%20-%20A%20critical%20analysis%20of%20the%20 Australian%20government_s%20rationale%20for.pdf.

39. Change.org petition to ask Australia's department of health to issue "condemnation of this travesty," https://www.change.org/p/simon-birmingham-stop-

the-university-of-wollongong-s-spread-of-disease-and-death-via-anti-vaccination -phd.

40. Kyler Loussikian, "Wollongong University accepts thesis on vaccine 'conspiracy,'" *The Australian*, January 13, 2016, https://www.theaustralian.com.au /higher-education/wollongong-university-accepts-thesis-on-vaccine-conspiracy /news-story/dbd57d8909779f4d82ece7b9ab8d520a.

41. "'As a leading research-intensive university, the University of Wollongong values intellectual openness, freedom of opinion, diversity of ideas, equity, and mutual respect,' a spokesperson from the University of Wollongong said in an official statement." Quoted in Andrea Booth, "Wollongong Uni Accepts Anti-Vaccination Thesis Citing 'Freedom of Opinion,'"*SBS News*, Jan. 14, 2016 https: //www.sbs.com.au/news/wollongong-uni-accepts-anti-vaccination-thesis -citing-freedom-of-opinion.

42. Brian Martin "News with a negative frame: a vaccination case study," March 4, 2016, http://www.bmartin.cc/pubs/16Loussikian.html.

43. Prime Minister Malcolm Turnbull on eliminating HPV virus via vaccination, http://www.skynews.com.au/news/national/2017/10/08/new-hpv-vaccine-to -be-rolled-out-in-schools.html.

44. Malcolm Turnbull, 2017. "Announcement of the Addition of Gardasil 9 to the National Immunisation Program." https://www.malcolmturnbull.com.au /media/announcement-of-the-addition-of-gardasil-9-to-the-national-immunisation -pro.

CHAPTER 19

1. "About Us," SaneVax, http://sanevax.org/media-about/about/.

2. Ibid.

3. S. H. Lee, "Detection of human papillomavirus (HPV) L1 gene DNA possibly bound to particulate aluminum adjuvant in the HPV vaccine Gardasil," *Journal of Inorganic Biochemistry*, 117: 85–92, 2012.

4. Norma Erickson, "SaneVax to FDA: Recombinant HPV DNA found in multiple samples of Gardasil," September 2, 2011, http://sanevax.org/sane -vax-to-fda-recombinant-hpv-dna-found-in-multiple-samples-of-gardasil/.

5. Walter J. Gardner, Office of Communication, Outreach and Development, Center for Biologics Evaluation and Research, letter to SaneVax, Inc., Sept. 23, 2011, http://sanevax.org/wp-content/uploads/2011/09/09.23.2011-FDA -response.pdf; *see also* FDA, 2011. "FDA Information on Gardasil–Presence of DNA Fragments Expected, No Safety Risk," https://www.fda.gov/Biologics BloodVaccines/Vaccines/ApprovedProducts/ucm276859.htm.

6. Ibid.

7. *See* April 19, 2006 Final Briefing Document, at 16, appended to the April 19, 2006 letter from Patrick Brill-Edwards, M.D., Merck's Director of Worldwide Regulatory Affairs for Vaccines/Biologics, to Christine Walsh, R.N. of the FDA's

CBER, archived at http://wayback.archive-it.org/7993/20180126170209/https://www.fda.gov/ohrms/dockets/ac/06/briefing/2006-4222B1.pdf.

8. Merck patent for the "Process for Purifying Human Papillomavirus Virus-Like Particles," Ex. 3, https://patents.google.com/patent/US6602697B1/en.

9. *See* Gardasil package insert, https://www.fda.gov/downloads/biologicsblood-vaccines/vaccines/approvedproducts/ucm111263.pdf.

10. "Macrophage," Dictionary.com, http://www.dictionary.com/browse/macrophage.

11. G. Arango Duque and A. Descoteaux, "Macrophage Cytokines: Involvement in Immunity and Infectious Diseases," *Frontiers in Immunology*, 5: 491, Oct. 7, 2014, https://www.ncbi.nlm.nih.gov/pmc/articles/PMC4188125/.

12. Norma Erickson, President of SaneVax, letter to Walter J. Gardner, Oct. 14, 2011, Re: Rebuttal to FDA response, http://sanevax.org/sane-vax-to-fda-recombinant-hpv-dna-found-in-multiple-samples-of-gardasil/.

13. Ibid.

14. Ibid.

15. Ibid.

16. Ibid.

17. FDA, "FDA Information on Gardasil-Presence of DNA Fragments Expected, No Safety Risk," note 5 above.

18. Ibid.

19. Ibid.

20. Norma Erickson and SaneVax, 2011, "FDA Information on Gardasil —Betrayal of the Public Trust?", http://sanevax.org/fda-information-on-gardasil-betrayal-of-the-public-trust/.

21. Ibid.

22. Ibid.

23. Copy of FOIA documents on file with authors.

24. Ibid.

25. S. H. Lee, "Detection of human papillomavirus L1 gene DNA fragments in postmortem blood and spleen after Gardasil vaccination—A case report," *Advances in Bioscience and Biotechnology*, 3:1214–24, 2012.

26. S. H. Lee, "Topological conformational changes of human papillomavirus (HPV) DNA bound to an insoluble aluminum salt – A study by low temperature PCR," *Advances in Biological Chemistry*, 3:76–85, 2013.

27. Ibid.

28. L. Bélec, H. Péré, C. Fayard, "Confirmation of the Creation of a Novel Molecule in Gardasil," presented at the 3rd International Symposium on Vaccines at the 9th International Congress on Autoimmunity, March 26, 2014, abstract previously available at http://autoimmunity.meetingxpert.net/AUTOIMMUNITY_475/poster_87049/program.aspx/anchor87049. A copy of this abstract is in the authors' files.

29. B. Baker, *et al.*, "The safety of human papilloma virus-blockers and the risk of triggering autoimmune disease," *Expert Opinion on Drug Safety*, 14(9):1387–1394 at 1391, 2015.

30. FDA, Summary Basis for Approval, Recombivax HB, archived at https://wayback.archive-it.org/7993/20170723025131/https://www.fda.gov/downloads/BiologicsBloodVaccines/Vaccines/ApprovedProducts/UCM244544.pdf; *see also* CDC, "Recommendations of the Immunization Practices Advisory Committee Update on Hepatitis B Prevention," *MMWR*, 36(23):353–366, June 19, 1987, https://www.cdc.gov/mmwr/preview/mmwrhtml/00019181.htm.

31. FDA, August 27, 1999 Approval Letter - Recombivax HB, to Merck, archived at https://wayback.archive-it.org/7993/20170723025129/https://www.fda.gov/BiologicsBloodVaccines/Vaccines/ApprovedProducts/ucm110129.htm.

32. S. Humphries, "What Biologically Plausible Mechanisms of Action are Health Agencies Ignoring?" AutismOne Media video, https://www.youtube.com/watch?v=jsVq0jWfHbM&t=1444s, at 35:49–36:25, published May 28, 2017 (Merck advised Medsafe New Zealand in 2000 that the description of the HepB vaccine should be changed to reflect AAHS, which Merck stated always had been in the vaccine).

33. Gardasil package insert, at 12 (sec. 11), https://www.fda.gov/downloads/biologics bloodvaccines/vaccines/approvedproducts/ucm111263.pdf

34. Recombivax HB package insert, at 6-7 (Sec. 11), https://www.merck.com/product/usa/pi_circulars/r/recombivax_hb/recombivax_pi.pdf.

35. Ibid.

36. S. R. Paludan and A. G. Bowie, "Immune sensing of DNA," *Immunity*, 38:870–80, 2013.

37. F. Steinhagen, *et al.*, "TLR-Based Immune Adjuvants," *Vaccine*, 29(17):3341–3355, April 12, 2011.

38. S. Gnjatic, *et al.*, "Toll-like receptor agonists: Are they good adjuvants?" *Cancer Journal*, 16(4): 382–391, July-August 2010.

39. P. M. Egan, *et al.*, "Relationship between tightness of binding and immunogenicity in an aluminum-containing adjuvant-adsorbed hepatitis B vaccine," *Vaccine*, 27(24):3175–80, May 21 ,2009.

40. A. M. Didierlaurent, *et al.*, "AS04, an aluminum salt- and TLR4 agonist-based adjuvant system, induces a transient localized innate immune response leading to enhanced adaptive immunity," *Journal of Immunology*, 83(10):6186–97, November 15, 2009.

41. S. R. Baratono, *et al.*, "Toll-like receptor 9 and interferon-receptor signaling suppress the B-cell fate of uncommitted progenitors in mice," *European Journal of Immunology*, 45(5):1313–25, May 2015.

42. Merck & Co., Inc. Polynucleaotide Vaccine Formulations. Patent no. CA2280839A1 filed Feb. 14, 1997, https://patents.google.com/patent/CA2280839A1/en

43. Ibid.

44. "Merck & Co., Inc. and Idera Pharmaceuticals Sign Collaboration Agreement Incorporating Idera's Toll-like Receptor Agonists in Merck's Vaccine Programs," *Business Wire*, December 11, 2006, https://www.businesswire.com /news/home/20061211005242/en/Merck-Idera-Pharmaceuticals-Sign- Collaboration-Agreement-Incorporating.

45. Dr. Lee posted his findings on PubMed Commons before the service was dis- continued in February 2018. A copy is in the authors' files.

CHAPTER 20

1. Transcript of "Workshop on Adjuvants and Adjuvanted Preventive and Therapeutic Vaccines for Infectious Disease Indications," Food and Drug Administration Center for Biologics Evaluation and Research, National Institutes of Health, National Institute of Allergy and Infectious Diseases, December 2, 2008, at 32, archived at https://web.archive.org/web/20170304081353 /https://www.fda.gov/downloads/biologicsbloodvaccines/newsevents/work shopsmeetingsconferences/ucm095708.pdf.

2. *See, e.g.,* "Vaccine Adjuvants," CDC, https://www.cdc.gov/vaccinesafety /concerns/adjuvants.html; *see also* "Aluminum in Vaccines: What You Should Know," Q&A from The Children's Hospital of Philadelphia, Vaccine Education Center, Vol. 5, at 2, Winter 2014, https://media.chop.edu/data/files/pdfs /vaccine-education-center-aluminum.pdf.

3. N. Baylor, *et al.*, "Aluminum salts in vaccines—U.S. perspective," *Vaccine*, 20:S18–S23, at S20, 2002.

4. Bert Ehgartner, "The Age of Aluminum," film by Janson Media, 2013, https: //www.videoproject.com/The-Age-of-Aluminum.html.

5. "Professor Chris Exley," Keele University profile, https://www.keele.ac.uk /aluminium/groupmembers/chrisexley/.

6. Chris Exley, "Human Exposure to Aluminium," *Environmental Science: Process & Impacts*, 15(10):1807–1816, at 1807, 2013.

7. Ibid.

8. P. O. Ganrot, "Metabolism and the Possible Health Effects of Aluminum," *Environmental Health Perspectives*, 65:363–441, at 363, 1986.

9. M. Kawahara and M. Kato-Negishi, "Link between Aluminum and the Pathogenesis of Alzheimer's Disease: The Integration of the Aluminum and Amyloid Cascade Hypotheses," *International Journal Alzheimer's Disease*, 2011, https://www.ncbi.nlm.nih.gov/pmc/articles/PMC3056430/pdf/IJAD2011- 276393.pdf.

10. Y. Shoenfeld, *et al.*, "Introduction," 1–7, *Vaccines & Autoimmunity*, at 2, Y. Schoenfeld, *et al.*, eds (Hoboken, NJ: Wiley Blackwell, 2015).

11. C. A. Janeway, "Approaching the Asymptote? Evolution and Revolution in Immunology," *Cold Spring Harbor Symposia on Quantitative Biology*, 54:1–13, at

6, 1989, reprinted in *Journal of Immunology*, 2013, http://www.jimmunol.org/content/191/9/4475.

12. Ibid.

13. Ibid.

14. G. Leroux-Roels, "Old and new adjuvants for hepatitis B vaccines," *Medical Microbiology and Immunology*, 204:69–78 at 71, 2015; *see also* C. Exley, *et al.*, "The immunobiology of aluminum adjuvants: how do they really work?" *Trends in Immunology*, 31(3):103–109, at 103, 2010; E. Israeli, *et al.*, "Role of Adjuvants in Infection and Autoimmunity," Chapter 1, 11–23, *Vaccines & Autoimmunity*, at 11.

15. Children's Hospital of Philadelphia, Vaccine Education Center, 2013, "Vaccines and Aluminum," reviewed by Dr. Paul Offit, archived at https://web.archive.org/web/20130528091723/http://www.chop.edu:80/service/vaccine-education-center/vaccine-safety/vaccine-ingredients/aluminum.html/.

16. C. Exley, qtd. in Marie-Ange Poyet, *Injecting Aluminum*, video by Cinéma Libre, at 0:40, https://vimeo.com/214102022.

17. Shoenfeld "Introduction," note 10 above, at 2; C. Perricone, *et al.*, "Autoimmune/inflammatory syndrome induced by adjuvants (ASIA) 2013: Unveiling the pathogenic, clinical and diagnostic aspects," *Journal of Autoimmunity*, 47:1–16, at 1, 2013; L. Tomljenovic and C. A. Shaw, "*Answers to Common Misconceptions Regarding the Toxicity of Aluminum Adjuvants in Vaccines*," Chapter 4, 43–55, *Vaccines & Autoimmunity*, note 10 above, at 43, 44.

18. S. J. Mandriota, *et al.*, "Aluminium chloride promotes tumorigenesis and metastasis in normal murine mammary gland epithelial cells," *International Journal of Cancer*, 139:2781–2790, 2016.

19. C. Exley, "Aluminum Should Now Be Considered a Primary Etiological Factor in Alzheimer's Disease," *Journal of Alzheimers Disease Reports*, 1:23–25, 2017.

20. I. Karakis, *et al.*, "Association between prenatal exposure to metals and neonatal morbidity," *Journal of Toxicology and Environmental Health Part A*, 77(21):1281–4, 2014; D. Fanni, *et al.*, "Aluminum exposure and toxicity in neonates: a practical guide to halt aluminum overload in the prenatal and perinatal periods," *World Journal of Pediatrics*,10(2):101–7, May 2014.

21. "Monograph on Occupational Exposures During Aluminum Production" International Agency for Research on Cancer, at 221, https://monographs.iarc.fr/ENG/Monographs/vol100F/mono100F-22.pdf.

22. "Aluminum is toxic to all life forms," video by Suzanne Humphries, https://www.youtube.com/watch?v=6WwKRokpEUM; Tomljenovic and Shaw, "Answers to Common Misconceptions Regarding the Toxicity of Aluminum Adjuvants in Vaccines," note 17 above, at 44.

23. "Aluminum salts, Report No. 43, NTIS Accession No. PB262655," FDA, Select Committee on GRAS Substances (SCOGS) Opinion,1975, archived at http://wayback.archive-it.org/7993/20170607022715/https://www.fda.gov

/Food/IngredientsPackagingLabeling/GRAS/SCOGS/ucm260848.htm; *see also* American Frozen Food Institute, Issue Brief: "Aluminum-Containing Food Additives," http://www.affi.org/sites/default/files/affi-issue-brief-aluminum-containing-food-additives-may-2015.pdf.

24. *See, e.g.*, P. A. Offit and R. K. Jew, "Addressing Parents' Concerns: Do Vaccines Contain Harmful Preservatives, Adjuvants, Additives, or Residuals?" *Pediatrics*, 112(6):1394–1401 at 1396, 2003; *see also* "Vaccine Ingredients – Aluminum," The Children's Hospital of Philadelphia, Vaccine Education Center, http://www.chop.edu/centers-programs/vaccine-education-center/vaccine-ingredients/aluminum; "Aluminum in Vaccines: What You Should Know," The Children's Hospital of Philadelphia, Vaccine Education Center, Q&A, Vol. 5, at 2, Winter 2014, https://media.chop.edu/data/files/pdfs/vaccine-education-center-aluminum.pdf.

25. P. A. Offit, "Is There a Difference Between Aluminum That Is Injected vs. Ingested?" http://www.chop.edu/centers-programs/vaccine-education-center/video/there-difference-between-aluminum-injected-vs-ingested.

26. The Agency for Toxic Substances and Disease Registry (ATSDR) found in its 2008 Toxicological Profile for Aluminum that there are significant findings in animal studies concerning oral toxicity of aluminum and its impact on, in particular, the central nervous system. ATSDR, Toxicological Profile for Aluminum (September 2008), https://www.atsdr.cdc.gov/toxprofiles/tp22.pdf; *see also* L. Tomljenovic and C. A. Shaw, "Aluminum Vaccine Adjuvants: Are they Safe?" *Current Medicinal Chemistry*, 18:2630–2637, at 2630, 2011. In 2016, French researchers published a study on the impact of aluminum on the gut, noting: "Although still poorly documented to date, the impact of oral exposure to aluminum in conditions relevant to real human exposure appears to be deleterious for gut homeostasis. Aluminum ingestion affects the regulation of the permeability, the microflora and the immune function of the intestine. Nowadays, several arguments are consistent with an involvement of aluminum as an environmental risk factor for inflammatory bowel disease." C. Vignal, *et al.*, "Gut: An underestimated target organ for Aluminum," *Morphologie*, 100(329):75–84, at 75, June 2016.

27. *See, e.g.*, G. Crépeaux, *et al.*, "Non-linear dose-response of aluminum hydroxide adjuvant particles: Selective low dose neurotoxicity," *Toxicology*, 375:48–57, at 55, 2017.

28. "ToxGuideTM for Aluminum," Agency for Toxic Substances and Disease Registry, https://www.atsdr.cdc.gov/toxguides/toxguide-22.pdf.

29. T. Z. Movsas, *et al.*, "Effect of Routine Vaccination on Aluminum and Essential Element Levels in Preterm Infants," *JAMA Pediatrics*, 167(9):870–872, September 2013.

30. 21 C.F.R. § 201.323(e).

31. *See, e.g.*, S. L. Hem and J. L. White, "Structure and Properties of Aluminum-Containing Adjuvants," in *Vaccine Design: The Subunit and Adjuvant Approach,*

249–276, at 249, eds. M. F. Powell and M. J. Newman (New York: Plenum Press, 1995); J.-D. Masson, *et al.*, "Critical analysis of reference studies on the toxicokinetics of aluminum-based adjuvants," *Journal of Inorganic Biochemistry*, 181:87–95, April 2018.

32. Transcript of "Department of Health and Human Services National Vaccine Program Office Presents: Workshop on Aluminum in Vaccines," May 11–12, 2000, San Juan Puerto Rico, at 35–36. A copy of this transcript is in the authors' files.

33. "Alum in Baking Powder: The Complete Text of the Trial Examiner's Report upon the Facts, including a Review of Scientific Testimony concerning Alum in Baking Powder and Its Physiological Effects," at 66 (1927). A copy of the testimony quoted herein is in the authors' files.

34. Ibid., 71.

35. "Department of Health and Human Services National Vaccine Program Office Presents: Workshop on Aluminum in Vaccines," note 32 above, at 35–36.

36. Ibid., 64.

37. "Workshop on Adjuvants and Adjuvanted Preventive and Therapeutic Vaccines for Infectious Disease Indications" note 1 above, at 105.

38. Masson, *et al.*, "Critical analysis of reference studies on the toxicokinetics of aluminum-based adjuvants," note 31 above.

39. Tomljenovic and Shaw, "Answers to Common Misconceptions Regarding the Toxicity of Aluminum Adjuvants in Vaccines," note 17 above, at 48.

40. Z. Khan *et al.*, "Slow CCL2-dependent translocation of biopersistent particles from muscle to brain," *BMC Medicine*, 11:99, at 2, 2013, https://bmcmedicine.biomedcentral.com/articles/10.1186/1741-7015-11-99.

41. Tomljenovic and Shaw, "Answers to Common Misconceptions Regarding the Toxicity of Aluminum Adjuvants in Vaccines," note 17 above, at 48.

42. C. A. Shaw, *et al.*, "Aluminum-Induced Entropy in Biological Systems: Implications for Neurological Disease," *Journal of Toxicology*, 2014, https://www.hindawi.com/journals/jt/2014/491316/; C. A. Shaw, *et al.*, "Aluminum's Role in CNS-immune System Interations leading to Neurological Disorders," *Immunome Research*, 2013, https://www.omicsonline.org/open-access/aluminums-role-in-cnsimmune-system-interactions-leading-to-neurological-disorders-14822-1745-7580-9-069.php?aid=20403.

43. "Department of Health and Human Services National Vaccine Program Office Presents: Workshop on Aluminum in Vaccines," note 32 above, at 95 (Dr. Harm HogenEsch). Dr. HogenEsch downplayed the possible role of adjuvants in increased reactivity to allergens by noting that there is an increased in allergic diseases recently but that aluminum-based adjuvants have been around for a long time. However, he failed to account for newer, more immune system stimulating adjuvants such as AAHS and AS04 as well as the increase in the vaccine schedule (and thus increase in exposure to aluminum adjuvants) in that time period, among other factors. Ibid., 115; *see also* E. Bergfors, *et al.*, "Contact

allergy to aluminum induced by commonly used pediatric vaccines," *Clinical and Translational Medicine*, 6:4, 2017, https://www.ncbi.nlm.nih.gov/pmc/articles/PMC5214894/pdf/40169_2016_Article_129.pdf.

44. Tomljenovic and Shaw, "Answers to Common Misconceptions Regarding the Toxicity of Aluminum Adjuvants in Vaccines," note 17 above, at 44-45, 48.

45. M. Mold, *et al.*, "Aluminium in brain tissue in autism," *Journal of Trace Elements in Medicine and Biology*, 46:76-82, at 81, 2018, https://doi.org/10.1016/j.jtemb .2017.11.012.

46. Ibid.

47. Ibid.

48. A. Mirza, *et al.*, "Aluminium in brain tissue in familial Alzheimer's disease," *Journal of Trace Elements in Medicine and Biology* 40:30-36, at 35, 2017.

49. "Department of Health and Human Services National Vaccine Program Office Presents: Workshop on Aluminum in Vaccines," note 32 above, at 3.

50. C. Exley, "Aluminium adjuvants and vaccine safety," *The Hippocratic Post*, October 2, 2016, https://www.hippocraticpost.com/pharmacy-drugs/aluminium -adjuvants-vaccine-safety/.

51. "Workshop on Adjuvants and Adjuvanted Preventive and Therapeutic Vaccines for Infectious Disease Indications," note 1 above, at 39, 40; "Common Ingredients in U.S. Licensed Vaccines," FDA, https://www.fda.gov/ BiologicsBloodVaccines/SafetyAvailability/VaccineSafety/ucm187810.htm ("When evaluating a vaccine for safety and efficacy, FDA considers adjuvants as a component of the vaccine; they are not licensed separately.").

52. "Workshop on Adjuvants and Adjuvanted Preventive and Therapeutic Vaccines for Infectious Disease Indications," note 1 above, at 40; "Guidelines on the non-clinical evaluation of vaccine adjuvants and adjuvanted vaccines," World Health Organization, at 7, 2013, http://www.who.int/biologicals/areas/vaccines /ADJUVANTS_Post_ECBS_edited_clean_Guidelines_NCE_Adjuvant_Final _17122013_WEB.pdf.

53. R. K. Gupta and B. E. Rost, "Aluminum Compounds as Vaccine Adjuvants," *Methods in Molecular Medicine*, Vol 42: Vaccine Adjuvants: Preparation Methods and Research Protocols, 65-89, at 66 (2000), ed. D. T. O'Hagan (New York: Humana Press, Inc., 2000).

54. F. Tavares Da Silva, *et al.*, "Safety Assessment of adjuvanted vaccines: Methodological considerations," *Human Vaccines & Immunotherapeutics*, 11(7): 1814-1824, at 1816, July 2015. At the time of publication, three of the authors were GSK employees and the fourth, a former GSK employee, was a patent holder in the following adjuvant systems: AS01, AS03, AS04, and AS15. Ibid., 1822.

55. 21 C.F.R. § 610.15.

56. 21 C.F.R. § 610.15(a)(1). With certain restrictions this amount can be increased to up to 1.25 mg ("The amount of aluminum in the recommended individual

dose of a biological product shall not exceed: . . . 1.25 milligrams determined by assay provided that data demonstrating that the amount of aluminum used is safe and necessary to produce the intended effect are submitted to and approved by the Director, Center for Biologics Evaluation and Research or the Director, Center for Drug Evaluation and Research . . . ." (21 C.F.R. § 610.15(a)(3))); *see also* Baylor US perspective, note 3 above, at S20, S21; J. T. Bryan, "Developing an HPV vaccine to prevent cervical cancer and genital warts," *Vaccine*, 25: 3001-3006, at 3002, 2007; "Study Reports Aluminum in Vaccines Poses Extremely Low Risk to Infants," FDA, archived at http://wayback.archive-it. org/7993/20171114195453/https://www.fda.gov/BiologicsBloodVaccines/ ScienceResearch/ucm284520.htm.

57. "Department of Health and Human Services National Vaccine Program Office Presents: Workshop on Aluminum in Vaccines," note 32 above, at 46-47.
58. Baylor, "Aluminum salts in vaccines—U.S. perspective," note 3 above, at S18.
59. Ibid.; *see also* Tomljenovic and Shaw, "Answers to Common Misconceptions Regarding the Toxicity of Aluminum Adjuvants in Vaccines," note 17 above, at 45.
60. World Health Organization, July 16, 2004, "Weekly Epidemiological Record," 79(29):265-272, at 269, http://www.who.int/wer/2004/en/wer7929.pdf?ua=1.
61. "Workshop on Adjuvants and Adjuvanted Preventive and Therapeutic Vaccines for Infectious Disease Indications," note 1 above.
62. *See, e.g.,* Ibid., 61, 65.
63. Ibid., 29.
64. Ibid., 31.
65. Ibid., 65.
66. Masson, *et al.*, "Critical analysis of reference studies on the toxicokinetics of aluminum-based adjuvants," note 31 above.
67. "Toxicokinetics," definition from Science Direct, https://www.sciencedirect .com/topics/pharmacology-toxicology-and-pharmaceutical-science/ toxicokinetics.
68. Masson, *et al.*, "Critical analysis of reference studies on the toxicokinetics of aluminum-based adjuvants," note 31 above.
69. Ibid.
70. G. Crépeaux, *et al.*, "Non-linear dose-response of aluminum hydroxide adjuvant particles: Selective low dose neurotoxicity," *Toxicology*, 375:48-57, 2017.
71. Ibid.
72. Ibid., 49.
73. Ibid.
74. Ibid., 55
75. Ibid.
76. J. Lyons-Weiler and R. Rickertson, "Reconsideration of the immunotherapeutic pediatric safe dose levels of aluminum," *Journal of Trace Elements in Medicine and*

Biology 48:67–73, July 2018, e-published in advance of print at https://www.sciencedirect.com/science/article/pii/S0946672X17300950.

77. A copy of Dr. Gherardi's June 15, 2017 letter is in the authors' files.
78. Ibid.
79. T. Jefferson, et al., "Adverse events after immunisation with aluminum-containing DTP vaccines: systematic review of the evidence," *Lancet Infectious Diseases*, 4:84–90, at 84, 90, February 2004.
80. Ibid.
81. Ibid., 90.
82. Ibid., 84.
83. C. Exley, "Aluminum-containing DTP vaccines," *Lancet Infectious Diseases*, 4:324, June 2004.
84. *See, e.g.*, Elizabeth Hart "Call for retraction of Jefferson et al's scientifically unsound review on aluminium and vaccine safety," March 20, 2018 email to Tom Jefferson, https://elizabethhart.files.wordpress.com/2018/03/call-for-retraction-of-jefferson-et-als-scientifically-unsound-review-on-aluminium-and-vaccine-safety.pdf; "Request for retraction of the Cochrane Vaccines Field systematic review re vaccine safety and aluminium," https://over-vaccination.net/2014/08/11/request-for-retraction-of-the-cochrane-vaccines-field-systematic-review-re-vaccine-safety-and-aluminium/.
85. Hart, "Call for retraction of Jefferson et al's scientifically unsound review on aluminium and vaccine safety,"
86. *See* Nordic Cochrane Centre, 2016, "Complaint to the European Medicines Agency (EMA) over maladministration at the EMA," https://nordic.cochrane.org/sites/nordic.cochrane.org/files/public/uploads/ResearchHighlights/Complaint-to-EMA-over-EMA.pdf.
87. S. Djurisic, *et al.*, "Aluminum adjuvants used in vaccines versus placebo or no intervention (Protocol)," Cochrane Database of Systematic Reviews 2017, Issue 9. Art. No.: CD012805, http://onlinelibrary.wiley.com/doi/10.1002/14651858.CD012805/pdf.
88. Ibid.
89. In the US, only aluminum salts and the adjuvant system AS04 are used, and in the EU, along with those adjuvants, MF59, AS03, and viromes are used. Ibid., 3.
90. Ibid.
91. Fed. Reg. Vol. 49, No. 107, at 23007 (June 1, 1984).
92. Khan, "Slow CCL2-dependent translocation of biopersistent particles from muscle to brain," note 40 above, at 16.
93. Exley, "Aluminum-containing DTP vaccines," note 83 above. According to Dr. Exley and his colleagues, immunologists have studied aluminum adjuvants, solely for their purpose as an immune stimulant, without taking into account their effect on other pathways in the human body following vaccination. Exley, *et al.* "The immunobiology of aluminum adjuvants: how do they really work?"

note 14 above, at 103. In fact, the efficacy of aluminum based adjuvants and the toxicity of aluminum may be two sides of the same coin. Whether aluminum is an effective adjuvant in potentiating the effect of the antigen in a vaccine and whether it can cause neurotoxic and other damage, particularly neurotoxic harm, are both impacted by the ability of aluminum to travel to points in the body away from the injection site. Khan, note 40 above.

94. "Department of Health and Human Services National Vaccine Program Office Presents: Workshop on Aluminum in Vaccines," note 32 above, at 10.

95. *See, e.g.,* M. J. Caulfield, *et al.,* "Effect of Alternative Aluminum Adjuvants on the Absorption and Immunogenicity of HPV 16 L1 VLPs in Mice," *Human Vaccines,* 3(4):139–145, at 141–142 (2007); W. Ruiz, *et al.,* "Kinetics and isotype profile of antibody responses in rhesus macaques induced following vaccination with HPV 6, 11, 16 and 18 L1-virus-like particles formulated with or without Merck Aluminum Adjuvant," *Journal of Immune Based Therapies and Vaccines,* 3:2 (2005), https://www.ncbi.nlm.nih.gov/pmc/articles /PMC1097753/pdf/1476-8518-3-2.pdf; S. L. Giannini, *et al.,* "Enhanced humoral and memory B cellular immunity using HPV16/18 L1 VLP vaccine formulated with the MPL/aluminium salt combination (AS04) compared to aluminium salt only," *Vaccine* 24(33–34):5937–5949, August 14, 2006. The adjuvants in Gardasil and Cervarix are very different compounds. Gardasil contains amorphous aluminum hydroxyphosphate sulfate (AAHS), an aluminum salt adjuvant that Merck claims is proprietary. In Cervarix, GSK employs a proprietary GSK product identified as AS04 (Adjuvant System 04), an emulsion of aluminum hydroxide and monophosphoryl lipid A (MPL), "a detoxified form of the lipopolysaccharide extracted from the Gram-negative bacterium Salmonellas Minnesota strain R595" which itself has immune stimulatory activity. *See* N. Garçon, *et al.,* "The safety evaluation of adjuvants during vaccine development: The AS04 experience," *Vaccine,* 29:4453–4459, at 4454, 2011. Cervarix seems to be the more immunogenic vaccine based on its adjuvant, which research suggests further activates the immune system by the inclusion of MPL. K. S. Kim, *et al.,* "Current status of human papillomavirus vaccines," *Clinical and Experimental Vaccine Research,* 3:168–175 (2014); M. Safaeian, *et al.,* "Durability of Protection Afforded by Fewer Doses of the HPV16/18 Vaccine: The CVT Trial," *Journal of the National Cancer Institute,* 110(2):djx158 (2018), https://academic.oup.com/jnci/article-abstract/110/2/djx158/4096545/ Durability-of-Protection-Afforded-by-Fewer-Doses?redirectedFrom=fulltext.

96. *See, e.g.,* Tavares, *et al.,* "Safety Assessment of adjuvanted vaccines: Methodological Considerations," *Human Vaccines & Immunotherapeutics,* note 54 above, at 1816, July 2015.

97. "Workshop on Adjuvants and Adjuvanted Preventive and Therapeutic Vaccines for Infectious Disease Indications," note 1 above, at 40.

98. Caulfield, *et al.* "Effect of Alternative Aluminum Adjuvants on the Absorption and Immunogenicity of HPV 16 L1 VLPs in Mice," note 95 above, at 141–42;

Gupta and Rost, "Aluminum Compounds as Vaccine Adjuvants," note 53 above, at 65.

99. *See, e.g.*, N. Petrovsky, "Comparative Safety of Vaccine Adjuvants: A Summary of Current Evidence and Future Needs," *Drug Safety*, 38(11):1059–1074, Nov. 2015; Caulfield, "Aluminum Compounds as Vaccine Adjuvants", note 95 above; "Guideline on Adjuvants in Vaccines for Human Use," European Medicines Agency, Committee for Medicinal Products for Human Use (CHMP), EMEA/CHMP/VEG/134716/2004, at 5, January 20, 2005, http://vaccine-safety-training.org/tl_files/vs/pdf/EMEA.pdf.

100. "Workshop on Adjuvants and Adjuvanted Preventive and Therapeutic Vaccines for Infectious Disease Indications," note 1 above, at 27; CHMP "Guideline on Adjuvants in Vaccines for Human Use," note 99 above, at 5.

101. "Workshop on Adjuvants and Adjuvanted Preventive and Therapeutic Vaccines for Infectious Disease Indications," note 1 above, at 433. While one cannot rely directly on the safety profile of one adjuvant/antigen combination to prove the safety of another, comparison can offer some insight. Recombivax HB, a Merck vaccine against Hepatitis B contains 0.25 mg (250 mcgs) of AAHS in the pediatric dose. As described below, the Recombivax data (taken from the package insert) should have raised concerns regarding AAHS. Recombivax HB package insert, at 6–7 (Sec. 11), https://www.merck.com/product/usa/pi_circulars/r/recombivax_hb/recombivax_pi.pdf. Adverse events reported after Recombivax HB are similar to those associated with Gardasil. The package insert notes that apnea has been observed in some premature infants following vaccination and also that in clinical trials systemic adverse reactions were reported in 10.4% of healthy children and infants. The clinical trials on healthy infants and children were small – only 147 infants and children up to age 10 – and they were only monitored for 5 days following each dose. A variety of systemic disorders, including musculoskeletal and connective tissue, cardiac, psychiatric, nervous system, and blood and lymphatic disorders were reported in clinical trials. Ibid.

In addition, post-marketing reports for Recombivax HB include many different systemic disorders, including a variety of immune system disorders, including systemic lupus erythematosus (SLE), lupus-like syndrome, dermatologic reactions, and others; nervous system disorders including Guillain-Barré syndrome, multiple sclerosis, myelitis, seizures and others; skin disorders; musculoskeletal and connective tissue disorders; psychiatric disorders; and cardiac disorders including syncope and tachycardia. These reported adverse events are similar to those seen after Gardasil. Ibid. While this similarity is not direct proof AAHS is causing any of these conditions, the similarities support the need for further exploration of the potential role of AAHS in adverse events from both vaccines.

102. Caulfield, "Effect of Alternative Aluminum Adjuvants on the Absorption and Immunogenicity of HPV 16 L1 VLPs in Mice," note 95 above, at 141–42.

103. Djurisic, *et al.*, "Aluminum adjuvants used in vaccines versus placebo or no intervention (Protocol)," note 87 above, at 3.

104. Ibid.

105. CHMP "Guideline on Adjuvants in Vaccines for Human Use," note 99 above, at 5.

106. FDA, 2009. "FDA Approves New Vaccine for Prevention of Cervical Cancer," https://web.archive.org/web/20160704055116/http://www.fda.gov /NewsEvents/Newsroom/PressAnnouncements/ucm187048.htm.

107. *See* N. Garçon, et al.,"The safety evaluation of adjuvants during vaccine development: The AS04 experience," note 95 above, at 4454. Further, GSK researchers noted no cardiac, respiratory, reproductive or female fertility results in the animal subjects but did note innate immune response at the injection site, which they characterize as expected because of the use of MPL. Ibid. The researchers (GSK employees) also reported that genotoxicity studies were negative but that carcinogenicity was not examined because of purported low risk of tumor induction. Ibid.

108. *See, e.g.*, J. T. Bryan, *et al.*, "Prevention of Cervical Cancer: Journey to Develop the First Human Papillomavirus Virus-like Particle Vaccine and the Next Generation Vaccine," *Current Opinion Chemical Biology*, 32:34–47, at 37, 2016; Bryan "Developing an HPV vaccine to prevent cervical cancer and genital warts," note 56 above, at 3002; Ruiz et. al., "Kinetics and isotype profile of antibody responses in rhesus macaques induced following vaccination with HPV 6, 11, 16 and 18 L1-virus-like particles formulated with or without Merck Aluminum Adjuvant," note 95 above, at 2.

109. Caulfield, *et al.*, "Effect of Alternative Aluminum Adjuvants on the Absorption and Immunogenicity of HPV 16 L1 VLPs in Mice," note 95 above, at 141–42.

110. Ruiz, *et al.*, "Kinetics and isotype profile of antibody responses in rhesus macaques induced following vaccination with HPV 6, 11, 16 and 18 L1-virus-like particles formulated with or without Merck Aluminum Adjuvant," note 95 above, at 2.

111. Transcript of FDA Center For Biologics Evaluation And Research VRBPAC Meeting, May 18, 2006, at 14, archived at https://wayback.archive-it.org /7993/20170404052136/https://www.fda.gov/ohrms/dockets/ac/06/transcripts /2006-4222t1.pdf

112. *See* "Workshop on Adjuvants and Adjuvanted Preventive and Therapeutic Vaccines for Infectious Disease Indications," note 1 above, at 267.

113. Drug Master Files for CBER-Regulated Products, https://www.fda.gov /BiologicsBloodVaccines/DevelopmentApprovalProcess/NewDrugApplication NDAProcess/ucm211604.htm, *see also* 21 C.F.R. 314.420.

114. A copy of the authors' correspondence with the FDA is in the authors' files.

115. "Scientific Discussion," European Medicines Agency, Committee for Medicinal Products for Human Use (CHMP), at 8, http://www.ema.europa.eu/docs /en_GB/document_library/EPAR_-_Scientific_Discussion/human/000703

/WC500021140.pdf; CHMP "Guideline on Adjuvants in Vaccines for Human Use."

116. *See* S. Shirodkar, *et al.*, "Aluminum compounds used as adjuvants in vaccines," *Pharmaceutical Research*, 7(12):1282–1288, 1990; Hem and White, "Structure and Properties of Aluminum-Containing Adjuvants," note 31 above, at 257. In 1990, Shirodkar and colleagues published results of their examination of three commercially available diphtheria and tetanus toxoids, U.S.P. (the "D" and the "T" from DTP vaccines), from Connaught, Schlavo and Wyeth. The Connaught sample (labeled potassium sulfate) was found to be similar to AAHS and the Wyeth sample (labeled aluminum phosphate) was found to be aluminum hydroxyphosphate (AAHS without the sulfate).

117. Whole-cell pertussis was eventually removed from vaccines in the United States but is still used in DTP and combination vaccines in lower resource countries. "Vaccine Market," WHO, http://www.who.int/immunization/programmes_systems/procurement/market/individual_vaccine/en/. A recently published Danish study of DTP vaccinated versus unvaccinated infants in Guinea-Bissau, West Africa in the 1980s found that "DTP was associated with 5-fold higher mortality than being unvaccinated . . . .It should be of concern that the effect of routine vaccinations on all-cause mortality was not tested in randomized trials. All currently available evidence suggests that DTP vaccine may kill more children from other causes than it saves from diphtheria, tetanus or pertussis." The study suggests that even if the DTP was protective against diphtheria, tetanus and pertussis, the vaccinated children were more vulnerable to other infections. S. W. Mogensen, *et al.*, "The Introduction of Diphtheria-Tetanus-Pertussis and Oral Polio Vaccine Among Young Infants in an Urban African Community: A Natural Experiment," *EBioMedicine*, 17:192–198, at 197, 2017, http://www.ebiomedicine.com/article/S2352-3964(17)30046-4/pdf. A follow-up published article further found that the increase in female mortality in particular was statistically significant (with a mortality hazard ratio [HR] of 2.60) (for boys it was raised (HR-1.71) but not above 2.0). P. Aaby, *et al.*, "Evidence of Increase in Mortality After Introduction of Diphtheria-Tetanus-Pertussis Vaccine to Children Aged 6–35 Months in Guinea-Bissau: A Time for Reflection?" *Frontiers In Public Health*, 6:79, March 19, 2018, https://www.frontiersin.org/articles/10.3389/fpubh.2018.00079/full. The researchers noted that "studies from low-income countries have been consistent in showing deleterious effect of DTP . . . Hence, it would seem to be high time to settle whether DTP has negative effects on overall child health and if it has negative effects to explore whether alternative vaccination schedules could remove the problem." Ibid.

118. S. Humphries, video: https://www.youtube.com/watch?v=jsVq0jWfHbM&t=1444s, at 30:20–35:40, published May 28, 2017.

119. Ibid.

120. *See, e.g.,* WHO, "Weekly Epidemiological Record," July 16, 2004, note 60 above, at 270; "Workshop on Adjuvants and Adjuvanted Preventive and Therapeutic Vaccines for Infectious Disease Indications," note 1 above, at 398–99 (Dr. Deborah Novicki, Novartis, discussing animal models); E. Y. Liu, *et al.,* "Quadrivalent human papillomavirus vaccination in girls and the risk of auto-immune disorders: the Ontario Grade 8 HPV Vaccine Cohort Study," *CMAJ,* 190(21):E648-E655, May 28, 2018; C. Chao, et al., "Surveillance of autoim-mune conditions following routine use of quadrivalent human papillomavirus vaccine," *Journal of Internal Medicine,* 271(2):193–203, February 2012, https://onlinelibrary.wiley.com/doi/epdf/10.1111/j.1365-2796.2011.02467.x. Both Liu *et al.* and Chao *et al.* are discussed at Chapter 22, note 14.

121. Masson *et al.,* "Critical analysis of reference studies on the toxicokinetics of aluminum-based adjuvants," note 31 above.

122. Ibid. (noting the lack of any "official experimental investigation" of aluminum adjuvants).

123. Tomljenovic and Shaw, "Aluminum Vaccine Adjuvants: Are They Safe?", note 26 above, at 2635.

124. Ibid.

CHAPTER 21

1. 21 C.F.R. § 610.15.

2. "Draft CHMP day 180 list of outstanding issues: Gardasil 9," European Medicines Agency, Dec. 12, 2014, at 23, https://www.scribd.com/document/367386166/Gardasil-9-Draft-Day-180-LoOI-Bortredigerad?secret_password=0JoPgqAzBrofjNI3hisU.

3. Ibid.

4. "Safety Data Sheet Polysorbate 80," Sigma Aldrich, https://www.sigmaaldrich.com/catalog/product/aldrich/w291706?lang=en&region=U.S.

5. 21 C.F.R. § 172.840(c).

6. Ibid., (c)(12) and (d)(1).

7. *See, e.g.,* P. Ramge, *et al.,* "Polysorbate-80 coating enhances uptake of polybutyl-cyanoacrylate (PBCA)-nanoparticles by human and bovine primary brain capil-lary endothelial cells," *European Journal of Neuroscience,* 12:1931–1940, 2000.

8. Ibid.

9. L. Tomljenovic and C. A. Shaw, "Death after Quadrivalent Human Papillomavirus (HPV) Vaccination: Causal or Coincidental?" *Pharmaceutical Regulatory Affairs,* 12:1–11, at 9, 2012.

10. *See, e.g.,* R. K. Gherardi, and F. J. Authier, "Macrophagic myofasciitis: character-ization and pathophysiology," *Lupus,* 21:184–189, 2012.

11. M.-R. Choi, *et al.,* "Delivery of nanoparticles to brain metastases of breast cancer using a cellular Trojan horse," *Cancer Nanotechnology,* 3:47–54, 2012.

12. "Safety Data Sheet Polysorbate 80," Sigma Aldrich, https://www.sigmaal drich.com/MSDS/MSDS/DisplayMSDSPage.do?country=U.S.&language =en&productNumber=W291706&brand=ALDRICH&PageToGoToURL =https%3A%2F%2Fwww.sigmaaldrich.com%2Fcatalog%2Fproduct %2Faldrich%2Fw291706%3Flang%3Den.

13. Ibid.

14. E. Torres-Arraut, *et al.*, "Electrophysiologic effects of Tween 80 in the myocardium and specialized conduction system of the canine heart," *Journal of Electrocardiology*, 17(2):145–151, April 1984; R. E. Cober, *et al.*, "Adverse Effects of Intravenous Amiodarone in 5 Dogs," *Journal of Veterinary Internal Medicine*, 23:657–661, 2009.

15. Torres-Arraut *et al.*, "Electrophysiologic effects of Tween 80 in the myocardium and specialized conduction system of the canine heart," note 14 above.

16. Ibid.

17. M. Gajdová, *et al.*, "Delayed effects of neonatal exposure to Tween 80 on female reproductive organs in rats," *Food and Chemical Toxicology*, 31(3):183–190, 1993, (delayed toxicity in rat ovaries); *see also* B. L. Oser and M. Oser, "Nutritional studies on rats of diets containing high levels of partial ester emulsifiers. II. Reproduction and lactation," *Journal of Nutrition*, 31:183–190, 1956 (ovarian toxicity in rats at high doses).

18. *See, e.g.*, D. T. Little and H. R. Ward, "Premature ovarian failure 3 years after menarche in a 16-year-old girl following human papillomavirus vaccination" *BMJ Case Reports*, September 30, 2012, https://www.ncbi.nlm.nih.gov/pmc /articles/PMC4543769/pdf/bcr-2012-006879.pdf; S. Colofrancesco, *et al.*, "Human papilloma virus vaccine and primary ovarian failure: another facet of the autoimmune/inflammatory syndrome induced by adjuvants," *American Journal of Reproductive Immunology*, 70:309–316, 2013; D. T. Little and H. R. Ward, "Adolescent Premature Ovarian Insufficiency Following Human Papillomavirus Vaccination: A Case Series Seen in General Practice," *Journal of Investigative Medicine High Impact Case Reports*, Oct.-Dec. 2014:1–12, https://www.ncbi.nlm. nih.gov/pmc/articles/PMC4528880/pdf/10.1177_2324709614556129.pdf.

19. E. Viennois, *et al.*, "Dietary emulsifier-induced low-grade inflammation promotes colon carcinogenesis," *Cancer Research*, November 7, 2016, http://cancerres .aacrjournals.org/content/early/2016/11/05/0008-5472.CAN-16-1359.full-text .pdf; B. Chassaing, *et al.*, "Dietary emulsifiers impact the mouse gut microbiota promoting colitis and metabolic syndrome," *Nature*, 5(7541):92–96, March 5, 2015.

20. I. Badiu, *et al.*, "Hypersensitivity reaction to human papillomavirus vaccine due to polysorbate 80," *BMJ Case Reports*, May 8, 2012, https://www.ncbi.nlm.nih .gov/pmc/articles/PMC3351639/pdf/bcr.02.2012.5797.pdf.

21. Ibid.

22. Ibid.

23. Ibid.

24. Ibid.

25. J. M. Brotherton, *et al.*, "Anaphylaxis following quadrivalent human papilloma-virus vaccination," *CMAJ*, 179(6):525–533, at 525, September 9, 2008.

26. Gardasil package insert, at 3 (Sec. 5.2), https://www.fda.gov/downloads/biologicsbloodvaccines/vaccines/approvedproducts/ucm111263.pdf; Gardasil 9 package insert, at 4 (Sec. 5.2), https://www.fda.gov/downloads/BiologicsBloodVaccines/Vaccines/ApprovedProducts/UCM426457.pdf.

27. N. A. Halsey, "The human papillomavirus vaccine and risk of anaphylaxis," *CMAJ*, 179(6):509–510, at 509, September 9, 2008.

28. L. W. Kang, *et al.*, "Hypersensitivity reactions to human papillomavirus vaccine in Australian schoolgirls: retrospective cohort study," *BMJ*, 337:a2642, 2008, http://www.bmj.com/content/bmj/337/bmj.a2642.full.pdf.

29. Ibid.

30. K. S. Özcan, *et al.*, "Anaphylactic shock associated with intravenous amiodarone," *Journal of Cardiology Cases*, 9:61–62, 2014, https://ac.els-cdn.com/S1878540913001333/1-s2.0-S1878540913001333-main.pdf?_tid=d733180d-0a32-47ec-9f4e-181877a19154&acdnat=1531058841_12176203ebdc647b008e5e06a9fdaf94.

31. Comvax, a combination Hib/HepB vaccine manufactured by Merck and dis-continued in 2014, also contained sodium borate.

32. "Vaccine Ingredients," The Immunisation Advisory Centre (New Zealand), August 2017, http://www.immune.org.nz/sites/default/files/resources/Written%20Resources/ConcernVaccineIngredients20170825V01Final.pdf.

33. "Borax (B4Na2O7.10H2O)" ECHA, European Chemicals Agency, Substance Information: "*Danger!* According to the classification provided by compa-nies to ECHA in CLP notifications this substance may damage fertility or the unborn child and causes serious eye irritation." https://echa.europa.eu/substance-information/-/substanceinfo/100.129.152.

34. "Borax 99% pure," Unguentarium sales page, https://www.unguentarium.eu/products/borax.

35. "Food Additive Status List," FDA, https://www.fda.gov/Food/IngredientsPackagingLabeling/FoodAdditivesIngredients/ucm091048.htm#ftnB.

36. "Re-evaluation of boric acid (E 284) and sodium tetraborate (E 285) as food ad-ditives," European Food Safety Authority (EFSA), Panel on Food Additives and Nutrient Sources added to Food (ANS), *EFSA Journal*, 11(10):3407, 2013, http://onlinelibrary.wiley.com/doi/10.2903/j.efsa.2013.3407/epdf.

37. Dana C. Leavitt, "Borax could be in your caviar depending on where you get it from," *CaviarStar.com*, November 15, 2017, http://www.caviarstar.com/caviar-truffles-and-specialty-products-blog/borax-could-be-in-your-caviar-depending-on-where-you-get-it-from/.

38. *See, e.g.,* "Borax," National Library of Medicine, ToxNet Toxicology Data Network, https://toxnet.nlm.nih.gov/cgi-bin/sis/search/a?dbs+hsdb:@term+@DOCNO+328.

39. "Material Safety Data Sheet Sodium borate MSDS," ScienceLab.com, http://www.sciencelab.com/msds.php?msdsId=9924968.

40. "Re-evaluation of boric acid (E 284) and sodium tetraborate (E 285) as food additives," European Food Safety Authority (EFSA), note 36 above, at 1.

41. "Human Health and Ecological Risk Assessment for Borax Final Report," US Forest Service, February 24, 2006, archived at https://web.archive.org/web/20090513232444/https://www.fs.fed.us/foresthealth/pesticide/pdfs/022406_borax.pdf.

42 Andrea Cespedes, "Does Corn on the Cob Provide All of the Essential Amino Acids?" *LiveStrong.com*, March 27, 2018, https://www.livestrong.com/article/427417-does-corn-on-the-cob-provide-all-of-the-essential-amino-acids/.

43. Ibid.

44. F. Vesunu and V. Raman, "Histamine: A Potential Therapeutic Agent for Breast Cancer Treatment?" *Cancer Biology & Therapy*, 5(11):1472–1473, November 2006.

45. Heidi Stevenson, "Gardasil Destroys Girl's Ovaries: It Should Have Been Predicted," *Gaia-Health.com*, http://gaia-health.com/conventional-medicine/vaccines/gardasil-destroys-girls-ovaries-it-should-have-been-predicted/.

46. Cespedes, "Does Corn on the Cob Provide All of the Essential Amino Acids?" note 42 above.

47. L. Maintz and N. Novak, "Histamine and histamine intolerance," *American Journal of Clinical Nutrition*, 85(5):1185–1196, May 2007, https://academic.oup.com/ajcn/article/85/5/1185/4633007; A. Myers, "Everything You Need To Know About Histamine Intolerance," https://www.amymyersmd.com/2017/10/everything-you-need-to-know-about-histamine-intolerance/.

48. *See, e.g.,* Maintz and Novak, "Histamine and histamine intolerance," note 47 above; Myers, "Everything You Need To Know About Histamine Intolerance," note 47 above; Healthline, "Histamine Intolerance," https://www.healthline.com/health/histamine-intolerance.

49. V501 Protocol/Amendment No: 015–00, at 32, https://www.scribd.com/document/367386168/V501-015-00-PRO-VD?secret_password=j4BXCUs76g4wRtDxk5cy.

50. M. Rinaldi, *et al.*, "Anti-*Saccharomyces cerevisiae* Autoantibodies in Autoimmune Diseases: from Bread Baking to Autoimmunity," *Clinical Reviews in Allergy and Immunology*, 45:152–161, at 152, 2013.

51. Ibid.

52. V501 Protocol/Amendment No: 015–00, note 49 above, at 32.

53. Merck Sharpe & Dohme Corp. (assignee), "Process for Purifying Human Papillomavirus-Like Particles," US Patent 6,602,697 B1, at 3 and 5, August 5, 2003, https://www.lens.org/images/patent/US/6602697/B1/US_6602697_B1.pdf.

54. The Benzonase brochure can be found at www.emdmillipore.com.

55. Ibid., 4.

56. Philip Boffey,"U.S. Approves a Genetically Altered Vaccine," *New York Times*, July 24, 1986, http://www.nytimes.com/1986/07/24/us/us-approves-a-genetically -altered-vaccine.html.

57. *See, e.g.*, C. M. Gallagher and M. S. Goodwin, "Hepatitis B vaccination of male neonates and autism diagnosis, NHIS 1997–2002," *Journal of Toxicology and Environmental Health, Part A*, 73(24):1665–77, 2010; C. M. Gallagher and M. S. Goodwin, "Hepatitis B Triple Series Vaccine and Developmental Disability in U.S. Children Aged 1–9 Years," *Toxicology and Environmental Chemistry*, 90(5): 997–1008, 2008.

58. "Medicines in Development: Vaccines, 2016 Vaccines in Development," Pharmaceutical Research and Manufacturers of America, Phrma.org, 2016, http: //phrma-docs.phrma.org/files/dmfile/medicines-in-development-drug-list -vaccines4.pdf; "Medicines in Development, Update 2017: Vaccines," Pharmaceutical Research and Manufacturers of America, Phrma.org, http: //phrma-docs.phrma.org/files/dmfile/MID_Vaccines_2017.PDF.

59. P. A. Offit, *Pandora's Lab: Seven Stories of Science Gone Wrong*, at Ch. 8.3 (Washington, DC: Nat'l Geographic, 2017).

60. *See, e.g.*, "Are You Concerned Over Genetically Modified Vaccines?" National Vaccine Information Center, *NVIC.org*, October 2, 2012, https://www.nvic .org/NVIC-Vaccine-News/October-2012/Are-You-Concerned-Over- Genetically-Modified-Vaccin.aspx#comments.

CHAPTER 22

1. D. Kanduc, "Quantifying the possible cross-reactivity risk of an HPV16 vaccine," *Journal of Experimental Therapeutics & Oncology*, 8:65–76, at 65, 2009.

2. L. Tomljenovic and C. A. Shaw, "Answers to Common Misconceptions Regarding the Toxicity of Aluminum Adjuvants in Vaccines," Chapter 4, 43– 55, *Vaccines & Autoimmunity*, at 46, eds.: Y. Shoenfeld *et. al.*, (Hoboken, NJ: Wiley Blackwell, 2015).

3. *See, e.g.*, M. J. Caulfield, *et al.*, "Effect of Alternative Aluminum Adjuvants on the Absorption and Immunogenicity of HPV 16 L1 VLPs in Mice," *Human Vaccines*, 3(4):139–145, at 143, 2007.

4. Tomljenovic and Shaw "Answers to Common Misconceptions Regarding the Toxicity of Aluminum Adjuvants in Vaccines," note 2 above, at 46; *see also* R. K. Gherardi, *et al.*, "Biopersistence and brain translocation of aluminum adjuvants of vaccines," *Frontiers in Neurology*, 6:art. 4, at 4, February 5, 2015, https:// www.frontiersin.org/articles/10.3389/fneur.2015.00004/full.

5. S. Humphries, "What Biologically Plausible Mechanisms of Action are Health Agencies Ignoring?" video from AutismOne Media, https://www.youtube.com /watch?v=jsVq0jWfHbM&t=1444s, at 24:23, published May 28, 2017.

6. R. K. Gherardi, *et al.*, "Aluminum adjuvants of vaccines injected into the muscle: Normal fate, pathology and associated disease," *Morphologie*, 100:85–94, at 86, 2016; Gherardi *et al.* "Biopersistence and brain translocation of aluminum adjuvants of vaccines," note 4 above, at 1; Tomljenovic and Shaw "Answers to Common Misconceptions Regarding the Toxicity of Aluminum Adjuvants in Vaccines," note 2 above, at 47; L. Tomljenovic and C. A. Shaw, "Aluminum Vaccine Adjuvants: Are they Safe?" *Current Medicinal Chemistry*, 18:2630–2637, at 2633, 2011. In related research, a 2012 study using a Chinese hepatitis B vaccine demonstrated that the vaccine, which included an aluminum hydroxide adjuvant, in mouse liver cells "leads to loss of mitochondrial integrity, apoptosis induction, and cell death." H. Hamza, *et al.*, "Hepatitis B vaccine induces apoptotic death in Hepa1-6 cells," *Apoptosis*, 17:516–27, at 516, 2012. The authors of that study noted that aluminum hydroxide adjuvants have been associated with MMF as well as recognize that aluminum can accumulate and cause central nervous system damage. The finding of apoptosis, or programmed cell death, is important because this phenomenon is associated with, among other things, inflammation, autoimmune conditions, and neurodegenerative conditions. Ibid., 516–17.

7. Y. Shoenfeld, *et al.*, "Introduction," 1–7, *Vaccines & Autoimmunity*, at 2 eds.: Y. Schoenfeld, *et al.* (Hoboken, NJ:Wiley Blackwell, 2015); C. Perricone, *et al.*, "Autoimmune/inflammatory syndrome induced by adjuvants (ASIA) 2013: Unveiling the pathogenic, clinical and diagnostic aspects," *Journal of Autoimmunity*, 47:1–16, at 1, 2013.

8. Shoenfeld, *et al.*, "Introduction" to *Vaccines & Autoimmunity*, note 7 above, at 3.

9. Perricone, *et al.*, "ASIA 2013," note 7 above, at 1.

10. Ibid., 2.

11. T. Verstraeten, *et al.*, "Analysis of adverse events of potential autoimmune aetiology in a large integrated safety database of AS04 adjuvanted vaccines," *Vaccine*, 26:6630–6638, at 6633, 6637, 2008.

12. Ibid., 6631.

13. Ibid., 6637.

14. A recently published study highlights this issue. The authors of a 2018 study in Ontario, Canada concluded that they did not see an increased risk of autoimmune disorders following HPV vaccination but it appears that only girls diagnosed with an autoimmune disorder between 7 and 60 days post-vaccination were even considered "exposed." E. Y. Liu, *et al.*, "Quadrivalent human papillomavirus vaccination in girls and the risk of autoimmune disorders: the Ontario Grade 8 HPV Vaccine Cohort Study," *CMAJ*, 190(21):E648-E655, May 28, 2018; *see also* C. Chao, *et al.*, "Surveillance of autoimmune conditions following routine use of quadrivalent human papillomavirus vaccine," *Journal of Internal Medicine*, 271(2):193–203, February 2012, https://onlinelibrary.wiley.com/doi/epdf/10.1111/j.1365-2796.2011.02467.x. In the Chao study, subjects

were followed only for 180 days after each Gardasil dose and only sixteen predetermined conditions appear to have been tracked.

15. Perricone, *et al.*, "ASIA 2013," note 7 above, at 1 and generally; M. Gatto, *et al.*, "Human papillomavirus vaccine and systemic lupus erythematosus," *Clinical Rheumatology*, 32:21301–1307, at 1304–05, 2013.

16. Perricone et al., "ASIA 2013," note 7 above, generally.

17. J. R. Schofield and J. E. Hendrickson, "Autoimmunity, Autonomic Neuropathy, and the HPV Vaccination: A Vulnerable Subpopulation," *Clinical Pediatrics*, 57(5):603–606, May 2018 (first published September 4, 2017).

18. Ibid.

19 M. Martínez-Lavín, "HPV Vaccination Syndrome: A Clinical Mirage, or a New Tragic Fibromyalgia Model," *Reumatología Clínica*, 14(4):211–214, July 27, 2018.

20. Schofield and Hendrickson, "Autoimmunity, Autonomic Neuropathy, and the HPV Vaccination: A Vulnerable Subpopulation," note 17 above.

21. B. Baker, *et al.*, "The safety of human papilloma virus-blockers and the risk of triggering autoimmune disease," *Expert Opinion on Drug Safety*, 14(9):1387–1394 at 1390, 2015.

22. Ibid.

23. Ibid.

24. I. Frazer, "Measuring serum antibody to human papillomavirus following infection or vaccination," *Gynecologic Oncology*, 118(1 Suppl):S8-11, at 9, June 2010; *see also* I. Frazer, "God's Gift to Women: The Human Papillomavirus Vaccine," *Immunity*, 25:179–184, at 183, 2006 (10-50-fold higher response from the vaccine).

25. N. B. Miller, "Clinical Review of Biologics License Application for Human Papillomavirus 6, 11, 16, 18 L1 Virus Like Particle Vaccine (S. cerevisiae) (STN 125126 GARDASIL), manufactured by Merck, Inc.," at 277 (Table 188) (Protocol 016 at Month 7), 312 (Table 221) (Protocol 018 at Month 7); 117 (Table 76) (Protocol 015, incl. data at Month 7), 179 (Table 122) (Protocol 013, including data at Month 7), June 8, 2006, archived at http://wayback. archive-it.org/7993/20161024002027/http://www.fda.gov/downloads/ BiologicsBloodVaccines/Vaccines/ApprovedProducts/UCM111287.pdf.

26. *See, e.g.*, R. S. Fujinami, *et al.*, "Molecular Mimicry, Bystander Activation, or Viral Persistence: Infections and Autoimmune Disease," *Clinical Microbiology Reviews*, 19(1):80–94, at 81, January 2006.

27. Baker, note 21 above, at 1390-91.

28. Ibid.

29. L. Tomljenovic and C. A. Shaw, "Death after Quadrivalent Human Papillomavirus (HPV) Vaccination: Causal or Coincidental?" *Pharmaceutical Regulatory Affairs*, 12:1–11, at 2–3, 9, 2012.

30. Ibid., 2–3, 8–9.

31. Ibid., 3.

32. Ibid.

33. "Talking About Vaccines with Dr. Paul Offit: News Briefs – August 2017 – HPV Vaccine and Chronic Diseases," Children's Hospital of Philadelphia (CHOP), video and transcript, http://www.chop.edu/video/talking-about-vaccines-dr-paul-offit-news-briefs-august-2017-hpv-vaccine-and-chronic-diseases.

34. Ibid.

35. Ibid.

36. Ibid.

37. Y. Segal, *et al.*, "Human Papilloma virus and lupus: the virus, the vaccine and the disease," *Current Opinion in Rheumatology*, 29:331–342, at Table 1, 2017; D. Kanduc and Y. Shoenfeld, "From HBV to HPV: Designing vaccines for extensive and intensive vaccination campaigns worldwide," *Autoimmunity Reviews*, 15:1054–1061, 2016; Kanduc, "Quantifying the possible cross-reactivity risk of an HPV16 vaccine," note 1 above.

38. Kanduc, "Quantifying the possible cross-reactivity risk of an HPV16 vaccine," note 1 above; Y. Segal and Y. Shoenfeld, "Vaccine-induced autoimmunity: the role of molecular mimicry and immune crossreaction," *Cellular & Molecular Immunology*, 14:1–9, 2018.

39. D. Kanduc, "Potential cross-reactivity between HPV 16 L1 protein and sudden death-associated antigens," *Journal of Experimental Therapeutics & Oncology*, 9:159–165, 2011.

40. Segal, "Human Papilloma virus and lupus: the virus, the vaccine and the disease," note 37 above, at 339 and Table 1.

41. Ibid.

42. Ibid.

43. "Talking About Vaccines with Dr. Paul Offit: News Briefs—August 2017—HPV Vaccine and Chronic Diseases," **CHOP**, note 33 above.

44. Ibid.

45. Segal, "Human Papilloma virus and lupus: the virus, the vaccine and the disease," note 37 above, at 339.

46. Baker, note 21 above, at 1390–91.

47. Transcript of Food and Drug Administration Center for Biologics Evaluation and Research, National Institutes of Health, National Institute of Allergy and Infectious Diseases "Workshop on Adjuvants and Adjuvanted Preventive and Therapeutic Vaccines for Infectious Disease Indications," December 2, 2008, at 34, archived at https://web.archive.org/web/20170304081353/https://www.fda.gov/downloads/biologicsbloodvaccines/newsevents/workshopsmeetings-conferences/ucm095708.pdf.

48. Kanduc and Shoenfeld, "From HBV to HPV: Designing vaccines for extensive and intensive vaccination campaigns worldwide," note 37 above; Segal, "Human Papilloma virus and lupus: the virus, the vaccine and the disease," note 37 above, at 339.

49. Koh, "A vaccine against cervical cancer for poor countries," No. 55, October 11, 2017, https://www.dkfz.de/en/presse/pressemitteilungen/2017/dkfz-pm-17-55-A-vaccine-against-cervical-cancer-for-poor-countries.php; "HPV: Neue Vakzine soll Impfquote steigern," April 12, 2018, https://www.gesundheitsstadt-berlin.de/hpv-neue-vakzine-soll-impfquote-steigern-12240/, translated at "HPV: New vaccine to increase vaccination rate," https://translate.googleusercontent.com/translate_c?depth=1&hl=en&ie=UTF8&prev=_t&rurl=translate.google.com&sl=de&sp=nmt4&tl=en&u=https://www.gesundheitsstadt-berlin.de/hpv-neue-vakzine-soll-impfquote-steigern-12240/print/&xid=17259,15700022,15700124,15700149,15700168,15700186,15700190,15700201,15700208&usg=ALkJrhgr7mQDwNk5KA_lHKu5iAY52kb-_Q.

Chapter 23

1. "Pap and HPV Testing," NCI, www.cancer.gov/types/cervical/pap-hpv-testing-fact-sheet#q4; "Cervical Cancer Screening," The American College of Obstetricians and Gynecologists (ACOG), 2017, www.acog.org/Patients/FAQs/Cervical-Cancer-Screening; Tara Parker-Pope, "New Guidelines Advise Less Frequent Pap Smears," *New York Times*, March 14, 2012, https://well.blogs.nytimes.com/2012/03/14/new-guidelines-advise-less-frequent-pap-smears.

2. ACOG, "Cervical Cancer Screening," note 1 above.

3. G. F. Sawaya and M. J. Huchko, "Cervical Cancer Screening," *Medical Clinics of North America*, 101:743–753, at 744, 2017.

4. W. K. Kinney and W. K. Huh, "Protection against cervical cancer versus decreasing harms from screening–What would u.s. patients and clinicians prefer and do their preferences matter?" *Preventative Medicine*, 98:31–32, may 2017.

5. G. Koliopoulos, *et al.*, "Cytology versus HPV Testing for Cervical Cancer Screening in the General Population," *Cochrane Database of Systematic Reviews*, Issue 8, 2017, http://cochranelibrary-wiley.com/doi/10.1002/14651858.CD008587.pub2/abstract;jsessionid=EDBFB3F3687C37D9E3342C-6C42DA8505.f01t03; *see also* M. Schiffman, *et al.*, "Carcinogenic human papillomavirus infection," *Nature Reviews Disease Primers*, 2:1–20, at 11, December 2016; Health Information and Quality Authority (HIQA), 2017 "HIQA advises a change to HPV testing as the primary cervical screening method for same benefits in fewer screenings," www.hiqa.ie/hiqa-news-updates/hiqa-advises-change-hpv-testing-primary-cervical-screening-method-same-benefits; Davis, Lauren, "So long, Pap Smears — HPV Screening Found to Be Better at Cancer Detection," *Lab+Life Scientists*, www.labonline.com.au/content/life-scientist/article/so-long-pap-smears-hpv-screening-found-to-be-better-at-cancer-detection-1299747981; McNeil, Donald, "DNA Test Outperforms Pap Smear," *New York Times*, April 6, 2009, www.nytimes.com/2009/04/07/health/07virus.html?mcubz=0.

6. Dr. Sin Hang Lee, interview with author, April 30, 2017.

7. A. J. Blatt, *et al.*, "Comparison of Cervical Cancer Screening Results Among 256,648 Women in Multiple Clinical Practices," *Cancer Cytopathology*, 282–288, at 286–87, May 2015.

8. C. Zhao, *et al.*, "Cytopathology and More: Evidence emerging for HPV-negative cervical cancer," January 2014, http://www.captodayonline.com/cytopathology-and-more-evidence-emerging-for-hpv-negative-cervical-cancer/.

9. *See, e.g.*, "FDA-Approved HPV Tests," LabCE, www.labce.com/spg761630_fda_approved_hpv_tests.aspx; "cobas® HPV Test," www.hpv16and18.com/index.html; Roche Molecular Diagnostics, "cobas® HPV Test," https://molecular.roche.com/assays/cobas-hpv-test/.

10. Schiffman, *et al.*, "Carcinogenic human papillomavirus infection," note 5 above; Tara Haelle, "Could Making Cancer Screening Simpler Increase Women's Risk?" *NPR.org*, www.npr.org/sections/health-shots/2017/10/11/556895389/could-making-cancer-screening-simpler-increase-womens-risk; HIQA, "HIQA advises a change to HPV testing as the primary cervical screening method for same benefits in fewer screenings," note 5 above; Christina Finn, "Explainer: Here's what you need to know about the new HPV test for cervical cancer," *TheJournal.ie*, May 3, 2018, http://www.thejournal.ie/explainer-hpv-test-3989627-May2018/; Davis, "So Long, Pap Smears," note 5 above; "The National Cervical Screening Program," Australian Clinical Labs, http://www.clinicallabs.com.au/doctor/testing-guide/hpv-screening-program/; Department of Health and Social Care (UK), "Changes to cervical cancer screening," July 6, 2016, https://www.gov.uk/government/news/changes-to-cervical-cancer-screening; Locke, Tim, "England Changes Cervical Cancer Screening: HPV Test First," *Medscape*, July 7, 2016, https://www.medscape.com/viewarticle/865837.

11. Haelle, "Could Making Cancer Screening Simpler Increase Women's Risk?" note 10 above.

12. Ibid.

13. Ibid.

14. Australian Clinical Labs, "The National Cervical Screening Program," note 10 above.

15. Ibid.

16. "Prevention of Cervical Cancer through Screening Using Visual Inspection with Acetic Acid (VIA) and Treatment with Cryotherapy," WHO, http://apps.who.int/iris/bitstream/10665/75250/1/9789241503860_eng.pdf?ua=1; "Screening still the 'best buy' for tackling cervical cancer," WHO, www.who.int/bulletin/volumes/89/9/11-030911/en/.

17. Jason Beaubein, "Botswana Doctors Stop Cervical Cancer With A Vinegar Swab," *NPR.org*, www.npr.org/sections/health-shots/2012/09/18/161264247/botswana-doctors-stop-cervical-cancer-with-a-vinegar-swab; C. Gallay, *et al.*, "Cervical cancer screening in low-resource settings: A smartphone image application as an alternative to colposcopy," *International Journal of Women's Health*,

9:455–461, June 22, 2017, www.dovepress.com/cervical-cancer-screening-in-low-resource-settings-a-smartphone-image--peer-reviewed-fulltext-article-IJWH; Amelia Martyn-Hemphill, "How 'cervical selfies' can help save lives," *BBC News* film, www.bbc.com/news/av/magazine-41553186/how-cervical-selfies-can-help-save-lives; *see also* M. Arbyn, *et al.*, "Low Cost versus Other Screening Tests to Detect Cervical Cancer or Precancer in Developing Countries (Protocol)," *Cochrane Database of Systematic Reviews* 22: Art. No. CD010186, 2012, http://onlinelibrary.wiley.com/doi/10.1002/14651858.CD010186/full.

18. Gallay, "Cervical cancer screening in low-resource settings: A smartphone image application as an alternative to colposcopy," note 17 above.

19. "Prevention of Cervical Cancer through Screening Using Visual Inspection with Acetic Acid (VIA) and Treatment with Cryotherapy," WHO, note 16 above.

20. P. Vassilakos, *et al.*, "Use of swabs for dry collection of self-samples to detect human papillomavirus among Malagasy women," *Infectious Agents and Cancer*, 11:13, March 17, 2016, www.ncbi.nlm.nih.gov/pmc/articles/PMC4794859/pdf/13027_2016_Article_59.pdf. These kits also are available in higher resource countries. *See, e.g.*, "Kit Questions," MyLab, www.mylabbox.com/resources/faq/; "Collecting Your Sample," uBiome, https://ubiome.com/smartjane-instructions/.

21. M. Kunckler, *et al.*, "Cervical cancer screening in a low-resource setting: A pilot study on an HPV-based screen-and-treat approach," *Cancer Medicine*, 6(7):1752–1761, 2017, https://onlinelibrary.wiley.com/doi/epdf/10.1002/cam4.1089; M. R. Zimmermann, *et al.*, "Cost-effectiveness of cervical cancer screening and preventative cryotherapy at an HIV treatment clinic in Kenya," *Cost Effectiveness and Resource Allocation*, 2017, https://resource-allocation.biomedcentral.com/track/pdf/10.1186/s12962-017-0075-6?site=resource-allocation.biomedcentral.com.

22. Australian Clinical Labs, "The National Cervical Screening Program," note 10 above.

23. T. Ngoma, *et al.*, "Downstaging cancer in rural Africa," *International Journal of Cancer*, 136:2875–2879, at 2875, 2879, 2015.

24. Ibid., 2877–78.

25. L. Gattoc, *et al.*, "Phase I dose-escalation trial of intravaginal curcumin in women for cervical dysplasia," *Open Access Journal of Clinical Trials*, 9:1–10, at 2–3, 2017, www.dovepress.com/phase-i-dose-escalation-trial-of-intravaginal-curcumin-in-women-for-ce-peer-reviewed-fulltext-article-OAJCT; P. Basu, *et al.*, "Clearance of cervical human papillomavirus infection by topical application of curcumin and curcumin containing polyherbal cream: a phase II randomized controlled study," *Asian Pacific Journal of Cancer Prevention*, 14(10):5753–5759, 2013, https://pdfs.semanticscholar.org/8461/4b5eba6dbdf034d35a6ed0ea5e2ff93b6682.pdf?_ga=2.46708263.1873140030.1529846340–1702088048.1529846340.

26. "Phase II Evaluation of AHCC for the Eradication of HPV Infections (AHCC4HPV)," ClinicalTrials.gov, https://clinicaltrials.gov/ct2/show/NCT02 405533?term=AHCC&rank=1.

27. Kristen Fischer, "In First Human Trial, Mushroom Extract Cures HPV Infections," *HealthLine.com*, November 6, 2014, www.healthline.com/health-news/mushroom-extract-cures-hpv-infections-110614; "Women's Health Integrative Medicine Research Program," University of Texas Health, Department of Obstetrics, Gynecology and Reproductive Sciences, https://med.uth.edu/obgyn/research/womens-health-integrative-medicine-research-program/; "Phase II Evaluation of AHCC for the Eradication of HPV Infections (AHCC4HPV)," ClinicalTrials.gov, note 26 above.

28. G. Shafi, *et al.*, "Induction of apoptosis in HeLa cells by chloroform fraction of seed extracts of *Nigella sativa*," *Cancer Cell International*, 9:29, November 27, 2009, https://cancerci.biomedcentral.com/track/pdf/10.1186/1475-2867-9-29; S. J. Ichwan, *et al.*, "Apoptotic Activities of Thymoquinone, an Active Ingredient of Black Seed (Nigella sativa), in Cervical Cancer Cell Lines," *Chinese Journal of Physiology*, 57(5):249-255, October 31, 2014; M. Imran, *et al.*, "Thymoquinone: A novel strategy to combat cancer: A review," *Biomedicine & Pharmacotherapy*, 106:390-402, June 29, 2018.

29. *See, e.g.*, J.-M. Gong, *et al.*, "The association between MTHFR polymorphism and cervical cancer," *Scientific Reports*, 8(1):7224, May 8, 2018, https://www.ncbi.nlm.nih.gov/pmc/articles/PMC5940696/pdf/41598_2018_Article_25726.pdf; H. Cunzhi, *et al.*, "Serum and tissue levels of six trace elements and copper/zinc ratio in patients with cervical cancer and uterine myoma," *Biological Trace Element Research*, 94(2):113-22, August 2003; L. Guo, *et al.*, "Associations between antioxidant vitamins and the risk of invasive cervical cancer in Chinese women: A case-control study," *Scientific Reports*, 5:13607, September 4, 2015, https://www.nature.com/articles/srep13607.pdf. .

30. *See, e.g.*, "Folic Acid Clinical Trial for the Prevention of Cervical Cancer," ClinicalTrials.gov, https://www.clinicaltrials.gov/ct2/show/NCT00703196; W. Zhao, "Association between folate status and cervical intraepithelial neoplasia," *European Journal of Clinical Nutrition*, 70:837-842, 2016, https://www.ncbi.nlm.nih.gov/pmc/articles/PMC4940925/pdf/ejcn201635a.pdf; C. J. Piyathilake, *et al.*, "Lower Risk of Cervical Intraepithelial Neoplasia in Women with High Plasma Folate and Sufficient Vitamin B12 in the Post-Folic Acid Fortification Era," *Cancer Prevention Research (Phila)*, 2(7):658-664, July 2009, http://cancerpreventionresearch.aacrjournals.org/content/2/7/658.long; M. Karamali, *et al.*, "The favourable effects of long-term selenium supplementation on regression of cervical tissues and metabolic profiles of patients with cervical intraepithelial neoplasia: a randomised, double-blind, placebo-controlled trial," *British Journal of Nutrition*, 114(12):2039-2045, December 28, 2015, https://www.cambridge.org/core/services/aop-cambridge-core/content/view/579B9F528040CA1CB94F0B61E59F46A4/S0007114515003852a.pdf/

favourable_effects_of_longterm_selenium_supplementation_on_regression
_of_cervical_tissues_and_metabolic_profiles_of_patients_with_cervical_in
traepithelial_neoplasia_a_randomised_doubleblind_placebocontrolled_trial
.pdf.

31. "If I Already Had the HPV Vaccine, Do I Need the HPV-9 Vaccine?" Children's Hospital of Philadelphia (CHOP), video and transcript (featuring P. A. Offit), http://www.chop.edu/video/if-i-already-had-hpv-vaccine-do-i-need-hpv-9-vaccine.

32. H. W. Chesson, *et al.*, "Impact and Cost-effectiveness of 3 Doses of 9-Valent Human Papillomavirus (HPV) Vaccine Among US Females Previously Vaccinated with 4-Valent HPV Vaccine," *Journal of Infectious Diseases*, 213:1694–1700, at 1698–99 (2016); D. M. Harper and L. R. DeMars, "HPV Vaccines—A Review of the First Decade," *Gynecologic Oncology*, 146(1):196–204, at 198, July 2017, https://www.gynecologiconcology-online.net/article/S0090-8258(17)30774-6/fulltext.

33. N. B. Miller, "Clinical Review of Biologics License Application for Human Papillomavirus 6, 11, 16, 18 L1 Virus Like Particle Vaccine (*S. cerevisiae*) (STN 125126 GARDASIL), manufactured by Merck, Inc.," at 12, June 8, 2006, archived at http://wayback.archive-it.org/7993/20161024002027/http://www.fda.gov/downloads/BiologicsBloodVaccines/Vaccines/ApprovedProducts/UCM111287.pdf.

34. J. T. Schiller and D. R. Lowy, "Developmental History of HPV Prophylactic Vaccines," in *History of Vaccine Development*, 265–284, at 266, ed.: S. A. Plotkin (Springer 2011) (referencing work of Rigoni-Stern); R. Gasparini and D. Panatto, "*Cervical Cancer: From Hippocrates through Rigoni-Stern to zur Hausen*," *Vaccine*, 27:A4-A5, 2009, at A4, May 29, 2009.

35. M. Griffiths, "'Nuns, Virgins, and Spinsters'. Rigoni-Stern and Cervical Cancer Revisited," September 23, 2011, www.physicianspractice.com/gynecological-oncology/nuns-virgins-and-spinsters-rigoni-stern-and-cervical-cancer-revisited; originally published in *British Journal of Obstetrics & Gynaecology*, 98:797–802, August 1991; Z. Liu, *et al.*, "Penises not Required: a Systemic Review of the Potential for Human Papillomavirus Horizontal Transmission that is Non-Sexual or Does not Include Penile Penetration," *Sexual Health*, 13:10–21, February 2016, http://www.publish.csiro.au/sh/SH15089.

36. D. Ferris, *et al.*, "Long-Term Study of a Quadrivalent Human Papillomavirus Vaccine," *Pediatrics*, 134(3):e657-e665, at e660, September 2014, http://pediatrics.aappublications.org/content/pediatrics/early/2014/08/12/peds.2013-4144.full.pdf.

37. E. M. Smith, *et al.*, "Evidence for Vertical Transmission of HPV from Mothers to Infants," *Infectious Diseases in Obstetrics & Gynecology*, Vol. 2010, at 1, 5–6, Article ID 326369, doi:10.1155/2010/326369; F. Bacopoulou, *et al.*, "Genital HPV in Children and Adolescents: Does Sexual Activity Make a Difference?" *Journal of Pediatric & Adolescent Gynecology*, 29(3):228-33, at 232, June 2016, http://daneshyari.com/article/preview/3961173.pdf.

38. *See* M. A. Rintala, *et al.*, "High-Risk Types of Human Papillomavirus (HPV) DNA in Oral and Genital Mucosa of Infants during Their First 3 Years of Life: Experience from the Finnish HPV Family Study," *Clinical Infectious Diseases*, 41:1728–1733, at 1731–32, 2005, https://academic.oup.com/cid/article/41/12/1728/344685. Rintala, *et al.* reported that 15% of infants tested at birth were positive for high-risk HPV in genital mucosal skin and 1.5% had persistent HPV infections at the end of the three-year follow-up period. *Ibid.* Additional studies of persistent HPV DNA have reported high concordance (37–83%) following birth up to about 6 months, whereas another study showed only 10% prevalence in babies at 24 months; Smith, "Evidence for Vertical Transmission of HPV from Mothers to Infants," note 37 above, at 1. Moreover, high-risk HPVs have been detected in 4%-15% of genital samples taken from infants who exhibit no symptoms. Bacopoulou, "Genital HPV in Children and Adolescents: Does Sexual Activity Make a Difference?", note 37 above, at 232.

39. Bacopoulou, "Genital HPV in Children and Adolescents: Does Sexual Activity Make a Difference?", note 37 above, at 232.

40. Ibid.

41. Ibid.

42. *See, e.g.*, D. J, Marais, *et al.*, "The Seroprevalence of IgG Antibodies to Human Papillomavirus (HPV) Types HPV-16, HPV-18, and HPV-11 Capsid-Antigens in Mothers and Their Children," *Journal of Medical Virology*, 79:1370–1374, 2007 (indicating multiple infection sources for children and that infection in children is a "factor which could be important in the assessment of candidates for future HPV vaccine strategies.").

43. *See, e.g.*, E. Petrosky, *et al.*, "Use of 9-Valent Human Papillomavirus (HPV) Vaccine: Updated HPV Vaccination Recommendations of the Advisory Committee on Immunization Practices," *Morbidity and Mortality Weekly Report*, 64(11):300–304, at 300, March 27, 2015, https://www.cdc.gov/mmwr/pdf/wk/mm6411.pdf; "Human papillomavirus (HPV) and cervical cancer," WHO, http://www.who.int/mediacentre/factsheets/fs380/en/; "African American Women May Benefit Less from Current HPV Vaccines for Cervical Cancer Prevention," American Association for Cancer Research (AACR), October 28, 2013, http://www.aacr.org/Newsroom/Pages/News-Release-Detail.aspx?ItemID=403#.WbFYVIqQyqA and http://mb.cision.com/Public/3069/9485752/be01030e2fc25ef5.pdf (comparing subtypes found in African-American and non-Hispanic white women with abnormal Pap tests).

44. "Basic Information about HPV and Cancer," CDC, https://www.cdc.gov/cancer/hpv/basic_info/index.htm; WHO HPV and Cervical Cancer, note 43 above; "HPV Type detect," Medical Diagnostic Laboratories L.L.C., 2007, archived at https://web.archive.org/web/20070927092931/http://www.mdlab.com/html/testing/hpv_typedetect.html; N. Munoz, *et al.*, "Epidemiological Classification of Human Papillomavirus Types Associated with Cervical Cancer," *NEJM*, 348:518–527, 2003; International Agency for Research on

Cancer (IARC) Monograph on Human Papillomaviruses, 255–313, at 259, http://monographs.iarc.fr/ENG/Monographs/vol100B/mono100B-11.pdf; "2013 Sexually Transmitted Diseases Surveillance," CDC, https://www.cdc .gov/std/stats13/default.htm; E. González-Bosquet, *et al.*, "Identification of vaccine human papillomavirus genotypes in squamous intraepithelial lesions (CIN2–3)," *Gynecologic Oncology*, 111:9–12, 2008.

45. *See, e.g.*, IARC Monograph on Human Papillomaviruses, note 44 above, at 259; *see also* S. Huang, *et al.*, "Human papillomavirus types 52 and 58 are prevalent in cervical cancers from Chinese women," *International Journal of Cancer*, 70:408–11, 1997; G. M. Clifford, *et al.*, "Worldwide distribution of human papillomavirus types in cytologically normal women in the International Agency for Research on Cancer HPV prevalence surveys: a pooled analysis," *Lancet*, 366:991–998, September 17, 2005; *see* note 44 above generally.

46. E. A. Burger, *et al.*, "Racial and Ethnic Disparities in Human Papillomavirus-Associated Cancer Burden With First-Generation and Second-Generation Human Papillomavirus Vaccines," *Cancer*, 122(13):2057–2066, July 1, 2016.

47. "Rate of New Cancers, Cervix, United States, 2015," CDC, https://gis.cdc. gov/cancer/USCS/DataViz.html; "Examples of Cancer Health Disparities," NIH, https://www.cancer.gov/about-nci/organization/crchd/about-health -disparities/examples.

48. A. C. Vidal, *et al.*, "What are the Implications of Distinct HPV Genotypes in Women of Different Ethnic/Racial Ancestry?" *Journal of Vaccines & Vaccination*, 5(3), 2014; *but see* NIH "Examples of Cancer Health Disparities," (noting that "[t]he disproportionate burden of cervical cancer in Hispanic/Latino and African American women is primarily due to a lack of screening.").

49. "African American Women May Benefit Less from Current HPV Vaccines for Cervical Cancer Prevention," AACR, note 43 above.

50. *See, e.g.*, Vidal, *et al.* "What are the Implications of Distinct HPV Genotypes in Women of Different Ethnic/Racial Ancestry?", note 48 above.

51. "African American Women May Benefit Less from Current HPV Vaccines for Cervical Cancer Prevention," AACR, note 43 above.

52. Ibid.

53. Ibid.

54. González-Bosquet *et al.*, "Identification of vaccine human papillomavirus genotypes in squamous intraepithelial lesions (CIN2–3)," note 44 above, at 9.

55. Ibid.

56. Ibid.

57. Ibid.

58. M. Stanley, "HPV vaccines," *Best Practice & Research Clinical Obstetrics & Gynaecology*, 20(2):279–293, at 287, 2006. Further confounding this issue, within each HPV type there are genomic variants and certain variants may be more or less prevalent in different populations. L. B. Freitas, *et al.*, "Human

Papillomavirus 16 Non-European Variants Are Preferentially Associated with High-Grade Cervical Lesions," *PLOS One*, 9(7) (July 2014), at 5, https://www.ncbi.nlm.nih.gov/pmc/articles/PMC4077691/pdf/pone.0100746.pdf; W. Lurchachaiwong, *et al.*, "Whole-genome sequence analysis of human papillomavirus type 18 from infected Thai women," *Intervirology*, 53: 161–6, 2010; M. M. Jelen, *et al.*, "Global Genomic Diversity of Human Papillomavirus 11 Based on 433 Isolates and 78 Complete Genomic Sequences," *Journal of Virology*, 90(11):5503–5513, June 2016; J. C. Prado, *et al.*, "Worldwide genomic diversity of the human papillomaviruses-53, 56, and 66, a group of high-risk HPVs unrelated to HPV 16 and HPV-18," *Virology*, 340:95–104, 2005; S. L. Arroyo, *et al.*, "Human Papillomavirus (HPV) genotype 18 variants in patients with clinical manifestations of HPV related infections in Bilbao, Spain," *Virology Journal*, 9:258, 2012.

59. *See, e.g.*, K. S. Cuschieri, *et al.*, "Multiple high risk HPV infections are common in cervical neoplasia and young women in a cervical screening population," *Journal of Clinical Pathology*, 57:68–72, 2004.

60. R. Senapati., *et al.*, "HPV genotypes co-infections associated with cervical carcinoma: Special focus on phylogenetically related and non-vaccine targeted genotypes," *PLOS One*, Nov. 21, 2017, http://journals.plos.org/plosone/article?id=10.1371/journal.pone.0187844.

61. Ibid.

62. Stanley, "HPV Vaccines," note 58 above; M. Stanley, *et al.*, "Chapter 12: Prophylactic HPV vaccines: Underlying mechanisms," *Vaccine*, 24S3:S3/106–S3/113, at 111, 2006.

63 T. R. Broker, Center for American Progress Special Presentation: "Preventing HPV, Easy as 1, 2, 3 Shots? Ensuring Access to the New Anti-Cancer Vaccines," January 27, 2006; https://web.archive.org/web/20081028100942/https://www.americanprogress.org/kf/hpv_event_transcript.pdf.

64. "Gardasil™ HPV Quadrivalent Vaccine May 18, 2006 VRBPAC Meeting," VRBPAC Background Document, at 25, archived at http://wayback.archive-it.org/7993/20180126170205/https://www.fda.gov/ohrms/dockets/ac/06/briefing/2006-4222B3.pdf.

65. Ibid., 13.

66. Ibid.

67. Norman W. Baylor, "June 8, 2006 Approval Letter - Human Papillomavirus Quadrivalent (Types 6, 11, 16, 18) Vaccine, Recombinant," FDA, http://wayback.archive-it.org/7993/20170722145339/https://www.fda.gov/BiologicsBloodVaccines/Vaccines/ApprovedProducts/ucm111283.htm.

68. L. Mirabello, *et al.*, "HPV16 E7 Genetic Conservation Is Critical to Carcinogenesis," *Cell*, 170(6):1164–1174, at 1164, 1166, September 7, 2017.

69. S. Fischer, *et al.*, "Shift in prevalence of HPV types in cervical cytology specimens in the era of HPV vaccinations," *Oncology Letters*, 12:601–610, at 608, 2016.

70. F. Guo, *et al.*, "Comparison of HPV prevalence between HPV-vaccinated and non-vaccinated young adult women (20–26 years)," *Human Vaccines & Immunotherapeutics*, 11(10):2337–2344, at 2338, October 2015.

71. Ibid., 2340; Fischer, *et al.*, "Shift in prevalence of HPV types in cervical cytology specimens in the era of HPV vaccinations," note 69 above, at 608.

72. L. E. Markowitz, *et al.*, "Prevalence of HPV After Introduction of the Vaccination Program in the United States," *Pediatrics*, 137(3):e20151968, at 7, March 2016, http://pediatrics.aappublications.org/content/pediatrics/early/2016/02/19/peds.2015-1968.full.pdf.

73. Ibid., 6.

74. Ibid.

75. J. Lyons-Weiler, "Biased Cochrane Report Ignores Flaws in HPV Vaccine Studies, and Studies of HPV Type Replacement," May 18, 2018, https://jameslyonsweiler.com/2018/05/18/biased-cochrane-report-ignores-flaws-in-hpv-vaccine-studies-and-studies-of-hpv-type-replacement/.

76. *See, e.g.*, Mirabello, "HPV16 E7 Genetic Conservation Is Critical to Carcinogenesis," at 1164–65, 1170, note 68 above; Freitas, *et al.* "Human Papillomavirus 16 Non-European Variants Are Preferentially Associated with High-Grade Cervical Lesions," note 58 above, at 5; M. Jiang, *et al.*, "Identification of recombinant human papillomavirus type 16 variants," *Virology*, 394:8011, at 9, 2009; M. Angulo and A. Carvajal-Rodríguez, "Evidence of recombination within human alpha-papillomavirus," *Virology Journal*, at 6, March 28, 2007, https://www.ncbi.nlm.nih.gov/pmc/articles/PMC1847806/pdf/1743-422X-4-33.pdf; Prado, *et al.*, "Worldwide genomic diversity of the human papillomaviruses-53, 56, and 66, a group of high-risk HPVs unrelated to HPV-16 and HPV-18," note 58 above.

77. T. Francis, "On the Doctrine of Original Antigenic Sin," in *Proceedings of the American Philosophical Society* (1960), at 572–578.

78. A. Vatti, *et al.*, "Original antigenic sin: A comprehensive review," *Journal of Autoimmunology*, 83:12–21, at 13–14, 2017.

79. S. Humphries and R. Bystrianyk, *Dissolving Illusions: Disease, Vaccines, and the Forgotten History*, at 323–327 (2013); Vatti, "Original antigenic sin: A comprehensive review," note 78 above, at 18–19.

80. Even Professor Ian Frazer raised the issue of OAS in 2006. Ian Frazer, "God's Gift to Women: The Human Papillomavirus Vaccine," *Immunity* 25:179–184, at 183, 2006.

81. Vatti, "Original antigenic sin: A comprehensive review," note 78 above, at 19.

82. IARC Monograph on Human Papillomaviruses at 257, note 44 above.

83. "HPV and Cancer," NCI, https://www.cancer.gov/about-cancer/causes-prevention/risk/infectious-agents/hpv-fact-sheet#r5.

84. IARC Monograph on Human Papillomaviruses at 257, note 44 above; "HPV and Cancer," NCI, note 83 above. Further, variants within an HPV type may have different biological and chemical properties that could impact the

importance or effect of certain risk factors, persistence of infection, disease progression and treatment response. For example, variants impacting the L1 proteins could effect immunogenicity and, similarly, changes that effect the E6 or E7 oncoproteins in a variant of a genotype could possibly change oncogenicity of that variant. Prado, note 76 above, at 104–05, 2005. In particular, some variants of HPV-16 appear to be associated with high-grade cervical lesions and recent research suggests that the E7 oncoprotein found in lesions and tumors is very consistent and this finding could create new pathways for research into determining who really is at risk for developing cervical cancer and in targeting treatments. Mirabello, *et al.*, "HPV16 E7 Genetic Conservation Is Critical to Carcinogenesis," note 68 above; Freitas, *et al.* "Human Papillomavirus 16 Non-European Variants Are Preferentially Associated with High-Grade Cervical Lesions," note 58 above.

85. G. D. Moschonas, *et al.*, "Association of codon 72 polymorphism of p53 with the severity of cervical dysplasia, E6-T350G and HPV16 variant lineages in HPV16-infected women," *Journal of Medical Microbiology*, 66(9):1358-1365, 2017; B. W. Stewart and C. P. Wild, "World Cancer Report 2014," at 474 (IARC 2014), http://publications.iarc.fr/Non-Series-Publications/World-Cancer-Reports/World-Cancer-Report-2014.

86. C. Zhao, *et al.*, "Cytopathology and More: Evidence emerging for HPV -negative cervical cancer," *CAP Today*, College of American Pathologists January 2014, http://www.captodayonline.com/cytopathology-and-more-evidence -emerging-for-hpv-negative-cervical-cancer/.

87. "United States Cancer Statistics Data Brief: Cancers associated with human papillomavirus, United States – 2010–2014," CDC, No. 1, December 2017, https://www.cdc.gov/cancer/hpv/pdf/USCS-DataBrief-No1-December2017-508.pdf.

88. H. zur Hausen, "Papillomaviruses in the causation of human cancers—a brief historical account," *Virology*, 384:260–265, at 261, 2009.

89. Ibid.

90. N. Erickson and P. H. Duesberg, "What if HPV does not cause cervical cancer?" *SaneVax.org*, January 20, 2015, http://sanevax.org/hpv-not-cause-cervical-cancer/.

91. "Chronic Inflammation," NCI, https://www.cancer.gov/about-cancer/causes -prevention/risk/chronic-inflammation.

92. M. Thabet, *et al.*, "Human papillomavirus (HPV) is not the main cause of pre-invasive and invasive cervical cancer among patients in Delta Region, Egypt," *Journal of Experimental Therapeutics and Oncology*, 10:247–253, at 252, 2014.

93. González-Bosquet et al., "Identification of vaccine human papillomavirus genotypes in squamous intraepithelial lesions (CIN2-3)," note 44 above, at 9.

94. A. McCormack, *et al.*, "Individual karyotypes at the origins of cervical carcinomas," *Molecular Cytogenetics*, 6:44, at 2, 20, 2013, https://molecularcytogenetics .biomedcentral.com/track/pdf/10.1186/1755-8166-6-44?site=molecularcytogenetics.biomedcentral.com.

95. Ibid., 2.

96. Ibid., generally.

97. Ibid., 16, 18–20.

98. Ibid., 2, 19.

99. J. T. Bryan, *et al.*, "Prevention of cervical cancer: journey to develop the first human papillomavirus virus-like particle vaccine and the next generation vaccine," *Current Opinion in Chemical Biology*, 32:34–47, at 38, 2016.

100. McCormack, "Individual karyotypes at the origins of cervical carcinomas," note 94 above, at 2–3, 19–20.

101. Ibid., 19.

102. Ibid.

103. "What Are the Risk Factors for Cervical Cancer?" American Cancer Society, https://www.cancer.org/cancer/cervical-cancer/causes-risks-prevention /risk-factors.html; McCormack, "Individual karyotypes at the origins of cervical carcinomas," note 94 above, at 19.

104. Larisa Brown and Michelle Nichols, "Home Fires: the World's Most Lethal Pollution," *Independent*, January 23, 2011, http://www.independent.co.uk/life-style/health-and-families/health-news/home-fires-the-worlds-most-lethal-pollution-2192000.html.

105. *See, e.g.*, A. A. Stepanenko and V. M. Kavsan, "Evolutionary karyotypic theory of cancer versus conventional cancer gene mutation theory," *Biopolymers & Cell*, 28(4):267–280, 2012.

106. Erickson and Duesberg, "What if HPV does not cause cervical cancer?", note 90 above.

CHAPTER 24

1. *Japan: Human Papillomavirus and Related Diseases Report.* HPV Information Centre. 2017, http://www.hpvcentre.net/statistics/reports/JPN.pdf.

2. Ibid.

3. Ryo Konno *et al.*, "Cervical Cancer Working Group Report," *Japanese Journal of Clinical Oncology* 40(1): i44-i50, Sept. 1, 2010 https://academic.oup.com/jjco /article/40/suppl_1/i44/947913/Cervical-Cancer-Working-Group-Report.

4. Sharon J.B. Hanley, *et al.*, "HPV vaccination crisis in Japan," *Lancet*, 385(9987):2571, June 27, 2015, http://www.thelancet.com/journals/lancet /article/PIIS0140-6736(15)61152-7/fulltext?rss%3Dyes.

5. Ibid.

6 "HPV Vaccine Raises Questions," *Japan Times editorial*, June 14, 2013, http: //www.japantimes.co.jp/opinion/2013/06/14/editorials/hpv-vaccine -raises-questions/.

7. Notification from MHLW on routine vaccination programme of HPV vaccine 2013.6.14 (in Japanese) (cited March 25, 2017); available http://www.mhlw.go .jp/stf/shingi2/0000091963.html.

8. WHO Global Advisory Committee on Vaccine Safety (GACVS), 2013. "Update on human papillomavirus vaccines." http://www.who.int/vaccine_safety/committee /topics/hpv/Jun_2013/en/.

9. R. Wilson, *et al.*, "The HPV Vaccination in Japan: Issues and Options," *Center for Strategic and International Studies*, at 8, May 2014, https://csis-prod. s3.amazonaws.com/s3fs-public/legacy_files/files/publication/140514_Wilson _HPVVaccination_Web.pdf.

10. Hanley *et al.*, "HPV vaccination crisis in Japan," note 4 above.

11. Wilson "The HPV Vaccination in Japan: Issues and Options," note 9 above, at 7.

12. T. Nakayama, "Vaccine chronicle in Japan," *Journal of Infection and Chemotherapy*, 19(5):787–798, July 9, 2013, https://www.ncbi.nlm.nih.gov/pmc/articles/ PMC3824286/.

13. Wilson 2014, "The HPV Vaccination in Japan: Issues and Options," note 9 above, at 7–8.

14. Ibid., 6.

15. Ibid.

16. Ibid.

17. S. Gilmour, "HPV vaccination programme in Japan," *Lancet*, 382(9894):743–832, August 31, 2013, http://www.thelancet.com/journals/lancet/article /PIIS0140-6736%2813%2961831-0/fulltext?rss=yes.

18. Ibid.

19. "HPV Vaccine Raises Questions," *Japan Times* editorial, June 14, 2013, https: //www.japantimes.co.jp/opinion/2013/06/14/editorials/hpv-vaccine-raises -questions/#.Wz_C-C2ZNuU.

20. Ibid.

21. Norma Erickson, "Japan and the HPV Controversy," *SaneVax, Inc.*, April 8, 2014, http://sanevax.org/japan-hpv-vaccine-controversy/.

22. Ibid.

23. S. Yokota, *et al.*, "General overview and discussion on hpv vaccine associated neuropathic syndrome," *Japan Medical Journal (Nihon Iji Shimpou)* 2015;4758:46–53 (in Japanese); "Dispute Over HPV Vaccinations," *Japan Times* editorial (English), July 29, 2016, https://www.japantimes.co.jp/opinion/2016/07/29 /editorials/dispute-over-hpv-vaccinations/#.Wz_ISy2ZNuU.

24. H. Beppu, *et al.*, "Lessons learnt in Japan from adverse reactions to the HPV vaccine: a medical ethics perspective," *Indian Journal of Medical Ethics*, 11(2):82–88, April-June 2017, http://ijme.in/wp-content/uploads/2017/04/252the82_lessons _learnt.pdf.

25. International symposium on HPV vaccines Feb 25–26, 2014, https://www .ft.dk/samling/20131/almdel/SUU/bilag/295/1340540.pdf.

26. Norma Erickson, "Japan and the HPV Controversy," *SaneVax, Inc.*, April 8, 2014, http://sanevax.org/japan-hpv-vaccine-controversy/.

27. "The Public Hearing on Adverse Events Following HPV Vaccine in Japan," Ministry of Health, Labour and Welfare, Transcript, February 26, 2014, https://www.mhlw.go.jp/stf/shingi/0000048229.html.

28. Ibid.

29. Ibid.

30. Ibid.

31. WHO Global Advisory Committee on Vaccine Safety, 2014. "Statement on the continued safety of HPV vaccination," http://www.who.int/vaccine_safety/committee/topics/hpv/GACVS_Statement_HPV_12_Mar_2014.pdf.

32. Sin Hang Lee, "Allegations of Scientific Misconduct by GACVS/WHO/CDC Representatives," SaneVax, Jan. 14, 2016. http://sanevax.org/wp-content/uploads/2016/01/Allegations-of-Scientific-Misconduct-by-GACVS.pdf.

33. Guidelines for symptom management post HPV vaccine, in Japanese, http://dl.med.or.jp/dl-med/teireikaiken/20150819_hpv.pdf.

34. "Guidelines for HPV symptom management," *Medscape*. https://www.medscape.com/viewarticle/850436. (Link requires a free login, copy on file with the authors.)

35. Yokota, "General overview and discussion on hpv vaccine associated neuropathic syndrome," *see* note 23 above.

36. Pain should not be described as "psychogenic," http://pj.jiho.jp/servlet/pjh/organization/detail/1226582212296.html.

37. "Guidelines for HPV symptom management," *Medscape*, *see* note 34 above.

38. Ibid.

39. Tomoyuki Fujii, "Declaration to Demand the Resumption of Recommendations for Human Papillomavirus (HPV) Vaccination for Cervical Cancer Prevention." Japan Society of Obstetrics and Gynecology, Aug. 29, 2015. http://www.jsog.or.jp/english/declaration_20150829.html.

40. "Guidelines for HPV symptom management," *Medscape*, note 34 above.

41. "Guidelines for HPV symptom management," *Medscape*, note 34 above.

42. "Guidelines for HPV symptom management," *Medscape*, note 34 above.

43. Dr. Riko Muranaka articles defending HPV vaccine, translated, https://translate.googleusercontent.com/translate_c?depth=1&hl=en&prev=search&rurl=translate.google.com&sl=ja&sp=nmt4&u=http://wedge.ismedia.jp/articles/-/5510%3Fpage%3D2&usg=ALkJrhjvOQwy4Q5_hY634MxhfDyYfMCsCA.

44. Ian Sample, "Doctor wins 2017 John Maddox prize for countering HPV vaccine misinformation," *The Guardian*, November 30, 2017, https://www.theguardian.com/science/2017/nov/30/doctor-wins-2017-john-maddox-prize-countering-hpv-vaccine-misinformation-riko-muranaka.

45. Justin McCurry, "Vaccine Battle Stakes are High," *The Foreign Correspondents Club of Japan*, December 28, 2016, http://www.fccj.or.jp/number-1-shimbun/item/892-vaccine-battle-stakes-are-high/892-vaccine-battle-stakes-are-high.html.

46. Riko Muranaka, "*Stopping The Spread of Japan's Antivaccine Panic,*" *Wall Street Journal,* November 28, 2016, https://www.wsj.com/articles/stopping-the-spread -of-japans-antivaccine-panic-1480006636.

47. "Japanese doctors take to courts in row over HPV vaccine," *Financial Times,* https://www.ft.com/content/f6f7b394-bba2-11e6-8b45-b8b81dd5d080.

48. McCurry, "Vaccine Battle Stakes are High," *see* note 45 above.

49. Ian Sample, "Doctor wins 2017 John Maddox prize for countering HPV vaccine misinformation," *see* note 44 above.

50. "Japanese doctors take to courts in row over HPV vaccine," *see* note 47 above.

51. K. Ozawa, *et al.,* "Suspected Adverse Effects After Human Papillomavirus Vaccination: A Temporal Relationship Between Vaccine Administration and the Appearance of Symptoms in Japan 2017," *Drug Safety,* 40(12):1219–1229, December 2017, https://link.springer.com/article/10.1007/s40264-017-0574-6.

52. Ibid.

53. H. J. Larson, *et al.,* "Tracking the global spread of vaccine sentiments: the global response to Japan's suspension of its HPV vaccine recommendation," *Human Vaccines & Immunotherapeutics,*10(9):2543–2550, 2014.

54. "Project Mission," Vaccine Confidence, http://www.vaccineconfidence.org /about/#mission.

55. R. Wilson, *et al.,* "HPV Vaccination in Japan: The Continuing Debate and Global Impacts," *Center for Strategic and International Studies,* April 2015, https://csis-prod.s3.amazonaws.com/s3fs-public/legacy_files/files/publica-tion/150422_Wilson_HPVVaccination2_Web.pdf. (2014 report does not dis-close funding.)

56. Wilson, "The HPV Vaccination in Japan: Issues and Options," *see* note 9 above.

57. "About Us," Center for Strategic and International Studies. https://www.csis .org/programs/about-us.

58. Wilson "HPV Vaccination in Japan: The Continuing Debate and Global Impacts," *see* note 55 above, at 7.

59. Ibid.

60. Ibid., 8.

61. Ibid., 2.

62. Ibid., 9.

63. Ibid., 9.

64. Ibid., 1.

65. Mizuho Aoki, "Suit Opens In Tokyo Court Over Cervical Cancer Vaccine Side Effects," *Japan Times,* February 13, 2007, https://www.japantimes.co.jp /news/2017/02/13/national/crime-legal/suit-opens-tokyo-court-cervical-cancer -vaccine-side-effects/#.W0DU4y2ZNuU.

66. H. Beppu, *et al.,* "Lessons learnt in Japan from adverse reactions to the HPV vaccine: a medical ethics perspective," note 24 above.

CHAPTER 25

1. "Human Papillomavirus and Related Diseases Report: Denmark." HPV Information Centre. July 27, 2017. http://www.hpvcentre.net/statistics/reports/DNK.pdf.

2. HPV vaccine available Matas cosmetic store, Denmark, https://www.matas.dk/danish-vaccination-service.

3. L. Amet, et al., "Changing the course of autism: The science and intervention," OA Autism, 2(1):1, January 10, 2014, http://www.oapublishinglondon.com/article/1138.

4. Signe Daugbjerg and Michael Bech ,The Vaccinated Girls, video–since removed from the internet, formerly available at https://www.youtube.com/watch?v=GO2i-r39hok.

5. L. Brinth, et al., "Suspected side effects to the quadrivalent human papilloma vaccine," Danish Medical Journal, 62(4):A5604, April 6, 2015, https://www.ncbi.nlm.nih.gov/pubmed/25872549; L. Brinth, et al., "Orthostatic intolerance and postural tachycardia syndrome as suspected adverse effects of vaccination against human papilloma virus," Vaccine, 33(22):2602–2605, May 21, 2015, https://www.ncbi.nlm.nih.gov/pubmed/25882168; L. Brinth, et al., "Is chronic fatigue syndrome/myalgic encephalomyelitis a relevant diagnosis in patients with suspected side effects to human papilloma virus vaccine?" International Journal of Vaccines & Vaccination, 1(1):00003, June 15, 2015.

6. Danish Health Authority "Our cooperation with EMA and the Syncope Centre at the Frederiksberg Hospital," https://www.sst.dk/en/news/2015/emas-new-assessment-of-the-hpv-vaccine-the-benefits-outweigh-the-risks/2-our-cooperation-with-ema-and-the-syncope-centre-at-frederiksberg-hospital.

7. Brinth, et al., "Suspected side effects to the quadrivalent human papilloma vaccine," note 5 above.

8. Danish Health Authority "Our cooperation with EMA and the Syncope Centre at the Frederiksberg Hospital," note 6 above.

9. "EMA's New Assessment of the HPV Vaccine: The Benefits Outweigh the Risks," Danish Health Authority, April 17, 2015, https://www.sst.dk/en/news/2015/emas-new-assessment-of-the-hpv-vaccine-the-benefits-outweigh-the-risks.

10. "Liselott Blixt, Chairperson of the Danish Health Committee," Danish Parliament website, https://www.thedanishparliament.dk/en/committees/committees/suu.

11. "Massive criticism: Liselott Blixt is grossly irresponsible in HPV cases," Altinget, December 8, 2015 (translated), https://translate.google.com/translate?hl=en&sl=da&u=https://www.altinget.dk/artikel/massiv-kritik-liselott-blixt-er-groft-uansvarlig-i-hpv-sag&prev=search.

12. Danish Medicines Agency, 2016, "Public funds allocated for research into possible adverse reactions from HPV vaccination," http://laegemiddelstyrelsen.dk/en

/news/2016/public-funds-allocated-for-research-into-possible-adverse-reactions
-from-hpv-vaccination/.

13. "Chronic Symptoms After HPV Vaccination: Danes Start Study," *Medscape*, November 13, 2015, https://www.medscape.com/viewarticle/854469.

14. "Suspected Gardasil Injured Girls Queue For Help In Denmark," *NewsVoice*, June 15, 2015 (translated), https://translate.google.com/translate?hl=en&sl=auto&tl=en&u=https%3A%2F%2Fnewsvoice.se%2F2015%2F06%2F15%2Fmis-stankt-gardasilskadade-flickor-koar-for-hjalp-i-danmark%2F.

15. K. Mølbak, "Methods to Study Serious Safety Signals – Examples of HPV Vaccinations in Denmark," *Statens Serum Institut*, https://www.escmid.org/escmid_publications/escmid_elibrary/material/?mid=44377.

16. Ibid., 9–10.

17. "After a dramatic decline in HPV vaccination coverage, it now seems that the trend is reversing," *Statens Serum Institut*, October 20, 2017, https://www.ssi.dk/English/News/News/2017/2017%20-%2010%20-%20EPI-NEWS%2041%20hpv.aspx.

18. Public discussion in Copenhagen at the Danish Society for Medical Philosophy, Ethics and Method in November 2016, video on file with authors.

19. Ibid.

20. Brinth, *et al.*, "Suspected side effects to the quadrivalent human papilloma vaccine," *see* note 5 above.

21. Assessment Report, HPV, November 11, 2015, http://www.ema.europa.eu/docs/en_GB/document_library/Referrals_document/HPV_vaccines_20/Opinion_provided_by_Committee_for_Medicinal_Products_for_Human_Use/WC500197129.pdf.

22. L. Brinth, "Responsum to Assessment Report," European Medicines Agency, November 26, 2015, http://hpv-bivirkningsramte.dk/sites/default/files/Responsum%20Louise%20Brinth%20Version%201.0.pdf.

23. Ibid., 55.

24. Ibid., 29.

25. Ibid., 26.

26. Uppsala Monitoring Centre official website, https://www.who-umc.org.

27. R. Chandler, "Current Safety Concerns with Human Papillomavirus Vaccine: A Cluster Analysis of Reports in VigiBase®," *Drug Safety*, 40(1):81–90, January 2017, https://link.springer.com/article/10.1007/s40264-016-0456-3.

28. Ibid.

29. Brinth, "Responsum to Assessment Report," note 22 above, at 29.

30. "The HPV Vaccine Then and Now," *Medscape*, August 1, 2016, http://www.medscape.com/viewarticle/866591_3 (Article available with free login.)

31. Danish Health Authority, 2016. "New HPV Vaccine in the Childhood Vaccination Programme," https://sundhedsstyrelsen.dk/en/news/2016/new-hpv-vaccine-in-the-childhood-vaccination-programme.

32. Ibid.
33. P. H. Andersen on behalf of the Consultancy Team, Department of Infectious Diseas Epidemiology and Prevention, "Status on the Coverage of the HPV Vaccination Programme," *Statens Serum Institut*, November 25, 2017, http://www.ssi.dk/English/News/EPI-NEWS/2017/No%2025%20-%202017.aspx.
34. "Denmark Campaign Rebuilds Confidence in HPV Vaccination," WHO, Feb. 2018 http://www.who.int/features/2018/hpv-vaccination-denmark/en/.
35. Cervarix indicated against anal cancer by EMA. "Cervarix," EMA, June 23, 2016, http://www.ema.europa.eu/ema/index.jsp?curl=pages/medicines/human/medicines/000721/smops/Positive/human_smop_001003.jsp&mid=WC0b01ac058001d127.
36. 6m Kroner 2013–2018 Future 2 Project, https://www.cancer.dk/dyn/resources/File/file/1/5801/1474015424/samarbejdsaftale-merck-sharp-et-dohme.hpv-vaccine-follow-up-2013-2018.pdf; FUTURE 9 Project, https://www.cancer.dk/dyn/resources/File/file/2/5802/1474015476/samarbejdsaftale-merck-sharp-et-dohme.nona-ltfu-2014-2024.pdf and https://www.cancer.dk/dyn/resources/File/file/3/5803/1474015516/samarbejdsaftale-merck-sharp-et-dohme.vip-3-dose-extension-2015-2017.pdf.
37. Danish Medicines Agency, 2016, "Public funds allocated for research into possible adverse reactions from HPV vaccination," *see* note 12 above.
38. Chandler, "Current Safety Concerns with Human Papillomavirus Vaccine: A Cluster Analysis of Reports in VigiBase®," *see* note 27 above.

CHAPTER 26

1. Evelyn Ring, "Vaccine Critics Using 'Emotional Terrorism' to Stop Take-up of Cervical Cancer Jab," *Irish Examiner*, August 31, 2017, https://www.irishexaminer.com/ireland/vaccine-critics-using-emotional-terrorism-to-stop-take-up-of-cervical-cancer-jab-458051.html.
2. "Information from FDA and CDC on the safety of Gardasil Vaccine," August 20, 2009, https://www.fda.gov/BiologicsBloodVaccines/SafetyAvailability/VaccineSafety/ucm179549.htm.
3. Gardasil package insert, warnings and precautions at 1, https://www.fda.gov/downloads/biologicsbloodvaccines/vaccines/approvedproducts/ucm111263.pdf.
4. "Cancer Factsheet," National Cancer Registry Ireland, https://www.ncri.ie/sites/ncri/files/factsheets/Factsheet%20cervix.pdf.
5. Steven Carroll, "Calls to reinstate plan for vaccine," *Irish Times*, December 11, 2008. http://www.irishtimes.com/news/calls-to-reinstate-plan-for-vaccine-1.922081.
6. Eithne Donnellan, "Roll-out of cervical cancer vaccine to start before school holidays," *Irish Times*, May 8, 2010, http://www.irishtimes.com/news/roll-out-of-cervical-cancer-vaccine-to-start-before-school-holidays-1.662349.
7. Mothers Alliance, letter to Mary Harney at Comelook.org, September 8, 2010, http://www.comelook.org/MA_letter.html.

8. Ibid.

9. Jennifer Hough, "Cancer Vaccine Warning," *Irish Examiner*, August 30, 2010 http://www.irishexaminer.com/ireland/health/cancer-vaccine-warning 129227 .html.

10. "HPV vaccine uptake in Ireland: 2011/2012," Health Protection Surveillance Centre http://www.hpsc.ie/az/vaccinepreventable/vaccination/immunisatio nuptakestatistics/hpvimmunisationuptakestatistics/File,14255,en.pdf.

11. HPV vaccine brochure, Health Service Executive (HSE) https://www.hse.ie /eng/health/immunisation/pubinfo/schoolprog/hpv/hpv-vaccine-information -for-parents.pdf.

12. *Consent to Medical Treatment in Ireland: an MPS Guide for Clinicians*, Medical Protection Society handbook https://www.medicalprotection.org/docs /default-source/pdfs/Booklet-PDFs/ireland-booklets/consent-to-medical-treat- ment-in-ireland—an-mps-guide-for-clinicians.pdf?sfvrsn=0.

13. "HPV vaccine Information materials," HSE official website, https://www.hse .ie/eng/health/immunisation/pubinfo/schoolprog/hpv/hpv-information -materials/.

14. Instructions not to send PIL home with parents, slide 10. Lesley Smith, "Human Papillomavirus (HPV) vaccination," presentation by the National Immunisation Office. https://web.archive.org/web/20161024142325/http: //www.hse.ie/eng/health/immunisation/hcpinfo/conference/hpv4.pdf.

15. "Literacy in Ireland," NALA, https://www.nala.ie/literacy/literacy-in-ireland.

16. "Guidelines For Staff, School Immunization Programme, 2015/2016," Health Products Regulatory Authority (HRPA) at 24, archived at https://web.archive .org/web/20160530061903/https://www.hse.ie/eng/health/immunisation /pubinfo/schoolprog/hpv/schoolguidelines.pdf.

17. Gardasil prescribing information, Ireland, at 4, https://www.hpra.ie/docs /default-source/vaccine-pils/gardasil-pil.pdf?sfvrsn=8.

18. "HPV vaccine Information materials," HSE official website, note 13 above.

19. Martin Healy, "Irish media consensus –'HPV vaccine fears put to rest with safety report,'" *ComeLook.Org*, October 10, 2011, http://www.comelook.org /Anaphylaxis.html.

20. Kim Robinson, "Gardasil, The Decision We Will Always Regret," *SaneVax.org*, February 4, 2014, http://sanevax.org/gardasil-decision-will-always-regret//.

21. Karen, "Gardasil: I Thought I Did Enough Research – I Was Wrong," *SaneVax.org*, February 7, 2015 http://sanevax.org/gardasil-thought-enough-research-wrong/.

22. Ann Fitzpatrick, "I Want My Daughter's Life Back The Way It Was Before Gardasil," *SaneVax.org*, August 7, 2015, http://sanevax.org/i-want -my-daughters-life-back-the-way-it-was-before-gardasil/.

23. REGRET website: www.regret.ie.

24. Fiona Dillon, "Cervical cancer vaccine has made my daughter ill," *Independent*, July 15, 2015, http://www.independent.ie/life/health-wellbeing/health-features /cervical-cancer-vaccine-has-made-my-daughter-ill-31378364.html.

25. Interview with members of REGRET, email on file with the authors.

26. "Cervical Cancer Vaccine: Is it Safe?" TV3 documentary, Dr. Connolly at 8 minutes, https://www.youtube.com/watch?v=m1QF9pdE2jQ&feature=youtu. be. Copy also on file with the authors.

27. "EMA meeting with REGRET spokesparents," video by TheVaxChannel, https://www.youtube.com/watch?v=ayOoDtkRnww.

28. EMA, November 5, 2015. "Review concludes evidence does not support that HPV vaccines cause CRPS or POTS." http://www.ema.europa.eu/docs/en_GB/document_library/Press_release/2015/11/WC500196352.pdf; Assessment Report, Pharmacovigilance Risk Assessment Committee (PRAC), November 11, 2015, http://www.ema.europa.eu/docs/en_GB/document_library/Referrals_document/HPV_vaccines_20/Opinion_provided_by_Committee_for_Medicinal_Products_for_Human_Use/WC500197129.pdf.

29. S. R. Dobson, et al., "Immunogenicity of 2 doses of HPV vaccine in younger adolescents vs 3 doses in young women: a randomized clinical trial," JAMA, 309(17):1793–802, May 1, 2013, https://www.ncbi.nlm.nih.gov/pubmed/23632723.

30. Email on file with the authors.

31. Elissa Meites, et al., "Use of a 2-Dose Schedule for Human Papillomavirus Vaccination—Updated Recommendations of the Advisory Committee on Immunization Practices," Morbidity and Mortality Weekly Report (MMWR), CDC, Dec. 16, 2016 https://www.cdc.gov/mmwr/volumes/65/wr/mm6549a5.htm.

32. Darragh O'Brien, http://www.darraghobrien.ie.

33. Anna Cannon, statement to Joint Committee on Health and Children, December 3, 2015, https://webarchive.oireachtas.ie/parliament/media/committees/healthandchildren/health2015/opening-statement-by-ms.-anna-cannon,-regret.pdf.

34. EMA, November 5, 2015. "Review concludes evidence does not support that HPV vaccines cause CRPS or POTS," see note 28 above.

35. "Cervical Cancer Vaccine: Is it Safe?" TV3 documentary, see note 26 above.

36. Ibid.

37. Dr. Brenda Corcoran, "HPV Vaccination Programme Ireland," HSE presentation, at slide 4, https://www.sabin.org/sites/sabin.org/files/2hpv_presentation_ireland_iaim_010217_corcoran.pdf.

38. Irish Cancer Society, 2016. "Irish Cancer Society Presents Facts About HPV Vaccine," https://www.cancer.ie/about-us/news/facts-about-hpv#sthash.Hc1Tuqht.dpbs.

39. "HPV vaccine uptake in Ireland: 2015/2016," HSE, http://www.hpsc.ie/az/vaccinepreventable/vaccination/immunisationuptakestatistics/hpvimmunisationuptakestatistics/File,16039,en.pdf.

40. Irish Cancer Society, 2016. "Irish Cancer Society Presents Facts About HPV Vaccine," note 38 above.

41. "Margaret Stanley (Virologist)," Wikipedia, https://en.wikipedia.org/wiki /Margaret_Stanley_(virologist).

42. Rebecca Hollidge and Dr. Margaret Stanley, R.E.G.R.E.T. Facebook video, with permission, August 24, 2016, https://www.facebook.com/REGRET.ie /videos/1266265963383958/.

43. Robert O'Connor, Irish Cancer Society, "Extremists, anti-vaccine campaigners" *The Michael Reade Show,* LMFM radio, August 31, 2016: 7.40 https://www .youtube.com/watch?v=wvXtyxKvrDg.

44. "Make Up Your Own Mind," REGRET video, with permission, August 31, 2016, https://www.facebook.com/REGRET.ie/videos/1273781345965753/.

45. "HPV vaccine uptake in Ireland: 2015/2016," HSE, note 39 above, at 4.

46. Paul Cullen, "Anti-HPV vaccine campaign will cause 40 deaths - O'Connell," *Irish Times,* November 10, 2016, https://www.irishtimes.com/news/health /anti-hpv-vaccine-campaign-will-cause-40-deaths-o-connell-1.2862677.

47. David Robert, "Impartial Journalism is Laudable. But False Balance is Dangerous," *Guardian,* November 8, 2016, https://www.theguardian.com/science /blog/2016/nov/08/impartial-journalism-is-laudable-but-false-balance-is -dangerous.

48. "The HPV Vaccine," *Alive and Kicking Radio Podcast,* October 16, 2016, archived at https://web.archive.org/web/20161020011543/http://www.new stalk.com:80/podcasts/Alive_and_Kicking/Alive_And_Kicking/162104 /The_HPV_Vaccine.

49. The Niall Boylan Show. Twitter post, May 4, 2017 https://twitter.com /niallboylan4fm/status/860217892578742272.

50. "Fighting the anti-vaxxers," *Irish Medical Times,* April 26, 2017, http://www.imt .ie/opinion/fighting-the-anti-vaxxers-26-04-2017/.

51. Ruairi Hanley, "Doctors Should Fight Irrational Movement Against Vaccination," *Irish Times,* June 13, 2017, https://www.irishtimes.com/opinion /doctors-should-fight-irrational-movement-against-vaccination-1.3116926.

52. Ibid.

53. Paul Cullen, "HSE Criticises Campaign Against HPV Vaccine and Accuses Opponents of Playing God," *Irish Times,* June 28, 2017, https://www.irishtimes .com/news/health/female-suicides-up-but-total-number-falls-to-lowest-in-22 -years-1.3136879.

54. Eilish O'Regan, "'Scaremongering' over HPV vaccine puts lives at risk: Harris," *Independent.ie,* April 23, 2017, http://www.independent.ie/irish-news/health /scaremongering-over-hpv-vaccine-puts-lives-at-risk-harris-35645734.html.

55. Ibid.

56. Irish Cancer Society, 2016. "Political Education Campaign - HPV vaccine," https: //www.cancer.ie/news/HPV-vaccine-political-education-campaign#sthash. D8dwob6y.dpbs.

57. $100k July 2015 page 5: http://www.msdresponsibility.com/wp-content/uploads/2017/03/FINAL-Charitable-2015-Transparency-Report-with-Vaccines-3.17.pdf and $100k contribution October 2016 page 5: http://www.msdresponsibility.com/wp-content/uploads/2017/03/FINAL-Charitable-2016-Full-Year-Transparency-Report-3.17.pdf.

58. "That is a Lie," video by REGRET with permission, August 24, 2016, https://www.facebook.com/REGRET.ie/videos/1743081085702441/.

59. Irish Cancer Society and HPV Alliance, 2017. "Urgent Action Required to Address Dramatic Fall in Uptake of Cancer Vaccine – HPV Vaccination Alliance." https://www.cancer.ie/about-us/news/hpv-vaccination-alliance#sthash.md5Tlb1B.dpbs.

60. Allison Bray, "Parents told to ignore 'fake news' over teen HPV jabs," *Independent.ie*, August 10, 2017, https://www.independent.ie/irish-news/health/parents-told-to-ignore-fake-news-over-teen-hpv-jabs-36017584.html.

61. KIRBY-V- HEALTH PRODUCTS REGULATORY AUTHORITY 2015 8185 P, http://highcourtsearch.courts.ie/hcslive/common.processNavigationButton.

62. Mary Carolan, "Court Told of 'Horrendous Adverse Effects of HPV Vaccine," *Irish Times*, March 15, 2016, https://www.irishtimes.com/news/crime-and-law/courts/high-court/court-told-of-horrendous-adverse-effects-of-hpv-vaccine-1.2414549.

63. "Judge Dismisses Legal Challenge over Cervical Cancer Vaccine," *Irish Times*, Mar. 15, 2016 https://www.irishtimes.com/news/crime-and-law/courts/high-court/judge-dismisses-legal-challenge-over-cervical-cancer-vaccine-1.2574391.

64. *Guidelines For Vaccinations In General Practice 2018*, HSE, at 17, https://www.hse.ie/eng/health/immunisation/infomaterials/pubs/guidelinesgp.pdf.

65. "Health Services Let This Happen," *Vaxxed TV*, May 8,2017, https://www.youtube.com/watch?v=yeP-eIyibQM&feature=youtu.be.

66. "How Jack & Jill Begun: The Story," The Jack & Jill Children's Foundation Website https://www.jackandjill.ie/about-jack-and-jill/.

67. Helen O'Callaghan, "Why the HPV-vaccine programme needs to be gender neutral," *Irish Examiner*, March 17, 2017, http://www.irishexaminer.com/lifestyle/healthandlife/why-the-hpv-vaccine-programme-needs-to-be-gender-neutral-445332.html.

68. "HIQA to research extending HPV vaccine to boys," RTE News, July 4, 2017, https://www.rte.ie/news/health/2017/0704/887592-hpv-vaccine/.

69. Ibid.

70. Health Information and Quality Authority (HIQA), 2018. "HIQA announces public consultation on extending HPV vaccination programme to include boys." https://www.hiqa.ie/hiqa-news-updates/hiqa-announces-public-consultation-extending-hpv-vaccination-programme-include.

71. RCPI, 2018: "The Opportunity To Eliminate HPV Cancers," https://www.imt.ie/events/opportunity-eliminate-hpv-cancers-royal-college-physicians-ireland-monday-9th-july-04-07-2018/.

72. RCPI, 2018, "The RCPI calls for boys to get the HPV vaccine," https://www. rcpi.ie/news/releases/the-royal-college-of-physicians-of-ireland-calls-for-boys-to-get-the-hpv-vaccine/.

73. Míheal Lehane, *RTE News* July 9, 2018, https://www.rte.ie/news/ politics/2018/0709/977474-hpv-protest/.

74. Twitter post of the RCPI honoring Professor Frazer with a fellowship, July 9, 2018, https://twitter.com/RCPI_news/status/1016415877703655424.

75. HSE, 2018, "HSE confirms nearly two in every three girls getting HPV Vaccine," https://www.hse.ie/eng/services/news/media/pressrel/hse-confirms-nearly-two-in-every-three-girls-getting-hpv-vaccine.html.

CHAPTER 27

1. EMA grants Cervarix approval, http://www.evaluategroup.com/Universal /View.aspx?type=Story&id=138540.

2. "Cervical Cancer Statistics," Cancer Research UK, http://www.cancerresearchuk .org/health-professional/cancer-statistics/statistics-by-cancer-type/cervical -cancer#heading-Zero.

3. "Jade Goody," *Wikipedia*, https://en.wikipedia.org/wiki/Jade_Goody.

4. Urmee Khan, "BBC Criticised Over Jade Goody Coverage." *Telegraph*, March 25, 2009, https://www.telegraph.co.uk/news/celebritynews/jade-goody/5045083 /BBC-criticised-over-Jade-Goody-coverage.html

5. S. Hilton and K. Hunt, "Coverage of Jade Goody's cervical cancer in UK newspapers: a missed opportunity for health promotion?" BMC *Public Health*, 10:368, June 24, 2010, https://bmcpublichealth.biomedcentral.com/articles /10.1186/1471-2458-10-368.

6. C. Millett, *et al.*, "Centers for Disease Control and Prevention: protecting the private good?" *BMJ*, 350:h2362, May 15, 2015, http://www.bmj.com/content /350/bmj.h2362/rr-3.

7. Hilton and Hunt, "Coverage of Jade Goody's cervical cancer in UK newspapers: a missed opportunity for health promotion?" note 5 above.

8. Paula Cocozza, "Whatever happened to the Jade Goody effect?," *Guardian*, January 21, 2018, https://www.theguardian.com/society/shortcuts/2018/jan /21/whatever-happened-to-the-jade-goody-effect.

9. Laura Donnelly, "Two thousand schoolgirls suffer suspected ill-effects from cervical cancer vaccine," *Telegraph*, September 12, 2009, https://www.telegraph .co.uk/news/health/news/6178045/Two-thousand-schoolgirls-suffer -suspected-ill-effects-from-cervical-cancer-vaccine.html.

10. Ibid.

11. Rachel Porter, "How Safe is the Cervical Cancer Jab?" *Daily Mail*, April 5, 2009, http://www.dailymail.co.uk/health/article-1167803/How-safe-cervical-cancer-jab-Five-teenagers-reveal-alarming-stories.html.

12. Ibid.

13. Chris Irvine, "14-year-old schoolgirl dies after being given cervical cancer jab," *Telegraph*, September 29, 2009, https://www.telegraph.co.uk/news/health /news/6241290/14-year-old-schoolgirl-dies-after-being-given-cervical-cancer-jab .html.

14. Ibid.

15. Ibid.

16. Daniel Martin, "NHS Trust suspends cervical cancer vaccinations after girl, 14, dies within hours of jab," *Daily Mail*, October 2, 2009, http://www.dailymail .co.uk/news/article-1216714/Schoolgirl-14-dies-given-cervical-cancer-jab.html.

17. Recall of Cervarix following death of Natalie Morton, https://www.cas.dh.gov .uk/ViewandAcknowledgment/ViewAlert.aspx?AlertID=101266.

18. "Tragic Natalie Morton sister has cervical cancer vaccine," *Coventry Telegraph*, February 24, 2010, http://www.coventrytelegraph.net/news/coventry-news /tragic-natalie-morton-sister-cervical-3069276.

19. Owen Bowcott, "Girl Who Died After Cervical Cancer Injection Had Tumour In Her Chest," *Guardian*, October 1, 2009, https://www.theguardian.com /society/2009/oct/01/cervical-cancer-vaccination-tumour-natalie-morton.

20. "Coventry cancer jab girl died of 'natural causes'," *BBC News*, April 30, 2010, http://news.bbc.co.uk/2/hi/uk_news/england/coventry_warwickshire /8654711.stm

21. "Tragic Natalie Morton sister has cervical cancer vaccine," *Coventry Telegraph*, note 18 above.

22. Ibid.

23. WHO, "Case Study C: How a Potential HPV Vaccination Crisis was Averted," http://vaccine-safety-training.org/c-public-perception.html.

24. "MHRA Public Assessment Report," 2010 at 22, http://www.mhra.gov.uk /home/groups/s-par/documents/websiteresources/con096797.pdf.

25. WHO, "Case Study C: How a Potential HPV Vaccination Crisis was Averted," note 23 above.

26. Ibid.

27. Stephen Adams, "Cervical Cancer Jab Left Girl, 13, In A Walking Coma," *Telegraph*, November 14, 2011, http://www.telegraph.co.uk/news/health /news/8889257/Cervical-cancer-jab-left-girl-13-in-waking-coma-claim-parents .html.

28. "Post Cervarix Syndrome: Lucy From The UK," *SaneVax.org*, February 18, 2013, http://sanevax.org/post-cervarix-syndrome-lucy-from-the-uk/.

29. Munchausen Syndrome By Proxy definition, https://en.wikipedia.org/wiki /Factitious_disorder_imposed_on_another.

30. Ibid.

31. Ibid.

32. "Factitious Disorder Imposed on Another (FDIA)," overview by the Cleveland Clinic official site, https://my.clevelandclinic.org/health/articles /munchausen-syndrome-by-proxy.

33. Gov.UK, 2012, "Human papillomavirus vaccine Cervarix: balance of risks and benefits remains clearly positive," https://www.gov.uk/drug-safety-update/human-papillomavirus-vaccine-cervarix-balance-of-risks-and-benefits-remains-clearly-positive.

34. "Vaccine Damage Payment: How to Claim," Gov.UK https://www.gov.uk/vaccine-damage-payment/how-to-claim.

35. Ibid.

36. UK Association of HPV Vaccine Injured Daughters, Facebook page https://www.facebook.com/AHVID.UK/.

37. Time For Action UK, website, http://timeforaction.org.uk.

38. "Yellow Card System," *Wikipedia*, https://en.wikipedia.org/wiki/Yellow_Card_Scheme.

39. "Case Series Drug Analysis" report for Cervarix and Gardasil through May 2018 from the MHRA, FOIA document, on file with the authors.

40. "Trends in UK spontaneous Adverse Drug Reaction (ADR) reporting between 2008 – 2012," MHRA report, at 37 (Table 5.1) and 37–39, http://webarchive.nationalarchives.gov.uk/20141206193208/http://www.mhra.gov.uk/home/groups/pl-p/documents/websiteresources/con408250.pdf.

41. Ibid., note 39 at 39.

42. Ibid., 39 (Table 5.2.3).

43. MHRA Public Assessment Report Cervarix 2008–2012, at 12, http://www.mhra.gov.uk/home/groups/s-par/documents/websiteresources/con213228.pdf.

44. Ibid., 15.

45. Nicola Blackwood, "Human Papillomavirus: Vaccination: Written question-70973," UK Parliament Written Questions and Answers, Apr. 24, 2017 https://www.parliament.uk/business/publications/written-questions-answers-statements/written-question/Commons/2017-04-13/70973.

46. "Trends in UK spontaneous Adverse Drug Reaction (ADR) reporting between 2008 – 2012," MHRA report, note 38 above, at 50.

47. "Case Series Drug Analysis" report for Cervarix and Gardasil, note 38 above.

48. Ibid.

49. Chris Smyth, "The backlash against the disgraced doctor Andrew Wakefield has shielded Britain from the worst of the "antivax" trend," *Guardian*, February 24, 2018, https://www.thetimes.co.uk/article/social-media-anti-vaxxers-fuel-mistrust-in-health-jabs-gf3jg25cf.

50. John Stone, "Damage Settlements Go From Hundreds to Zero In Four Decades, *Age of Autism*, August 21, 2017, http://www.ageofautism.com/2017/08/hit-and-run-vaccine-policy-of-the-british-government-revealed-damage-settlements-go-from-hundreds-to-zero-in-four-decades.html.

51. "Human Papillomavirus (HPV) Vaccination Coverage in Adolescent Females in England: 2016/17," Public Health England report, https://assets.publishing.service.gov.uk/government/uploads/system/uploads/attachment_data/file

/666087/HPV_vaccination_coverage_in_adolescent_females_in_England_2016_to_2017.pdf.

52. A.-B. Moscicki, J. M. Palefsky, "HPV in Men: An Update," *Journal of Lower Genital Tract Disease*, 15(3):231–234, July 15, 2011, https://www.ncbi.nlm.nih.gov/pmc/articles/PMC3304470/.

53. M. Stanley, "Vaccinate boys too," *Nature*, 488(7413):S10, August 30, 2012, https://www.nature.com/articles/488S10a.

54. Ibid.

55. Ibid.

56. Robin McKie, "Fears For Women's Health As Parents Reject The HPV Vaccine," *Guardian*, December 2, 2017, https://www.theguardian.com/society/2017/dec/03/hpv-vaccine-fears-women-health-take-up-falls.

57. www.hpvaction.org.

58. Groups represented by HPVAction.org, http://www.hpvaction.org/members.html.

59. "MSD Supports Jabs for the Boys Campaign," *PMLive*, December 18, 2017, http://www.pmlive.com/pharma_news/msd_supports_jabs_for_the_boys_campaign_1214595.

60. "Throat Cancer Foundation," OCR Filing, https://www.oscr.org.uk/about-charities/search-the-register/charity-details?number=SC043439#results.

61. "Our Team," Throat Cancer Foundation archived at http://web.archive.org/web/20160808132917/http:/www.throatcancerfoundation.org/about/our_team/the_team.

62. Current team, Throat Cancer Foundation, http://www.throatcancerfoundation.org/about/our_team/the_team.

63. JVCI, July 2017, "JCVI Interim Statement on Extending HPV Vaccination to Adolescent Boys," https://assets.publishing.service.gov.uk/government/uploads/system/uploads/attachment_data/file/630125/Extending_HPV_Vaccination.pdf.

64. Ibid.

65. HPVAction, Nov. 2017, "HPV Action Response to JCVI Postponed Decision Regarding Boys Receiving the Human Papillomavirus (HPV) Vaccination," http://www.hpvaction.org/news/hpv-action-response-to-jcvi-postponed-decision-regarding-boys-receiving-the-human-papillomavirus-hpv-vaccination.

66. David Rose, "The HPV Backlash: Leading Throat Cancer Charity Says it'll Sue NHS if it Persists in Refusal to Offer Boys as Well as Girls Jab that can Prevent Killer Virus." *Daily Mail*, Feb. 10, 2018, http://www.dailymail.co.UK/health/article-5377077/Campaigners-urge-vaccinating-boys-against-HPV-Virus.html.

67. JCVI, July 2018. "Statement on HPV Vaccination," https://assets.publishing.service.gov.uk/government/uploads/system/uploads/attachment_data/file/726319/JCVI_Statement_on_HPV_vaccination_2018.pdf.

68. Ibid., 10.

69. Ibid., 7.

Chapter 28

1. N. Muñoz and L. E. Bravo, "Epidemiology of Cervical Cancer in Colombia," *Colombia Medica (Cali)*, 43(4):298–304, December 30, 2012, https://www.ncbi.nlm.nih.gov/pubmed/24893303.

2. Ibid.

3. Bill 1626 in Spanish, title translated to English as "THROUGH WHICH THE FREE AND COMPULSORY VACCINATION IS GUARANTEED TO THE COLOMBIAN POPULATION OBJECTED THEREOF, INTEGRAL MEASURES ARE ADOPTED FOR THE PREVENTION OF UTERINE CERVICAL CANCER AND OTHER PROVISIONS ARE DICTATED," https://www.invima.gov.co/images/pdf/normatividad/medicamentos/leyes/Ley%201626%20de%2030%20de%20Abril%20de%202013.pdf.

4. *Human Papillomavirus and Related Diseases Report: Colombia*, IARC http://www.hpvcentre.net/statistics/reports/COL.pdf.

5. P. C. Webster, "Health in Colombia: a system in crisis," *CMAJ*, 184(6):E289–E290, April 3, 2012, https://www.ncbi.nlm.nih.gov/pmc/articles/PMC3314050/.

6. "Gardasil the Vaccine the Kills," http://www.escritoresyperiodistas.com/NUMERO63/mario.htm. English translation, https://translate.google.com/translate?hl=en&sl=es&u=http://www.escritoresyperiodistas.com/NUMERO65/mario.html&prev=search.

7. Ibid.

8. "Letter to the Blog Director Of *El Tiempo*," May 27, 2013, English translation, https://translate.google.com/translate?hl=en&sl=es&u=http://www.escritoresyperiodistas.com/NUMERO65/mario.html&prev=search.

9. Rebuttal by Mario Lamo July 2013, http://www.escritoresyperiodistas.com/NUMERO65/mario.html. English translation, https://translate.google.com/translate?hl=en&sl=es&u=http://www.escritoresyperiodistas.com/NUMERO65/mario.html&prev=search.

10. Ibid.

11. Norma Erickson, "HPV Vaccination Program in Colombia: Undermining the Truth?" *SaneVax*, Nov. 12, 2014http://sanevax.org/hpv-vaccination-program-colombia-undermining-truth/.

12. "Hundreds of teenage girls in Colombia struck by mystery illness," Associated Press, August 27, 2014, http://globalnews.ca/news/1530883/hundreds-of-teenage-girls-in-colombia-struck-by-mystery-illness/.

13. Ibid.

14. Facebook footage from Carmen De Bolivar following vaccination, https://www.facebook.com/AVPHMEX/videos/1479482689044091/.

15. "Hundreds of Colombian girls hospitalized after vaccinations," CGTN America September 1, 2014, https://www.youtube.com/watch?v=1307z5xltrU.

16. Ibid.

17. M. Pompilio, MD, "Karen Durán-Cantor: A Colombian girl and Gardasil victim dies," June 4, 2015: https://pompiliomartinez.wordpress.com/2015/06/04/karen-duran-cantor-a-colombian-girl-and-gardasil-victim-dies/.

18. Ibid.

19. Ibid.

20. "Colombia 2017: Fue el Gardasil" ("Gardasil Did It"), VaxTV, English subtitles beginning at 2:45, https://www.youtube.com/watch?v=RS72EeILlqY.

21. Ibid.

22. "Constitutional Court asks for Accounts for Vaccine against Human Papollomavirus," *La Semana*, Feb. 2, 2016 (in Spanish), http://www.semana.com/nacion/articulo/corte-constitucional-pide-cuentas-por-vacuna-contra-el-virus-del-papiloma-humano/459467. English translation, https://translate.google.com/translate?hl=en&sl=auto&tl=en&u=https%3A%2F%2Fwww.semana.com%2Fnacion%2Farticulo%2Fcorte-constitucional-pide-cuentas-por-vacuna-contra-el-virus-del-papiloma-humano%2F459467.

23. Ibid.

24. Kenji Doku, "Court rules in favor of girl from Carmen De Bolivar," *El Heraldo*, November 15, 2014 (in Spanish), https://www.elheraldo.co/local/ordenan-minsalud-estudiar-caso-de-menor-vacunada-contra-el-vph-174133. English translation, https://translate.google.com/translate?hl=en&sl=auto&tl=en&u=https%3A%2F%2Fwww.elheraldo.co%2Flocal%2Fordenan-minsalud-estudiar-caso-de-menor-vacunada-contra-el-vph-174133.

25. Norma Erickson, "HPV Vaccine Controversy In Colombia Continues," *Natural Blaze*, January 12, 2015, https://www.naturalblaze.com/2015/01/hpv-vaccine-controversy-in-colombia.html.

26. Ibid.

27. "Attorney General asks for transparency re HPV Vaccine," *Caracol Radio*, December 5, 2014 (in Spanish), http://caracol.com.co/radio/2014/12/05/nacional/1417779780_538932.html. Translated in English: https://translate.google.com/translate?hl=en&sl=auto&tl=en&u=http%3A%2F%2Fcaracol.com.co%2Fradio%2F2014%2F12%2F05%2Fnacional%2F1417779780_538932.html.

28. Ibid.

29. "Attorney General Ordóñez ordered out," *Bogota Post*, September 16, 2016: https://thebogotapost.com/2016/09/16/attorney-general-ordonez-ordered-out/.

30. Nubia Muñoz Calero, "La Vacuna Contra el VPH Salva Muchas Vidas," *El País*, Oct. 5, 2014 (in Spanish) http://www.elpais.com.co/colombia/la-vacuna-contra-el-vph-salva-muchas-vidas-nubia-munoz-calero.html.

31. Ibid.

32. Vicente Arcieri, "They want to throw two shovels of earth to the case of the girls of El Carmen," *El Heraldo*, January 6, 2015 (in Spanish), https://www.elheraldo.co/bolivar/quieren-echarle-dos-palas-de-tierra-al-caso-de-las-ninas-de-el-carmen-179516. English translation, https://translate.google.com/

translate?hl=en&sl=auto&tl=en&u=https%3A%2F%2Fwww.elheraldo.co%2F-
bolivar%2Fquieren-echarle-dos-palas-de-tierra-al-caso-de-las-ninas-de-el-car-
men-179516.

33. Norma Erickson, "Controversy in Colombia," *SaneVax.org*, April 11, 2015,
http://sanevax.org/hpv-vaccines-colombian-controversy-continues/.

34. Ibid.

35 Adrián Marcelo Buitrago Gallego, "Yes there are risks for HPV," *El
Mundo,* February 16, 2015 (in Spanish), http://www.elmundo.com/portal
/vida/salud/si_hay_riesgos__por_vacuna_contra_vph.php#.W0VZ_y3Mz67.

36. M. Pompilio, MD, "Colombian National Academy of Medicine asks for a change
in current HPV vaccine application protocols," March 14, 2016, https://pompil-
iomartinez.wordpress.com/2016/03/21/colombian-national-academy-of-medi-
cine-asks-for-a-change-in-current-hpv-vaccine-application-protocols/.

37. M. Pompilio, MD, "Motor and sensory clinical findings in girls vaccinated
against the human papillomavirus from Carmen de Bolivar, Colombia," https://
pompiliomartinez.wordpress.com/2016/03/04/motor-and-sensory-clinical
-findings-in-girls-vaccinated-against-the-human-papillomavirus-from-carmen
-de-bolivar-colombia/.

38. Ibid.

39. Lorayne Solano Naizzir, "The Attorney General's Office asks the
Constitutional Court to rule against the application of the HPV vaccine in
Cali," *El Heraldo*, July 10, 2016 (in Spanish), https://www.elheraldo.co/noticias
/procuraduria-pide-corte-constitucional-que-haga-regir-fallo-contra-aplicacion
-de-la-vacuna. English translation, https://translate.google.com/translate?hl
=en&sl=auto&tl=en&u=https%3A%2F%2Fwww.elheraldo.co%2Fnoticias
%2Fprocuraduria-pide-corte-constitucional-que-haga-regir-fallo-contra-aplicacion
-de-la-vacuna.

40. Norma Erickson, "Protesting Parents," *SaneVax.org*, July14, 2014, http://sanevax
.org/gardasil-colombia-protesting-parents-progress/.

41. Ibid.

42. "The meeting will be today in the Government of Bolivar. The cessation of
activities in the schools of this municipality completes four days," *El Heraldo*,
July 14, 2016 (in Spanish), https://www.elheraldo.co/bolivar/madres-de-ninas
-afectadas-de-el-carmen-aceptan-dialogo-con-minsalud-271658.

43. Erickson, note 40 above.

44. Ibid.

45. Ibid.

46. Alejandro Gaviria, Twitter message, Aug. 9, 2015 https://twitter.com/agaviriau
/status/630525443700051968.

47. Alejandro Gaviria, Twitter message, Dec. 30, 2015 https://twitter.com/
agaviriau/statuses/682296143049523201.

48. "Colombia: Decreasing HPV vaccination coverage: mapping roles of different stakeholders and societal-historical factors," *Vaccine Confidence Project*, June 2017, http://www.vaccineconfidence.org/wp-content/uploads/2017/01/Colombia -final-country-poster05062017corII.pdf.

49. Ibid.

50. Carlos Guevara, "Class Action Lawsuit Against HPV Vaccine Filed in Colombia," *Medscape*, August 7, 2017, https://www.medscape.com/viewarticle /883873 (available after free login).

51. Ibid.

52. Office Attorney General, August 10, 2017: "Preliminary investigation to protect the rights of minors affected by human papilloma vaccine in Bolívar" (in Spanish), https://www.procuraduria.gov.co/portal/Indagacion-preliminar-vacuna-papiloma.news.

53. "Vaccine against human papillomavirus can not be mandatory: Constitutional Court," August 27, 2017 (in Spanish), http://www.elespectador.com/noticias /judicial/vacuna-contra-el-virus-del-papiloma-humano-no-puede-ser-obligatoria-corte-constitucional-articulo-710196.

54. Ibid.

55. Ibid.

INDEX